Mayo Clinic Case Review for Pulmonary and Critical Care Boards

MAYO CLINIC SCIENTIFIC PRESS

Mayo Clinic Atlas of Regional Anesthesia and Ultrasound-Guided Nerve Blockade
Edited by James R. Hebl, MD, and
Robert L. Lennon, DO

Mayo Clinic Preventive Medicine and Public Health Board Review
Edited by Prathibha Varkey, MBBS, MPH, MHPE

Mayo Clinic Infectious Diseases Board Review
Edited by Zelalem Temesgen, MD

Just Enough Physiology
By James R. Munis, MD, PhD

Mayo Clinic Cardiology: Concise Textbook,
Fourth Edition
Edited by Joseph G. Murphy, MD, and
Margaret A. Lloyd, MD

Mayo Clinic Electrophysiology Manual
Edited by Samuel J. Asirvatham, MD

Mayo Clinic Gastrointestinal Imaging Review,
Second Edition
By C. Daniel Johnson, MD

Arrhythmias in Women: Diagnosis and Management
Edited by Yong-Mei Cha, MD,
Margaret A. Lloyd, MD, and
Ulrika M. Birgersdotter-Green, MD

Mayo Clinic Body MRI Case Review
By Christine U. Lee, MD, PhD, and
James F. Glockner, MD, PhD

Mayo Clinic Gastroenterology and Hepatology Board Review, Fifth Edition
Edited by Stephen C. Hauser, MD

Mayo Clinic Guide to Cardiac Magnetic Resonance Imaging, Second Edition
Edited by Kiaran P. McGee, PhD, Eric E. Williamson, MD, and Matthew W. Martinez, MD

Mayo Clinic Critical Care Case Review
Edited by Rahul Kashyap, MBBS,
J. Christopher Farmer, MD, and
John C. O'Horo, MD

Mayo Clinic Medical Neurosciences,
Sixth Edition
Edited by Eduardo E. Benarroch, MD, Jeremy K. Cutsforth-Gregory, MD, and
Kelly D. Flemming, MD

Mayo Clinic Principles of Shoulder Surgery
By Joaquin Sanchez-Sotelo, MD

Mayo Clinic Essential Neurology, Second Edition
By Andrea C. Adams, MD

Mayo Clinic Antimicrobial Handbook: Quick Guide, Third Edition
Edited by John W. Wilson, MD, and
Lynn L. Estes, PharmD

Mayo Clinic Critical and Neurocritical Care Board Review
Edited by Eelco F. M. Wijdicks, MD, PhD,
James Y. Findlay, MB, ChB,
William D. Freeman, MD, and Ayan Sen, MD

Mayo Clinic Internal Medicine Board Review,
Twelfth Edition
Edited by Christopher M. Wittich, MD, PharmD,
Thomas J. Beckman, MD, Sara L. Bonnes, MD,
Nerissa M. Collins, MD, Nina M. Schwenk, MD,
Christopher R. Stephenson, MD, and
Jason H. Szostek, MD

Mayo Clinic Strategies for Reducing Burnout and Promoting Engagement
By Stephen J. Swensen, MD, and
Tait D. Shanafelt, MD

Mayo Clinic General Surgery
By Jad M. Abdelsattar, MBBS,
Moustafa M. El Khatib, MB, BCh,
T. K. Pandian, MD, Samuel J. Allen, and
David R. Farley, MD

Mayo Clinic Neurology Board Review,
Second Edition
Edited by Kelly D. Flemming, MD

Mayo Clinic Illustrated Textbook of Neurogastroenterology
By Michael Camilleri, MD

Mayo Clinic Cases in Neuroimmunology
Edited by Andrew McKeon, MB, BCh, MD,
B. Mark Keegan, MD, and
W. Oliver Tobin, MB, BCh, BAO, PhD

Mayo Clinic Infectious Diseases Case Review
Edited by Larry M. Baddour, MD,
John C. O'Horo, MD, MPH, Mark J. Enzler, MD,
and Rahul Kashyap, MBBS

Mayo Clinic Case Review for Pulmonary and Critical Care Boards

Editors

Alice Gallo de Moraes, MD

*Consultant, Division of Pulmonary
& Critical Care Medicine
Mayo Clinic, Rochester, Minnesota
Associate Professor of Medicine
Mayo Clinic College of Medicine and Science*

Diana J. Kelm, MD

*Consultant, Division of Pulmonary
& Critical Care Medicine
Mayo Clinic, Rochester, Minnesota
Assistant Professor of Medicine
Mayo Clinic College of Medicine and Science*

Kannan Ramar, MBBS, MD

*Consultant, Division of Pulmonary
& Critical Care Medicine
Mayo Clinic, Rochester, Minnesota
Professor of Medicine
Mayo Clinic College of Medicine and Science*

MAYO CLINIC SCIENTIFIC PRESS

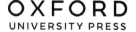

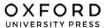

Oxford University Press is a department of the University of Oxford. It furthers the University's objective of excellence in research, scholarship, and education by publishing worldwide. Oxford is a registered trade mark of Oxford University Press in the UK and certain other countries.

Published in the United States of America by Oxford University Press
198 Madison Avenue, New York, NY 10016, United States of America.

© Mayo Foundation for Medical Education and Research 2024

Oxford is a registered trademark of Oxford University Press.

CIP data is on file at the Library of Congress

ISBN 978–0–19–775587–7

DOI: 10.1093/med/9780197755877.001.0001

Printed by Marquis Book Printing, Canada

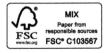

We would like to thank our families for their unconditional support.

Preface

Yet another board examination. More studying. More stress. More money. This is the typical life cycle of all physicians-in-training.

In 2016, we were again facing this obstacle, but this time it was the Pulmonary Disease board examination. We were hoping to study as we had in the past—by using a good board review study book. We recalled many prior board review books that we annotated with notes in the margins, highlighted nearly entire pages with a yellow marker, and carried around with us at all times to study for even just a few minutes while we waited for a bus. You can call us "old school," but we wanted *that* board review book.

Unfortunately, we did not find *that* book. We searched online. We asked prior graduates. But no luck. We were left without a board review book. As others did in the past, we relied on the available multiple-choice question banks, which were helpful. But they were not a board review book.

Don't worry—we did fine. We are board certified in both Pulmonary Disease and Critical Care Medicine, so we passed our board examinations without *that* book. Yet we still wanted it, and when asking around, we weren't alone in that desire.

But we wanted to do it differently than most other board review books. Reading about various disease processes is great and is what we do a majority of the time in medicine. But what is the best way to learn about pulmonary and critical care medicine? Many of us would say, "Through our patients." Fortunately, we had the support of Dr. Kannan Ramar, our program director at that time, to pursue this passion project.

If that is true, why isn't there a board review book with a focus on case-based learning? At our institution, the Division of Pulmonary and Critical Care Medicine has the longest successfully running conference. The reason for its success is that it is focused solely on patient cases. A fellow or faculty member presents a case they saw in the clinic or the intensive care unit, but the fun part is that they ask questions related to the case to another fellow or faculty member. There is great discussion between the presenter and the discussant. And after the case presentation, the presenter leaves us with some high-yield teaching pearls.

At the end of this conference, we always left feeling a little smarter than when we had entered. The goal of this book is to do the same for our readers as they prepare for their own board examination.

Diana Kelm
Alice Gallo de Moraes

Table of Contents

Section VIII
Interventional Pulmonology
(Cases 44 and 45)

Section IX
Transplantation (Cases 46–48)

Section X
Vascular Diseases (Cases 49–51)

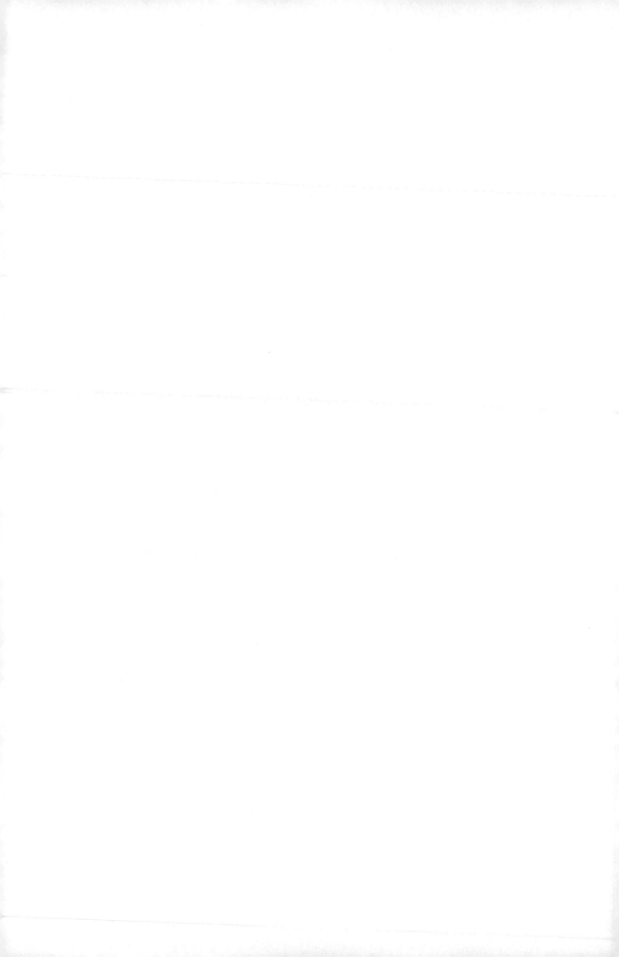

Contributors

Vaibhav Ahluwalia, MBBS
Research Collaborator in Pulmonary & Critical Care Medicine, Mayo Clinic School of Graduate Medical Education, Mayo Clinic College of Medicine and Science, Rochester, Minnesota; now with Nazareth Hospital, Philadelphia, Pennsylvania

Timothy R. Aksamit, MD
Consultant, Division of Pulmonary & Critical Care Medicine, Mayo Clinic, Rochester, Minnesota; Professor of Medicine, Mayo Clinic College of Medicine and Science

Hasan A. Albitar, MD
Fellow in Pulmonary & Critical Care Medicine, Mayo Clinic School of Graduate Medical Education and Assistant Professor of Medicine, Mayo Clinic College of Medicine and Science, Rochester, Minnesota; now with Deaconess Healthcare, Evansville, Indiana

Faysal K. Al-Ghoula, MB, BCh
Resident in Pulmonary & Critical Care Medicine, Mayo Clinic School of Graduate Medical Education, Mayo Clinic College of Medicine and Science, Rochester, Minnesota

Phanindra Antharam, MD
Research Trainee, Division of Pulmonary & Critical Care Medicine, Mayo Clinic, Rochester, Minnesota; now with University of North Dakota School of Medicine and Health Sciences, Fargo, North Dakota

Catarina N. Aragon Pinto, MD
Research Fellow in Pulmonary & Critical Care Medicine, Mayo Clinic, School of Graduate Medical Education, Mayo Clinic College of Medicine and Science, Rochester, Minnesota

Luiza Azevedo Gross, MD
Telehealth Consultant, Telehealth Program, Federal University of Rio Grande do Sul, Porto Alegre, Rio Grande do Sul, Brazil

Misbah Baqir, MBBS
Consultant, Division of Pulmonary & Critical Care Medicine, Mayo Clinic, Rochester, Minnesota; Assistant Professor of Medicine, Mayo Clinic College of Medicine and Science

Michael Bourne, MD
Fellow in Pulmonary & Critical Care Medicine, Mayo Clinic School of Graduate Medical Education, Mayo Clinic College of Medicine and Science, Rochester, Minnesota; now with Oregon Clinic Pulmonary West, Portland, Oregon

Cassandra M. Braun, MD
Consultant, Division of Pulmonary & Critical Care Medicine, Rochester, Minnesota; Assistant Professor of Medicine, Mayo Clinic College of Medicine and Science

Scott M. Canepa, MD
Fellow in Pulmonary & Critical Care Medicine, Mayo Clinic School of Graduate Medical Education, Mayo Clinic College of Medicine and Science, Rochester, Minnesota

Matthew J. Cecchini, MD, PhD
Fellow in Laboratory Medicine & Pathology, Mayo Clinic School of Graduate Medical Education, Mayo Clinic College of Medicine and Science, Rochester, Minnesota; now with Schulich School of Medicine & Dentistry, Western University, London, Ontario, Canada

Sarah J. Chalmers, MD
Senior Associate Consultant, Division of Pulmonary & Critical Care Medicine, Mayo Clinic, Rochester, Minnesota; Assistant Professor of Medicine, Mayo Clinic College of Medicine and Science

Jeremy M. Clain, MD
Consultant, Division of Pulmonary & Critical Care Medicine, Mayo Clinic, Rochester, Minnesota; Assistant Professor of Medicine, Mayo Clinic College of Medicine and Science

Ryan D. Clay, MD
Fellow in Pulmonary & Critical Care Medicine, Mayo Clinic School of Graduate Medical Education, Mayo Clinic College of Medicine and Science, Rochester, Minnesota; now with Northwest Permanente Physicians and Surgeons, PC, Vancouver, Washington

Craig E. Daniels, MD
Consultant, Division of Pulmonary & Critical Care Medicine, Mayo Clinic, Rochester, Minnesota; Professor of Medicine, Mayo Clinic College of Medicine and Science

Kathryn T. del Valle, MD
Fellow in Pulmonary & Critical Care Medicine, Mayo
Clinic School of Graduate Medical Education and
Assistant Professor of Medicine, Mayo Clinic College of
Medicine and Science, Rochester, Minnesota

Daniel A. Diedrich, MD
Chair, Division of Critical Care Medicine Anesthesia,
Mayo Clinic, Rochester, Minnesota; Assistant Professor
of Anesthesiology, Mayo Clinic College of Medicine and
Science

Hilary M. DuBrock, MD
Consultant, Division of Pulmonary & Critical Care
Medicine, Mayo Clinic, Rochester, Minnesota;
Associate Professor of Medicine, Mayo Clinic College of
Medicine and Science

Jennifer D. Duke, MD
Fellow in Pulmonary & Critical Care Medicine, Mayo
Clinic School of Graduate Medical Education, Mayo Clinic
College of Medicine and Science, Rochester, Minnesota

William F. Dunn, MD
Emeritus Member, Division of Pulmonary & Critical
Care Medicine, Mayo Clinic, Rochester, Minnesota;
Emeritus Associate Professor of Medicine, Mayo Clinic
College of Medicine and Science

Kara L. Dupuy-McCauley, MD
Consultant, Division of Pulmonary & Critical Care
Medicine, Mayo Clinic, Rochester, Minnesota; Assistant
Professor of Medicine, Mayo Clinic College of Medicine
and Science

Eric S. Edell, MD
Consultant, Division of Pulmonary & Critical Care
Medicine, Mayo Clinic, Rochester, Minnesota;
Professor of Medicine, Mayo Clinic College of Medicine
and Science

Ashley M. Egan, MD
Consultant, Division of Pulmonary & Critical Care
Medicine, Mayo Clinic, Rochester, Minnesota; Assistant
Professor of Medicine, Mayo Clinic College of Medicine
and Science

Samuel F. Ekstein
Medical Student, Mayo Clinic Alix School of
Medicine, Mayo Clinic College of Medicine and
Science, Rochester, Minnesota; now with Concentra
Occupational Health, Minneapolis, Minnesota

Jamie R. Felzer, MD, MPH
Fellow in Pulmonary & Critical Care Medicine,
Mayo Clinic School of Graduate Medical Education and
Assistant Professor of Medicine, Mayo Clinic College of
Medicine and Science, Rochester, Minnesota

Xavier E. Fonseca Fuentes, MD
Research Collaborator in Pulmonary & Critical Care
Medicine, Mayo Clinic School of Graduate Medical
Education, Mayo Clinic College of Medicine and
Science, Rochester, Minnesota; now with Henry Ford
Medical Center, Taylor, Michigan

Alice Gallo de Moraes, MD
Consultant, Division of Pulmonary & Critical Care
Medicine, Mayo Clinic, Rochester, Minnesota;
Associate Professor of Medicine, Mayo Clinic College of
Medicine and Science

Phillip J. Gary, MD
Fellow in Pulmonary & Critical Care Medicine, Mayo
Clinic School of Graduate Medical Education, Mayo
Clinic College of Medicine and Science, Rochester,
Minnesota

Kavitha Gopalratnam, MBBS
Research Collaborator, Mayo Clinic School of
Graduate Medical Education, Mayo Clinic College of
Medicine and Science, Rochester, Minnesota; now with
Bridgeport Hospital, Bridgeport, Connecticut

Michelle B. Herberts, MD
Resident in Internal Medicine, Mayo Clinic School of
Graduate Medical Education, Mayo Clinic College of
Medicine and Science, Rochester, Minnesota

Tyler L. Herzog, MD
Resident in Internal Medicine, Mayo Clinic School of
Graduate Medical Education, Mayo Clinic College of
Medicine and Science, Rochester, Minnesota

Sara E. Hocker, MD
Chair, Division of Critical Care and Hospital
Neurology, Mayo Clinic, Rochester, Minnesota;
Professor of Neurology, Mayo Clinic College of
Medicine and Science

Sumedh S. Hoskote, MBBS
Consultant, Division of Pulmonary & Critical Care
Medicine, Mayo Clinic, Rochester, Minnesota; Assistant
Professor of Medicine, Mayo Clinic College of Medicine
and Science

Vivek N. Iyer, MD, MPH
Associate Professor, Division of Pulmonary & Critical
Care Medicine, Mayo Clinic, Rochester, Minnesota;
Associate Professor of Medicine, Mayo Clinic College of
Medicine and Science

Amjad N. Kanj, MD, MPH
Fellow in Pulmonary & Critical Care Medicine, Mayo
Clinic School of Graduate Medical Education, Mayo
Clinic College of Medicine and Science, Rochester,
Minnesota

Rahul Kashyap, MBBS, MBA
Research Scientist, Department of Anesthesiology
and Perioperative Medicine, Mayo Clinic, Rochester,
Minnesota; Assistant Professor of Anesthesiology,
Mayo Clinic College of Medicine and Science; now with
HCA Healthcare, Brentwood, Tennessee

Bryan T. Kelly, MD
Fellow in Pulmonary & Critical Care Medicine,
Mayo Clinic School of Graduate Medical Education
and Instructor in Medicine, Mayo Clinic College of
Medicine and Science, Rochester, Minnesota; now in
private practice, Grapevine, Texas

Diana J. Kelm, MD
Consultant, Division of Pulmonary & Critical Care
Medicine, Mayo Clinic, Rochester, Minnesota; Assistant
Professor of Medicine, Mayo Clinic College of Medicine
and Science

Cassie C. Kennedy, MD
Consultant, Division of Pulmonary & Critical Care
Medicine, Mayo Clinic, Rochester, Minnesota;
Associate Professor of Medicine, Mayo Clinic College of
Medicine and Science

Ryan M. Kern, MD
Consultant, Division of Pulmonary & Critical Care
Medicine, Mayo Clinic, Rochester, Minnesota; Assistant
Professor of Medicine, Mayo Clinic College of Medicine
and Science

Matthew Koslow, MD
Fellow in Pulmonary & Critical Care Medicine, Mayo
Clinic School of Graduate Medical Education, Mayo
Clinic College of Medicine and Science, Rochester,
Minnesota; now with National Jewish Health, Denver,
Colorado

Richard D. Koubek, MD
Research Collaborator in Pulmonary & Critical Care
Medicine, Mayo Clinic School of Graduate Medical
Education, Mayo Clinic College of Medicine and
Science, Rochester, Minnesota

Rachana Krishna, MBBS
Fellow in Pulmonary & Critical Care Medicine, Mayo
Clinic School of Graduate Medical Education, Mayo
Clinic College of Medicine and Science, Rochester,
Minnesota; now with Medical University of South
Carolina, Charleston, South Carolina

Aahd F. Kubbara, MBBS
Associate Consultant, Division of Pulmonary & Critical
Care Medicine, Mayo Clinic, Rochester, Minnesota;
Assistant Professor of Medicine, Mayo Clinic College
of Medicine and Science; now with Aspirus Wausau
Hospital, Reno, Nevada

Jessica Lau, MD
Fellow in Pulmonary & Critical Care Medicine, Mayo
Clinic School of Graduate Medical Education, Mayo
Clinic College of Medicine and Science, Rochester,
Minnesota; now with Vancouver Clinic, Vancouver,
Washington

Heyi Li, MD
Fellow in Pulmonary & Critical Care Medicine,
Mayo Clinic School of Graduate Medical Education
and Instructor in Medicine, Mayo Clinic College of
Medicine and Science, Rochester, Minnesota; now with
Montefiore Medical Center, Bronx, New York

Kaiser G. Lim, MD
Consultant, Division of Pulmonary & Critical Care
Medicine, Mayo Clinic, Rochester, Minnesota;
Professor of Medicine, Mayo Clinic College of Medicine
and Science

Andrew H. Limper, MD
Consultant, Division of Pulmonary & Critical Care
Medicine, Mayo Clinic, Rochester, Minnesota; Professor
of Medicine and of Biochemistry and Molecular Biology,
Mayo Clinic College of Medicine and Science

Cameron M. Long, MD, MS
Fellow in Pulmonary & Critical Care Medicine,
Mayo Clinic School of Graduate Medical Education
and Instructor in Medicine, Mayo Clinic College of
Medicine and Science, Rochester, Minnesota; now with
the Oregon Clinic, Portland, Oregon

Paige K. Marty, MD
Fellow in Pulmonary & Critical Care Medicine, Mayo
Clinic School of Graduate Medical Education, Mayo
Clinic College of Medicine and Science, Rochester,
Minnesota; now with Cleveland Clinic, Cleveland, Ohio

Amanda J. McCambridge, MD
Fellow in Pulmonary & Critical Care Medicine,
Mayo Clinic School of Graduate Medical Education
and Instructor in Medicine, Mayo Clinic College of
Medicine and Science, Rochester, Minnesota; now with
Park Nicollet Pulmonary Medicine, St. Louis Park,
Minnesota

David E. Midthun, MD
Consultant, Division of Pulmonary & Critical Care
Medicine, Mayo Clinic, Rochester, Minnesota;
Professor of Medicine, Mayo Clinic College of Medicine
and Science

Teng Moua, MD
Consultant, Division of Pulmonary & Critical Care
Medicine, Mayo Clinic, Rochester, Minnesota; Assistant
Professor of Medicine, Mayo Clinic College of Medicine
and Science

Harsha V. Mudrakola, MD, MS
Fellow in Pulmonary & Critical Care Medicine,
Mayo Clinic School of Graduate Medical Education
and Instructor in Medicine, Mayo Clinic College of
Medicine and Science, Rochester, Minnesota; now with
Summa Health, Akron, Ohio

John J. Mullon, MD
Consultant, Division of Pulmonary & Critical Care
Medicine, Mayo Clinic, Rochester, Minnesota;
Associate Professor of Medicine, Mayo Clinic College of
Medicine and Science

Melissa K. Myers, MD
Senior Associate Consultant, Division of Critical Care
Medicine, Mayo Clinic Health System—Southwest
Wisconsin, La Crosse, Wisconsin; Instructor in
Medicine, Mayo Clinic College of Medicine and
Science, Rochester, Minnesota

Darlene R. Nelson, MD, MHPE
Consultant, Division of Pulmonary & Critical Care
Medicine, Mayo Clinic, Rochester, Minnesota; Assistant
Professor of Medicine, Mayo Clinic College of Medicine
and Science

Kianna M. Nguyen
MD-PhD Student, Mayo Clinic Graduate School, Mayo
Clinic College of Medicine and Science, Rochester,
Minnesota

Alexander S. Niven, MD
Consultant, Division of Pulmonary & Critical Care
Medicine, Mayo Clinic, Rochester, Minnesota;
Professor of Medicine, Mayo Clinic College of Medicine
and Science

Mark S. Norton, MD
Senior Associate Consultant, Pulmonology and
Critical Care Medicine, Mayo Clinic Health System—
Southwest Wisconsin, La Crosse, Wisconsin; Instructor
in Medicine, Mayo Clinic College of Medicine and
Science, Rochester, Minnesota

Yewande E. Odeyemi, MBBS
Consultant, Division of Pulmonary & Critical Care
Medicine, Mayo Clinic, Rochester, Minnesota; Assistant
Professor of Medicine, Mayo Clinic College of Medicine
and Science

Richard A. Oeckler, MD, PhD
Consultant, Division of Pulmonary & Critical Care
Medicine, Mayo Clinic, Rochester, Minnesota;
Associate Professor of Medicine and of
Physiology, Mayo Clinic College of Medicine
and Science

John C. O'Horo, MD, MPH
Consultant, Divisions of Infectious Diseases and
Pulmonary & Critical Care Medicine, Mayo Clinic,
Rochester, Minnesota; Professor of Medicine, Mayo
Clinic College of Medicine and Science

Emily M. Olson, MD
Special Clinical Fellow in Internal Medicine, Mayo
Clinic School of Graduate Medical Education and
Instructor in Medicine, Mayo Clinic College of
Medicine and Science, Rochester, Minnesota; now with
Northwestern University Pulmonary & Critical Care
Medicine Fellowship Program, Chicago, Illinois

Govind Panda, MD
Senior Associate Consultant, Departments of
Critical Care Medicine and Neurology, Mayo Clinic,
Jacksonville, Florida

Ashokakumar M. Patel, MD
Consultant, Division of Pulmonary & Critical Care
Medicine, Mayo Clinic, Rochester, Minnesota;
Associate Professor of Medicine, Mayo Clinic College of
Medicine and Science

Bhavesh M. Patel, MD
Consultant, Department of Critical Care Medicine,
Mayo Clinic Hospital, Phoenix, Arizona; Assistant
Professor of Anesthesiology, of Medicine, and of
Neurology, Mayo Clinic College of Medicine and
Science

Tobias Peikert, MD
Consultant, Division of Pulmonary & Critical Care
Medicine, Mayo Clinic, Rochester, Minnesota;
Associate Professor of Medicine, Mayo Clinic College of
Medicine and Science

Kelly M. Pennington, MD
Senior Associate Consultant, Division of Pulmonary
& Critical Care Medicine, Mayo Clinic, Rochester,
Minnesota; Assistant Professor of Medicine, Mayo
Clinic College of Medicine and Science

Steve G. Peters, MD
Consultant, Division of Pulmonary & Critical Care
Medicine, Mayo Clinic, Rochester, Minnesota;
Professor of Medicine, Mayo Clinic College of Medicine
and Science

Daniel O. Pfeifle, MD
Resident in Internal Medicine, Mayo Clinic School
of Graduate Medical Education, Mayo Clinic,
Rochester, Minnesota; now Resident Appointee with
Indiana University School of Medicine, Indianapolis,
Indiana

Laura Piccolo Serafim
Research Trainee, Division of Pulmonary & Critical Care Medicine, Mayo Clinic, Rochester, Minnesota; now with MedStar Health-Georgetown/Washington Hospital Center Residency Program, Washington, DC

Gautam Raju Mehta, MBBS
Fellow in Critical Care Medicine, Mayo Clinic School of Graduate Medical Education and Instructor, Mayo Clinic College of Medicine and Science, Rochester, Minnesota; now with Advocate Aurora Heath, Oak Lawn, Illinois

Muhammad A. Rishi, MBBS
Consultant, Division of Pulmonary & Critical Care Medicine, Mayo Clinic Health System—Northwest Wisconsin, Eau Claire, Wisconsin; Assistant Professor of Medicine, Mayo Clinic College of Medicine and Science, Rochester, Minnesota; now with Indiana University Health, Indianapolis, Indiana

Anja C. Roden, MD
Consultant, Department of Laboratory Medicine & Pathology, Mayo Clinic, Rochester, Minnesota; Professor of Laboratory Medicine & Pathology, Mayo Clinic College of Medicine and Science

Jay H. Ryu, MD
Consultant, Division of Pulmonary & Critical Care Medicine, Mayo Clinic, Rochester, Minnesota; Professor of Medicine, Mayo Clinic College of Medicine and Science

Swathi S. Sangli, MD
Fellow in Critical Care Medicine, Mayo Clinic School of Graduate Medical Education, Mayo Clinic College of Medicine and Science, Rochester, Minnesota; now with Allegheny Health Network, Pittsburgh, Pennsylvania

Paul D. Scanlon, MD
Emeritus Member, Division of Pulmonary & Critical Care Medicine, Mayo Clinic, Rochester, Minnesota; Emeritus Professor of Medicine, Mayo Clinic College of Medicine and Science

Dante N. Schiavo, MD
Consultant, Division of Pulmonary & Critical Care Medicine, Mayo Clinic, Rochester, Minnesota; Assistant Professor of Medicine, Mayo Clinic College of Medicine and Science

Bernardo J. Selim, MD
Consultant, Division of Pulmonary & Critical Care Medicine, Mayo Clinic, Rochester, Minnesota; Associate Professor of Medicine, Mayo Clinic College of Medicine and Science

Gaja F. Shaughnessy, MD
Fellow in Pulmonary & Critical Care Medicine, Mayo Clinic School of Graduate Medical Education, Mayo Clinic College of Medicine and Science, Rochester, Minnesota; now with NCH Healthcare System, Naples, Florida

Joseph H. Skalski, MD
Consultant, Division of Pulmonary & Critical Care Medicine, Mayo Clinic, Rochester, Minnesota; Assistant Professor of Medicine, Mayo Clinic College of Medicine and Science

Ulrich Specks, MD
Consultant, Division of Pulmonary & Critical Care Medicine, Mayo Clinic, Rochester, Minnesota; Professor of Medicine, Mayo Clinic College of Medicine and Science

Gregory R. Stroh, MD
Fellow in Pulmonary & Critical Care Medicine, Mayo Clinic School of Graduate Medical Education and Assistant Professor of Medicine, Mayo Clinic College of Medicine and Science, Rochester, Minnesota; now with Essentia Health, Duluth, Minnesota

Yosuf W. Subat, MD
Fellow in Pulmonary & Critical Care Medicine, Mayo Clinic School of Graduate Medical Education and Assistant Professor of Medicine, Mayo Clinic College of Medicine and Science, Rochester, Minnesota; now with Montage Medical Group, Monterey, California

Tara Tarmey, MB, BCh, BAO
Fellow in Cardiothoracic Imaging, Mayo Clinic School of Graduate Medical Education, Mayo Clinic College of Medicine and Science, Rochester, Minnesota; now with University Hospital, Galway, Ireland

Taylor T. Teague, MD
Fellow in Pulmonary & Critical Care Medicine, Mayo Clinic School of Graduate Medical Education, Mayo Clinic College of Medicine and Science, Rochester, Minnesota; now with UT Health, Tyler, Texas

Charles F. Thomas Jr, MD
Consultant, Division of Pulmonary & Critical Care Medicine, Mayo Clinic, Rochester, Minnesota; Associate Professor of Medicine, Mayo Clinic College of Medicine and Science

Gwen E. Thompson, MD
Research Collaborator in Pulmonary & Critical Care Medicine, Mayo Clinic School of Graduate Medical Education, Mayo Clinic College of Medicine and Science, Rochester, Minnesota; now with Sanford Health, Fargo, North Dakota

James P. Utz, MD
Consultant, Division of Pulmonary & Critical Care
Medicine, Mayo Clinic, Rochester, Minnesota; Associate
Professor of Medicine, Mayo Clinic College of Medicine
and Science

Cyril Varghese, MD, MS
Consultant, Division of Pulmonary & Critical Care
Medicine, Mayo Clinic Hospital, Phoenix, Arizona;
Assistant Professor of Medicine, Mayo Clinic College of
Medicine and Science

Kirtivardhan Vashistha
Research Trainee, Multidisciplinary Epidemiology and
Translational Research in Intensive Care (METRIC)
Project; Divisions of Infectious Diseases Department
& Pulmonary & Critical Care Medicine, Mayo Clinic,
Rochester, Minnesota; now with Allegheny Health
Network, Pittsburgh, Pennsylvania

Robert Vassallo, MD
Consultant, Division of Pulmonary & Critical Care
Medicine, Mayo Clinic, Rochester, Minnesota; Professor
of Medicine, Mayo Clinic College of Medicine and Science

Naresh K. Veerabattini, MD
Resident in Internal Medicine, University of Nevada,
Reno School of Medicine, Reno, Nevada

Ann N. Vu, MD
Fellow in Pulmonary & Critical Care Medicine, Mayo
Clinic School of Graduate Medical Education, Mayo
Clinic College of Medicine and Science, Rochester,
Minnesota; now with Holy Cross Medical Group, Fort
Lauderdale, Florida

Catherine Wegner Wippel
Research Trainee, Division of Gastroenterology &
Hepatology, Mayo Clinic, Rochester, Minnesota;
now with Internal Medicine Residency Program,
Washington University School of Medicine, St. Louis,
Missouri

Michael E. Wilson, MD
Senior Associate Consultant, Division of Pulmonary
& Critical Care Medicine, Mayo Clinic, Rochester,
Minnesota; Assistant Professor of Medicine, Mayo
Clinic College of Medicine and Science;
now with Department of Internal Medicine, Division of
Critical Care Medicine, Halifax Health, Daytona Beach,
Florida

Mark E. Wylam, MD
Consultant, Division of Pulmonary & Critical Care
Medicine, Mayo Clinic, Rochester, Minnesota;
Associate Professor of Medicine and of Pediatrics, Mayo
Clinic College of Medicine and Science

Hemang Yadav, MBBS
Consultant, Division of Pulmonary & Critical Care
Medicine, Mayo Clinic, Rochester, Minnesota; Assistant
Professor of Medicine, Mayo Clinic College of Medicine
and Science

Zhenmei Zhang, MD
Senior Associate Consultant, Division of Pulmonary
& Critical Care Medicine, Mayo Clinic, Rochester,
Minnesota; Assistant Professor of Medicine, Mayo Clinic
College of Medicine and Science

Obstructive Lung Disease

A 45-Year-Old Man With Chronic Cough and Dyspnea on Exertion

Emily M. Olson, MD, and Diana J. Kelm, MD

Case Presentation

A 45-year-old man presented to the outpatient clinic for evaluation of uncontrolled asthma. Over the past 4 years, he had progressive nonproductive cough and dyspnea on exertion. The cough was exacerbated with any activity, including talking, and he had several episodes of posttussive syncope. Nocturnal cough and postnasal drainage occurred frequently. These symptoms started shortly after he was exposed to chemicals while working for an oil company; however, most recently he worked in an office. Since the initial diagnosis of asthma, he had been using prednisone in a cyclical fashion, but the symptoms recurred whenever prednisone was discontinued. New symptoms in the previous 3 months included weight loss of 13.5 kg (30 lb), left leg paresthesias, a nonpruritic rash over the elbows, diarrhea, and occasional bright red blood from the rectum. He did not have fevers, hemoptysis, orthopnea, or night sweats.

The patient's past medical history included chronic rhinosinusitis that involved 2 previous sinus surgeries, a recent diagnosis of colonic ulcers, and a remote history of smoking cigarettes (a 4-pack-year history with no smoking in the past 20 years). His medications included cetirizine, clobetasol 0.05% cream twice daily, fluticasone-salmeterol inhaler (500-50 mcg) 1 puff twice daily, fluticasone 220-mcg inhaler 2 puffs twice daily, fluticasone nasal spray, prednisone 10 mg daily, and saline nasal rinse daily. He did not have a family history of lung disease, and he had not traveled outside the US. He had a hot tub, which he cleaned regularly, and he spent time with woodworking. He did not have animal or bird exposure.

On physical examination, the patient was afebrile with a normal heart rate, blood pressure, and oxygen saturation. Breath sounds were clear bilaterally. No oral or nasal ulcers were apparent. Each elbow had multiple violaceous nodules (Figure 1.1).

Laboratory test results (and reference ranges) included the following: elevated eosinophil count, 1.73×10^9/L; immunoglobulin (Ig)E, 655 kU/L (<214 kU/L); IgA, 357 mg/dL (61-356 mg/dL); and urine leukotriene, 670 pg/mg creatinine (<104 pg/mg creatinine). Results were unremarkable for the complete blood cell count, complete metabolic panel, C-reactive protein level, sedimentation rate, and urinalysis. Results were negative for antineutrophil cytoplasmic autoantibody (ANCA), *Aspergillus* antigen, *Blastomyces* antibody, *Coccidioides* antibody, *Cryptococcus* antigen, and *Histoplasma* antibody.

Pulmonary function testing showed mixed restriction and obstructive disease with decreased diffusing capacity for carbon monoxide (64% of the predicted value). Total lung capacity was 79% of the predicted value, residual volume was 134%

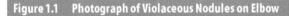

Figure 1.1   Photograph of Violaceous Nodules on Elbow

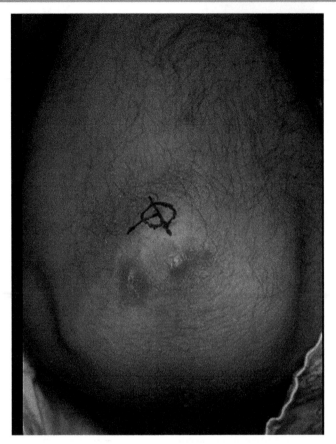

Nodules were present on each elbow, and biopsy results were consistent with granuloma.

of the predicted value, and the ratio of forced expiratory volume in the first second of expiration (FEV$_1$) to forced vital capacity (FVC) was 83% of the predicted value. After bronchodilator administration, the FEV$_1$ improved from 43% to 57% of the predicted value. The exhaled nitric oxide test results were normal.

Computed tomography (CT) of the chest showed diffuse thickening of the bronchial wall with innumerable micronodules and scattered tree-in-bud opacities, primarily in the inferior upper lobes and both lower lobes, and interlobular septal thickening at the bases (Figure 1.2). CT of the sinuses showed diffuse sinus mucosal thickening and hyperdense material within the right maxillary and frontal sinuses (Figure 1.3).

To rule out active infection, bronchoscopy was performed. The cell count from bronchoalveolar lavage (BAL) was 6% neutrophils, 46% eosinophils, 46% alveolar macrophages, and 2% lymphocytes. Results were negative for *Aspergillus* antigen, *Pneumocystis* polymerase chain reaction (PCR), *Legionella* PCR, and adenovirus PCR. BAL cultures had no growth.

Figure 1.2   CT of the Chest

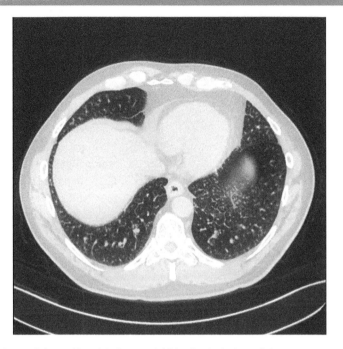

Axial view shows micronodules and interlobular septal thickening in the lower lobes.

Figure 1.3   CT of the Sinuses

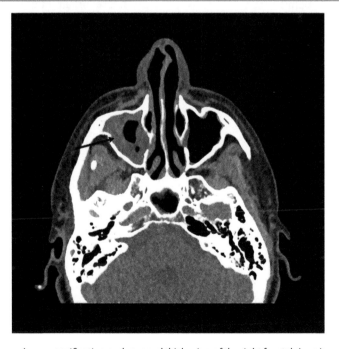

Axial view shows hyperdense opacification and mucosal thickening of the right frontal sinus (arrow).

Questions

Multiple Choice (choose the best answer)

1.1. For the patient described above, which of the following would be diagnostically useful?
a. IgE level
b. Asthma diagnosis
c. ANCA result
d. Lung biopsy findings
e. Eosinophilia on BAL

1.2. Which sinus manifestation is most commonly associated with the condition in the patient described above?
a. Epistaxis
b. Nasal ulcers
c. Rhinosinusitis
d. Nasal polyps
e. Nasal cartilage destruction

1.3. Which diagnostic test is important for determination of the prognosis of all patients with this condition?
a. Colonoscopy
b. Echocardiography
c. Electromyography (EMG)
d. Kidney biopsy
e. Magnetic resonance imaging (MRI) of the brain

1.4. Which statement best describes the disease course for this condition?
a. After completing cyclophosphamide induction, a minority of patients require daily corticosteroids for ongoing asthma symptoms
b. Patients have a higher risk for relapse if they are transitioned to mepolizumab compared to placebo
c. Most patients die of cardiac disease within 5 years
d. Gastrointestinal tract symptoms are the most difficult to control and require high doses of corticosteroids
e. Compared to patients with negative results for ANCA, patients with positive results for ANCA have underlying glomerulonephritis more frequently

1.5. Which of the following is the best way to track clinical remission?
a. Birmingham Vasculitis Activity Score (BVAS)
b. Serum eosinophil level
c. Serum IgG4 level
d. Use of an oral corticosteroid dose equivalent to less than 20 mg prednisone
e. When daily use of an inhaled corticosteroid is no longer required

Case Follow-up and Outcome

A diagnosis of eosinophilic granulomatosis with polyangiitis (EGPA) was established on the basis of the following: history of asthma and rhinosinusitis, peripheral eosinophilia, and high level of IgE. Skin biopsy findings included palisading granulomatous inflammation with dermal collagen necrosis (Figure 1.4). EMG provided confirmation of mild length-dependent axonal neuropathy. A thorough evaluation for extrapulmonary involvement was pursued. Transthoracic echocardiography and electrocardiography did not show any abnormalities. Results from pathology review of colonic ulcers were consistent with EGPA involvement.

Treatment was started with a high dose of prednisone and cyclophosphamide. Over the next 3 months, the patient's cough resolved. Results from follow-up pulmonary function testing were normal, and the peripheral eosinophilia resolved. The patient has subsequently transitioned to azathioprine for maintenance therapy, and he is treated with a low dose of prednisone and lower amounts of inhaled corticosteroids.

Discussion

Patients with refractory asthma, as defined in the 2000 report of the American Thoracic Society Workshop on Refractory Asthma (1), are those who used oral corticosteroids continuously or nearly continuously (>50% of the time) in the previous year or used high doses of inhaled corticosteroids in the previous year. In addition, these patients must have met 2 of the following minor criteria in the previous year: 1) need for an additional daily control medication; 2) need for a short-acting β-agonist daily or nearly daily for symptoms; 3) persistent airway obstruction (FEV$_1$ <80% of the predicted value and diurnal peak expiratory flow variability >20%); 4) need

for at least 3 oral corticosteroid bursts; 5) prompt deterioration with a decreased dose of oral or inhaled corticosteroid; 6) at least 1 urgent care visit for asthma; or 7) a nearly fatal asthma event (requiring hospitalization, intensive care unit stay, or mechanical ventilation).

The differential diagnosis for uncontrolled eosinophilic asthma is broad and includes EGPA, allergic bronchopulmonary aspergillosis (ABPA), hypereosinophilic syndrome, Löffler syndrome, and acute and chronic eosinophilic pneumonia. Notably, asthma and sinus involvement are less likely in patients with hypereosinophilic syndrome. The patient's history may prompt consideration of other independent causes for uncontrolled asthma or hypereosinophilia, such as medication adverse effects or helminthic infections, such as strongyloidiasis (2).

The most common infectious cause of uncontrolled asthma is ABPA, which is a hypersensitivity reaction to airway colonization by *Aspergillus*. Evaluation of serum *Aspergillus* antigens is recommended as part of the diagnostic evaluation for eosinophilic asthma (2). IgE levels are nearly always elevated, so they are typically measured during screening. Diagnosis is made when patients who have asthma, hypereosinophilia, and fleeting pulmonary opacities on chest imaging also have high levels of *Aspergillus* antigens and IgE. Typically, symptoms are controlled with 6 weeks of oral corticosteroids. However, occasionally patients require antifungal therapy (eg, itraconazole) if they have frequent flares or if corticosteroids alone do not control symptoms. If disease control becomes challenging, other comorbid diagnoses should be considered (3).

Upper airway obstruction, such as from vocal cord dysfunction or a tumor, can also cause asthma to worsen or be difficult to control (4). If patients have inspiratory wheezing that is not responsive to typical asthma therapy, functional airway obstruction from paradoxical adduction of the vocal cords should be a strong consideration. Vocal cord dysfunction can occur

Figure 1.4 Skin Biopsy of the Elbow

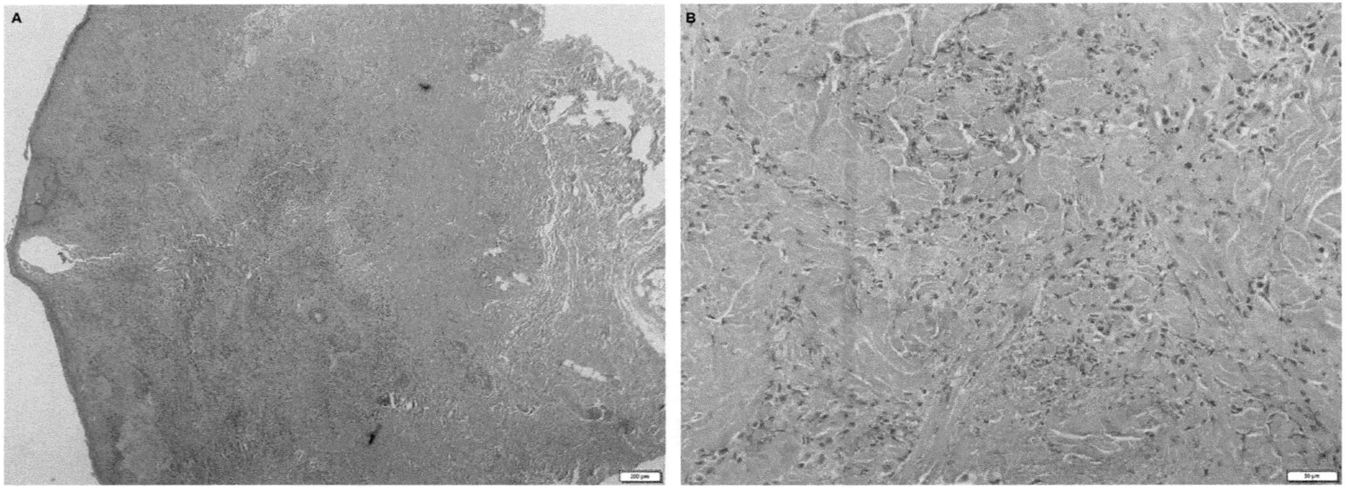

A and B, Histopathology findings included granulomatous inflammation with dermal collagen necrosis (A and B, hematoxylin–eosin).

independently of asthma or coexist with it (5). Laryngoscopy can be helpful in the diagnosis. Treatment requires therapy with a speech-language pathologist.

As with the patient described above, if eosinophilic asthma is accompanied by systemic symptoms, evaluation for EGPA should be undertaken. A lack of underlying allergies should increase clinical suspicion for EGPA (6). However, the converse is not true, and patients who have EGPA and atopy have a considerably higher risk for severe or uncontrolled asthma (7). EGPA is a small-vessel vasculitis that typically occurs with a primary syndrome of asthma and accompanying eosinophilia. Disease presentation is heterogeneous, and other common symptoms include rhinosinusitis, peripheral neuropathies, and granulomatous skin disease (8).

EGPA has 2 commonly described clinical phenotypes: eosinophilic-predominant EGPA and vasculitic-predominant EGPA. Early in the disease course, patients primarily have asthma and sinusitis before they have systemic symptoms secondary to eosinophilic infiltration. Years later, a third disease phase may occur and be characterized by vasculitis with inflammation outside the sinopulmonary system, such as glomerulonephritis, palpable purpura, and mononeuritis multiplex (9,10). However, these phases and phenotypes are fluid and commonly overlap.

Imaging, pulmonary function testing, and laboratory analysis are all essential in the diagnostic evaluation for EGPA. High-resolution CT of the chest often shows patchy migratory consolidations, and noncaseating nodules. Rarely, patients have diffuse alveolar hemorrhage or pleural effusions (11). Although ANCA is not sensitive or specific for EGPA, ANCA should be evaluated as recommended in an international consensus (9). Patients tend to have myeloperoxidase antibodies, and the patients who have them also have the vasculitic phenotype (9,10). In other words, patients who have EGPA and test positive for ANCA have a higher

risk for glomerulonephritis or neuropathy and a lower risk for eosinophilic infiltrative disease such as cardiomyopathy or gastrointestinal tract ulcers (11).

The Five-Factor Score (FFS) establishes the risk of mortality and drives additional evaluation for involvement of the kidneys, gastrointestinal tract, heart, or central nervous system. Additionally, an FFS greater than 1 predicts risk of relapse (12). Cardiac disease from eosinophilic infiltration is an independent risk factor, so all patients should undergo cardiac evaluation with electrocardiography and imaging with echocardiography or cardiac MRI. Similarly, patients should undergo routine evaluation for kidney involvement.

Patients with multisystem involvement typically require high doses of corticosteroids in addition to another immunosuppressant for disease remission. Cyclophosphamide is usually a first-line induction agent; however, recent studies suggest that rituximab is safe and efficacious for both induction and maintenance (13). This is especially true for patients who have EGPA and myeloperoxidase antibodies. Patients who use cyclophosphamide or rituximab are typically transitioned to either azathioprine or methotrexate for maintenance therapy in combination with low doses of corticosteroids (2). Asthma symptoms often flare with decreased doses of glucocorticoid, and many patients require lifelong therapy with glucocorticoids. Even if symptoms improve, the results of pulmonary function tests often do not change (14). In a recent systematic review, Basta et al (15) identified omalizumab as an effective option for decreasing corticosteroid doses for patients who have asthma-predominant disease. However, about one-third of patients have symptom relapse that requires using higher doses of corticosteroids or adding other agents such as an inhibitor of interleukin 5 (eg, mepolizumab) (16).Other agents targeting interleukin 5, such as benralizumab and reslizumab, are being studied.

Summary

The differential diagnosis for uncontrolled asthma is broad and includes vasculitis, eosinophilic pneumonia, structural abnormalities such as vocal cord dysfunction, and infectious causes such as ABPA among many others. EGPA should be considered when patients have uncontrolled asthma, eosinophilia and rhinosinusitis, and systemic symptoms such as neuropathy, skin lesions, or glomerulonephritis. Glucocorticoids are the mainstay of management, and often patients require long-term therapy with prednisone for asthma control.

Answers

1.1. Answer b.

Asthma is critical for the diagnosis of EGPA. The 1990 American College of Rheumatology criteria continue to evolve, but the criteria have a high specificity for the diagnosis of EGPA when patients meet 4 or more of the following 6 criteria: asthma, eosinophilia (>10% eosinophils) on the leukocyte count, mononeuropathy, migratory pulmonary infiltrates, sinus abnormality, and biopsy results that identify eosinophilia in the extravascular space. Alternatively, all 3 Lanham criteria can be applied (asthma, peripheral eosinophilia [eosinophils >1.5×10^9/L], and systemic vasculitis involving ≥2 extrapulmonary organs). Not all patients have elevated IgE levels or positive ANCA results, so they are not part of the diagnostic criteria. Biopsy is not required for diagnosis, and lung biopsy would be a high-risk procedure. However, when the diagnosis is in question, biopsies of affected extrapulmonary organs may prove helpful and are encouraged by the EGPA Consensus Task Force. Eosinophilia on BAL is a nonspecific finding. Additional information is available in the medical literature (2,17,18).

1.2. Answer c.

A majority of patients with EGPA have rhinosinusitis. Epistaxis is not a primary presentation of EGPA sinus disease. Although nasal polyps can occur, polyps are not the most common presentation. Nasal ulcers and nasal cartilage destruction (saddle nose deformity) occur in granulomatosis with polyangiitis but not with EGPA. Additional information is available in the medical literature (8).

1.3. Answer b.

Cardiac complications are the most feared because they increase mortality, so a European consensus task force suggests that all patients with EGPA undergo cardiac imaging (eg, echocardiography). Although routine monitoring for kidney involvement is suggested, this can be accomplished through routine monitoring of serum creatinine levels and urinalyses to evaluate for proteinuria. Evaluation for gastrointestinal tract and nervous system involvement should be considered on the basis of patient symptoms; thus colonoscopy, EMG, and MRI of the brain are not indicated for all patients. Additional information is available in the medical literature (2,19).

1.4. Answer e.

Compared to patients with negative results for ANCA, patients with positive results for ANCA are more likely to have a vasculitis-predominant presentation, including glomerulonephritis, mononeuritis multiplex, and skin manifestations. Most patients require a low dose of corticosteroids long-term for management of symptoms, and asthma symptoms are the most difficult to control. Use of mepolizumab can decrease relapse rates among patients with EGPA. Patients with EGPA have a good prognosis; the 5-year mortality is less than 10%. Additional information is available in the medical literature (2,7,9,11,16,19,20).

1.5. Answer a.

The BVAS can be used to monitor symptoms. Disease is considered to be in remission if the BVAS is zero while the patient's dosage of prednisone is less than 7.5 mg daily. Although the disease course typically corresponds with the degree of serum eosinophilia and the IgG4 level, these findings are not part of the definition of disease remission. Patients typically have an ongoing need for inhaled corticosteroids and a low dose of oral corticosteroids for asthma control and thus clinical remission. Additional information is available in the medical literature (2,21,22).

References

1. Proceedings of the ATS workshop on refractory asthma: current understanding, recommendations, and unanswered questions. American Thoracic Society. Am J Respir Crit Care Med. 2000;162(6):2341–51.
2. Groh M, Pagnoux C, Baldini C, Bel E, Bottero P, Cottin V, et al. Eosinophilic granulomatosis with polyangiitis (Churg-Strauss) (EGPA) Consensus Task Force recommendations for evaluation and management. Eur J Intern Med. 2015;26(7):545–53.
3. Kanj A, Abdallah N, Soubani AO. The spectrum of pulmonary aspergillosis. Respir Med. 2018;141:121–31.
4. Valerio MP, Sousa S, Costa J, Rodrigues DM, Ferreira C, Martins Y, et al. Difficult to treat asthma: the importance of thoracic imaging. Respir Med Case Rep. 2020;30:101127.
5. Vertigan AE, Kapela SL, Gibson PG. Laryngeal dysfunction in severe asthma: a cross-sectional observational study. J Allergy Clin Immunol Pract. 2021;9(2):897–905.
6. Bottero P, Bonini M, Vecchio F, Grittini A, Patruno GM, Colombo B, et al. The common allergens in the Churg-Strauss syndrome. Allergy. 2007;62(11):1288–94.
7. Berti A, Volcheck GW, Cornec D, Smyth RJ, Specks U, Keogh KA. Severe/uncontrolled asthma and overall survival in atopic patients with eosinophilic granulomatosis with polyangiitis. Respir Med. 2018;142:66–72.
8. Low CM, Keogh KA, Saba ES, Gruszczynski NR, Berti A, Specks U, et al. Chronic rhinosinusitis in eosinophilic granulomatosis with polyangiitis: clinical presentation and antineutrophil cytoplasmic antibodies. Int Forum Allergy Rhinol. 2020;10(2):217–22.
9. Moiseev S, Bossuyt X, Arimura Y, Blockmans D, Csernok E, Damoiseaux J, et al. International Consensus on ANCA testing in eosinophilic granulomatosis with polyangiitis. Am J Respir Crit Care Med. 2020.
10. Trivioli G, Terrier B, Vaglio A. Eosinophilic granulomatosis with polyangiitis: understanding the disease and its management. Rheumatology (Oxford). 2020;59(Suppl 3):iii84–iii94.
11. Chang HC, Chou PC, Lai CY, Tsai HH. Antineutrophil cytoplasmic antibodies and organ-specific manifestations in eosinophilic granulomatosis with polyangiitis: a systematic review and meta-analysis. J Allergy Clin Immunol Pract. 2021;9(1):445–52 e6.
12. Kim DS, Song JJ, Park YB, Lee SW. Five factor score of more than 1 is associated with relapse during the first 2 year-follow up in patients with eosinophilic granulomatosis with polyangiitis. Int J Rheum Dis. 2017;20(9):1261–8.
13. Casal Moura M, Berti A, Keogh KA, Volcheck GW, Specks U, Baqir M. Asthma control in eosinophilic granulomatosis with polyangiitis treated with rituximab. Clin Rheumatol. 2020;39(5):1581–90.
14. Berti A, Cornec D, Casal Moura M, Smyth RJ, Dagna L, Specks U, et al. Eosinophilic granulomatosis with polyangiitis: clinical predictors of long-term asthma severity. Chest. 2020;157(5):1086–99.
15. Basta F, Mazzuca C, Nucera E, Schiavino D, Afeltra A, Antonelli Incalzi R. Omalizumab in eosinophilic granulomatosis with polyangiitis: friend or foe? A systematic literature review. Clin Exp Rheumatol. 2020;38 Suppl 124(2):214–20.
16. Wechsler ME, Akuthota P, Jayne D, Khoury P, Klion A, Langford CA, et al. Mepolizumab or placebo for eosinophilic granulomatosis with polyangiitis. N Engl J Med. 2017;376(20):1921–32.
17. Masi AT, Hunder GG, Lie JT, Michel BA, Bloch DA, Arend WP, et al. The American College of Rheumatology 1990 criteria for the classification of Churg-Strauss syndrome (allergic granulomatosis and angiitis). Arthritis Rheum. 1990;33(8):1094–100.
18. Wu EY, Hernandez ML, Jennette JC, Falk RJ. Eosinophilic granulomatosis with polyangiitis: Clinical Pathology Conference and Review. J Allergy Clin Immunol Pract. 2018;6(5):1496–504.
19. Comarmond C, Pagnoux C, Khellaf M, Cordier JF, Hamidou M, Viallard JF, et al. Eosinophilic granulomatosis with polyangiitis (Churg-Strauss): clinical characteristics and long-term followup of the 383 patients enrolled in the French Vasculitis Study Group cohort. Arthritis Rheum. 2013;65(1):270–81.
20. Samson M, Puechal X, Devilliers H, Ribi C, Cohen P, Stern M, et al. Long-term outcomes of 118 patients with eosinophilic granulomatosis with polyangiitis (Churg-Strauss syndrome) enrolled in two prospective trials. J Autoimmun. 2013;43:60–9.
21. Mukhtyar C, Lee R, Brown D, Carruthers D, Dasgupta B, Dubey S, et al. Modification and validation of the Birmingham Vasculitis Activity Score (version 3). Ann Rheum Dis. 2009;68(12):1827–32.
22. Vaglio A, Strehl JD, Manger B, Maritati F, Alberici F, Beyer C, et al. IgG4 immune response in Churg-Strauss syndrome. Ann Rheum Dis. 2012;71(3):390–3.

A 59-Year-Old Woman With Episodic Dyspnea

Paige K. Marty, MD, and Alexander S. Niven, MD

2

Case Presentation

A 59-year-old woman presented for evaluation of progressive episodic dyspnea over the past 3 years. She had been healthy until the preceding 3 years, when progressive, waxing and waning dyspnea developed and was accompanied by cough, sinus congestion, and postnasal drainage. She was given a diagnosis of asthma and treated with an inhaled corticosteroid, a long-acting β-agonist, and albuterol as needed. Her symptoms remained uncontrolled. Six months before presentation, she underwent a pulmonary evaluation at another medical facility. That evaluation included extensive laboratory testing and bronchoscopy, but the results were unremarkable. Findings were also unremarkable from bronchoalveolar lavage and transbronchial biopsy. For rhinosinusitis, the patient underwent functional endoscopic sinus surgery and septoplasty 5 months before presentation; the cough, sinus congestion, and postnasal drainage improved, but the symptoms of dyspnea did not.

At presentation, the patient reported that she had shortness of breath after walking several blocks but did not have wheezing or nocturnal respiratory symptoms. She also reported that she had abrupt episodes when she had difficulty taking a deep breath. Those episodes were not associated with exertion, but they were accompanied by throat tightness, stridor, and changes in her voice. The symptoms did not improve with short courses of prednisone and antibiotics and a prolonged trial of omeprazole.

Her past medical history included chronic lymphocytic thyroiditis (also called Hashimoto disease) treated with levothyroxine, chronic urticaria, and episodic peripheral eosinophilia. She had never smoked and had a remote history of exposure to tuberculosis. She did not report any occupational exposure to irritants or a family history of pulmonary disease.

On physical examination, she coughed intermittently but seemed comfortable. Her vital signs were normal, and oxygen saturation as measured by pulse oximetry was 98% while she breathed room air. She had bilateral nasal turbinate erythema, dried nasal secretions, and oropharyngeal erythema with cobblestoning. The lungs were clear on auscultation, and heart sounds were normal.

Radiography of the chest did not show abnormalities. Computed tomography of the sinuses showed widely patent postsurgical changes and mild chronic mucosal thickening. Results were normal for spirometry and diffusing capacity of the lung for carbon monoxide, and the oral exhaled nitric oxide level was high (133 ppb). Results were normal for a complete blood cell count and a differential count, a basic metabolic profile, thyroid studies, and autoimmune serology cascade. Other recent test results were normal or negative for quantitative serum immunoglobulins, fungal antibodies, antineutrophil cytoplasmic autoantibodies, immunoglobulin E, *Aspergillus*-specific antibodies, and sputum cultures for acid-fast bacilli.

Questions

Multiple Choice (choose the best answer)

2.1. You suspect that the patient may have inducible laryngeal obstruction (ILO), also known as vocal cord dysfunction. What element of the patient's past medical history is most commonly associated with ILO?
a. Recurrent infections
b. Chronic urticaria
c. Asthma
d. Tuberculosis exposure
e. Hypothyroidism

2.2. Which of the following tests is most likely to be diagnostic for this condition?
a. pH impedance testing
b. Methacholine challenge testing (bronchoprovocation testing)
c. Exercise bronchoprovocation testing
d. Cardiopulmonary exercise testing
e. Rhinolaryngoscopy

2.3. Which of the following pulmonary function testing abnormalities is associated with ILO?
a. Flattening of the inspiratory limb of the flow-volume loop
b. Flattening of the expiratory limb of the flow-volume loop
c. Flattening of both the inspiratory and the expiratory limbs of the flow-volume loop
d. A scooped appearance on the expiratory limb of the flow-volume loop
e. A sawtooth pattern on the expiratory limb of the flow-volume loop

2.4. Which of the following rhinolaryngoscopic findings is most closely associated with a diagnosis of ILO?
a. Adduction of the anterior vocal cords during inspiration
b. Adduction of the anterior vocal cords during early expiration
c. Adduction of the anterior vocal cords at the end of expiration
d. Posterior oropharyngeal cobblestoning
e. Vocal cord erythema and edema

2.5. Which of the following treatments decreases ILO symptoms most effectively?
a. Positive airway pressure
b. Inhaled corticosteroids
c. Targeted antibiotic treatment
d. Speech-behavioral therapy
e. Inhaled mixture of helium and oxygen (heliox)

Case Follow-up and Outcome

Flexible fiberoptic rhinolaryngoscopy showed extensive mucosal inflammation and cobble-stoning in both nares and the posterior oro-pharynx with clear mucus pooling. The arytenoid cartilages, true vocal cords, and vocal folds were erythematous and edematous. Provocative maneuvers elicited paradoxical anterior vocal cord adduction during inspiration and repro-duced the patient's shortness of breath and stridor; those responses were consistent with ILO. The patient was treated with nasal saline rinses twice daily, an intranasal corticosteroid, and an oral antihistamine. Her inhaler technique was sub-optimal, so additional education was provided with observed practice. She was also referred to a speech-language pathologist for voice therapy techniques to prevent and treat the ILO episodes. In follow-up, her asthma and rhinosinusitis symptoms were well controlled, and the episodes of dyspnea and stridor had greatly improved.

Discussion

Dyspnea is a common and complex problem that can be due to several organic and psychosocial factors. Patients with unexplained dyspnea have symptoms for at least 3 weeks from a cause that cannot be identified from the initial medical his-tory, physical examination, and screening tests. More than 1 cause is present in up to one-third of patients, and evaluation should start with a clinical assessment that guides the stepwise selec-tion of tests for accurate detection or exclusion of commonly associated conditions (1).

The clinical syndrome of *vocal cord dysfunc-tion* was first described by Christopher et al (2) in a series of patients who presented with episodic wheezing and shortness of breath that had previously been diagnosed as asthma. Their symptoms were caused by paradoxical vocal fold motion in combination with functional laryngeal obstruction, now more commonly described as ILO. Epidemiologic studies of ILO have identified a female predominance (>70% in some series) and triggers that include exertion (particularly in children); irritants (eg, smoke and strong odors, gastroesophageal reflux, and rhinosinusitis); psychiatric disorders (eg, con-version or factitious disorder, anxiety, or depres-sion); and emotional stress (3-5). ILO has been identified as the primary cause of exertional dyspnea in 10% to 15% of young patients, with approximately one-third having a misdiagnosis of asthma and being referred for further evalu-ation after having no improvement with aggres-sive therapy (6). In a large series, 35% to 56% of patients with ILO had objective evidence of asthma, which underscores that these conditions are not mutually exclusive, as illustrated with the patient in the case described above (7,8). Patients with ILO often have a history of physical or psychologic abuse and frequent use of health care. Correct diagnosis and therapy often de-crease the frequency with which these patients seek medical attention (9).

Common symptoms of ILO include wheezing (36%), stridor (28%), cough (25%), chest tight-ness (25%), throat tightness (22%), and voice changes (12%). Patients may also have symptoms of hyperventilation, such as light-headedness, changes in vision, and numbness and tingling in the extremities (4). Physical examination findings are often normal unless the patient is acutely symptomatic at presentation. Therefore, careful evaluation is required for identification of findings that may suggest triggers (eg, allergic rhinitis) or concomitant conditions.

When patients have acute symptoms of ILO, the inspiratory limb of the flow-volume loop may flatten in a pattern consistent with vari-able extrathoracic obstruction (10-13). The fre-quency of this finding among patients with ILO has not been evaluated prospectively but is low in our clinical experience, and it may be dem-onstrated more frequently during methacholine bronchoprovocation testing. An important point is that many other conditions can cause variable extrathoracic obstruction (eg, upper airway tumors, vocal cord paralysis, airway strictures, or granulomatosis with polyangiitis), and this pattern is not specific for ILO (4,11,14).

Fiberoptic rhinolaryngoscopy is commonly performed to evaluate for upper airway abnormalities in patients who present with stridor, dysphonia, and wheezing. This procedure allows for assessment of the location of obstruction throughout the respiratory cycle (15). During a normal respiratory cycle, the vocal cords abduct on inspiration and slightly adduct on exhalation (3). The typical findings in patients who have ILO are adduction of the vocal cords on inspiration, which is usually confined to the anterior two-thirds of the vocal cords, and a diamond-shaped posterior glottic chink (Figure 2.1) (16,17). This assessment can be made while the patient is inspiring deeply or sniffing or while the patient is exposed to

a common trigger (eg, perfume) (18). The obstruction can also be identified in the supraglottic area, which includes the epiglottis, arytenoid cartilages, and false vocal folds (15). Patients with symptoms of ILO on exertion can undergo continuous videolaryngoscopic examination during a cardiopulmonary exercise test to establish the diagnosis (19).

Management of ILO may require multispecialty collaboration for targeted treatment of contributing conditions such as allergic rhinitis, asthma, and gastroesophageal reflux. Patients should avoid common triggers and irritants if possible. Therapy with a speech-language pathologist is important in the prevention and treatment of ILO with techniques that focus on vocal hygiene and phonation training (5,20). Many patients, particularly those with a history of abuse or psychiatric conditions, may also need relief of underlying

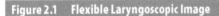

Figure 2.1   Flexible Laryngoscopic Image

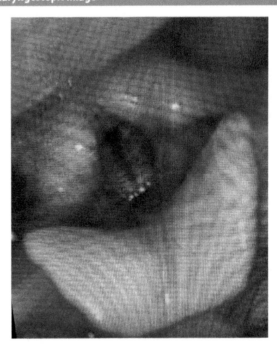

This image shows paradoxical adduction of the vocal cords during inspiration and a posterior glottic chink. These findings suggest ILO.

psychodynamic stressors, cognitive behavioral therapy, and treatment of concomitant mood disorders by a behavioral health specialist. Botulinum toxin injection into the larynx has been used in refractory cases of ILO with variable efficacy (12,21).

The approach to management of an acute episode of ILO is multifactorial and often challenging. Initial strategies include reassurance and breathing exercises, such as panting, exhaling through pursed lips, or breathing through a straw (5,12,22). Anxiolytic medication may be used in patients who have anxious features and no response to these measures. The use of continuous positive airway pressure devices has also been used with some success if patients present with severe respiratory distress, although evidence is limited (22,23). Inhaled helium-oxygen mixture (heliox) has also been used during acute episodes of ILO although without definite evidence of benefit (24). Hypoxemia or respiratory arrest do not occur in patients with uncomplicated ILO (12).

Summary

Dyspnea is a symptom with many possible causes, including upper airway pathology. ILO should be considered when patients have acute-onset episodic dyspnea, stridor, and difficulty with inspiration. The diagnosis of ILO is established when patients present with an appropriate clinical history and laryngoscopic examination shows adduction of the vocal cords resulting in symptomatic, transient upper airway obstruction. During pulmonary function testing of such patients, the inspiratory limb of the flow-volume loop may be flattened, but this sign is insensitive and is not required for diagnosis. ILO can coexist in patients who have other conditions that cause cough and dyspnea, including rhinosinusitis and asthma, and ILO is also associated with psychiatric disorders. The mainstays of treatment include optimization of other upper airway pathologic findings, speech-behavioral therapy, and management of behavioral health conditions if identified.

Answers

2.1. Answer c.

The patient's history of asthma would be the element most commonly associated with ILO. ILO can also be associated with gastroesophageal reflux disease, exertion, rhinosinusitis, and psychiatric disorders. The other diagnoses listed are not typically associated with ILO. Additional information is available in the medical literature (14).

2.2. Answer e.

The most appropriate study would be flexible rhinolaryngoscopy for a definitive diagnosis of ILO. The pH impedance test is performed to assess for gastroesophageal reflux disease and can be considered for patients presenting with chronic cough. Methacholine challenge tests and exercise bronchoprovocation tests can be helpful for identifying bronchial hyperresponsiveness and diagnosing asthma. However, the frequency with which this testing provokes ILO symptoms and produces flow-volume loop findings of variable extrathoracic obstruction is not well defined and is low in our experience. A cardiopulmonary exercise test may give insight into other causes of exercise limitation and dyspnea, but without concomitant rhinolaryngoscopy, exercise testing is unlikely to be diagnostic for ILO. Additional information is available in the medical literature (15).

2.3. Answer a.

ILO may produce a flattening of the inspiratory limb of the flow-volume loop during pulmonary function testing in a pattern consistent with a variable extrathoracic obstruction. Flattening of the expiratory limb of the flow-volume loop is associated with a variable intrathoracic obstruction (eg, diffuse obstructive pathology of intrathoracic airways or an endobronchial tumor), whereas flattening of both the inspiratory limb and the expiratory limb of the flow-volume loop indicates a fixed obstruction (eg, tracheal stenosis). A scooped appearance of the expiratory limb of the flow-volume curve indicates dynamic airflow obstruction (eg, chronic obstructive pulmonary disease or asthma). A sawtooth pattern on the expiratory flow-volume loop has been described when patients have obstructive sleep apnea. Additional information is available in the medical literature (11).

2.4. Answer a.

The characteristic finding of ILO on rhinolaryngoscopy is adduction of the anterior vocal cords during inspiration. A diamond-shaped opening near the posterior glottis (the *posterior glottic chink*) may be present. Patients with ILO can also present with chronic rhinosinusitis, leading to the findings of rhinitis, oropharyngeal cobblestoning, and vocal cord edema and erythema. Mild adduction of the vocal cords during expiration is a normal finding. Additional information is available in the medical literature (17).

2.5. Answer d.

Speech-behavioral therapy is an important intervention for prevention and treatment of paradoxical vocal fold motion through breathing and phonation exercises. Positive airway pressure and heliox have been used anecdotally during acute, severe episodes of ILO, but their use is not standard for treatment or prevention (for lack of evidence). Inhaled corticosteroids (in the treatment of asthma) and targeted antibiotics (in the treatment of sinusitis) do not affect ILO symptoms. Additional information is available in the medical literature (20).

References

1. Niven AS, Weisman IM. Diagnosis of unexplained dyspnea. In: Mahler DA, O'Donnell DE, editors. Dyspnea: mechanisms, measurement and management. Lung biology in health and disease. 2nd ed. New York (NY): Marcel Dekker; 2005. p. 207–63. (Lung biology in health and disease.)
2. Christopher KL, Wood RP 2nd, Eckert RC, Blager FB, Raney RA, Souhrada JF. Vocal-cord dysfunction presenting as asthma. N Engl J Med. 1983; 308(26):1566–70.
3. Forrest LA, Husein T, Husein O. Paradoxical vocal cord motion: classification and treatment. Laryngoscope. 2012;122(4):844–53.
4. Morris MJ, Christopher KL. Diagnostic criteria for the classification of vocal cord dysfunction. Chest. 2010;138(5):1213–23.
5. Petrov AA. Vocal cord dysfunction: the spectrum across the ages. Immunol Allergy Clin North Am. 2019;39(4):547–60.
6. Morris MJ AP, Perkins PJ. Vocal cord dysfunction: etiologies and treatment. Clin Pulm Med. 2006; 13(2):73–86.
7. Newman KB, Mason UG, 3rd, Schmaling KB. Clinical features of vocal cord dysfunction. Am J Respir Crit Care Med. 1995;152(4 Pt 1):1382–6.
8. O'Connell MA, Sklarew PR, Goodman DL. Spectrum of presentation of paradoxical vocal cord motion in ambulatory patients. Ann Allergy Asthma Immunol. 1995;74(4):341–4.
9. Mikita J, Parker J. High levels of medical utilization by ambulatory patients with vocal cord dysfunction as compared to age- and gender-matched asthmatics. Chest. 2006;129(4):905–8.
10. Scanlon PD. Respiratory function: mechanisms and testing. In: Goldman L, Schafer AI, editors. Goldman-Cecil medicine. 25th ed. Philadelphia (PA): Elsevier; 2016. p. 539–45.
11. Dempsey TM, Scanlon PD. Pulmonary function tests for the generalist: a brief review. Mayo Clin Proc. 2018;93(6):763–71.
12. Wood RP 2nd, Milgrom H. Vocal cord dysfunction. J Allergy Clin Immunol. 1996;98(3):481–5.
13. Dunn NM, Katial RK, Hoyte FCL. Vocal cord dysfunction: a review. Asthma Res Pract. 2015;1:9.
14. Lee J, Denton E, Hoy R, Tay TR, Bondarenko J, Hore-Lacy F, et al. Paradoxical vocal fold motion in difficult asthma is associated with dysfunctional breathing and preserved lung function. J Allergy Clin Immunol Pract. 2020;8(7):2256–62.
15. Christensen PM, Heimdal JH, Christopher KL, Bucca C, Cantarella G, Friedrich G, et al. ERS/ELS/ACCP 2013 international consensus conference nomenclature on inducible laryngeal obstructions. Eur Respir Rev. 2015;24(137):445–50.
16. George S, Suresh S. Vocal cord dysfunction: analysis of 27 Cases and updated review of pathophysiology & management. Int Arch Otorhinolaryngol. 2019;23(2):125–30.
17. Christopher KL, Morris MJ. Vocal cord dysfunction, paradoxic vocal fold motion, or laryngomalacia? Our understanding requires an interdisciplinary approach. Otolaryngol Clin North Am. 2010;43(1):43–66.
18. Powell DM, Karanfilov BI, Beechler KB, Treole K, Trudeau MD, Forrest LA. Paradoxical vocal cord dysfunction in juveniles. Arch Otolaryngol Head Neck Surg. 2000;126(1):29–34.
19. Lim K, Li JT. Exertional dyspnea and inspiratory stridor of 2 years' duration: a tale of 2 wheezes. J Allergy Clin Immunol. 2011;128(5):1135-6 e1-10.
20. Patel RR, Venediktov R, Schooling T, Wang B. Evidence-based systematic review: effects of speech-language pathology treatment for individuals with paradoxical Vocal Fold Motion. Am J Speech Lang Pathol. 2015;24(3):566–84.
21. Altman KW, Mirza N, Ruiz C, Sataloff RT. Paradoxical vocal fold motion: presentation and treatment options. J Voice. 2000;14(1):99–103.
22. Denipah N, Dominguez CM, Kraai EP, Kraai TL, Leos P, Braude D. Acute management of paradoxical vocal fold motion (vocal cord dysfunction). Ann Emerg Med. 2017;69(1):18–23.
23. Heiser JM, Kahn ML, Schmidt TA. Functional airway obstruction presenting as stridor: a case report and literature review. J Emerg Med. 1990;8(3):285–9.
24. Slinger C, Slinger R, Vyas A, Haines J, Fowler SJ. Heliox for inducible laryngeal obstruction (vocal cord dysfunction): a systematic literature review. Laryngoscope Investig Otolaryngol. 2019;4(2):255–8.

A 77-Year-Old Man With Chronic Cough and Recurrent Pneumonia

Faysal K. Al-Ghoula, MB, BCh, and Timothy R. Aksamit, MD

3

Case Presentation

A 77-year-old man, a nonsmoker, was evaluated for chronic productive cough and recurrent pneumonia. The cough was intermittent and produced copious amounts of yellow sputum that sometimes contained blood streaks. His symptoms were associated with fatigue and intermittent nocturnal sweats over the past year and a half. The patient was very active, and he did not have shortness of breath, fevers, frank hemoptysis, or chest pain.

His past medical history was notable for stage IV follicular lymphoma for which he was beginning to receive cyclophosphamide, doxorubicin, vincristine, and prednisone (CHOP) therapy. Over the past 20 years, the patient had recurrent pneumonia for which he received multiple courses of antibiotics.

On physical examination, the patient was cachectic but not in acute respiratory distress; his oxygen saturation was 94% while breathing room air. On auscultation, he had coarse breath sounds with rare, soft expiratory wheezes but no rubs or bronchial breathing. He did not have clubbing, cyanosis, or pitting edema. The patient underwent computed tomography (CT) of the chest and bronchoscopy, including bronchoalveolar lavage with the immunocompromised host protocol, which grew *Mycobacterium avium* complex (MAC).

Questions

Multiple Choice (choose the best answer)

3.1. For the patient described above, which test should *not* be performed next?
a. Sweat chloride testing
b. Total immunoglobulin level
c. α_1-Antitrypsin serum (AAT) level
d. *Aspergillus*-specific immunoglobulin (Ig) E
e. Screening for the *CFTR* gene sequence variation

3.2. What is the typical distribution or location of cylindrical bronchiectasis associated with nodular infiltrates due to MAC?
a. Diffuse
b. Lingula and right middle lobe
c. Right lower lobe
d. Left lower lobe
e. Apices

3.3. What is the first-line treatment of MAC lung disease?
a. Azithromycin, moxifloxacin, and rifampin
b. Amikacin, azithromycin, and moxifloxacin

c. Azithromycin, ethambutol, and rifampin
d. Azithromycin, clofazimine, and rifampin
e. Amoxicillin-clavulanic acid, azithromycin, and metronidazole

3.4. Which of the following factors would affect treatment decisions for a patient with MAC?
a. Cavitary lung disease
b. Sex of patient
c. Iron replacement therapy
d. Kidney impairment
e. Lung function test results

3.5. For how long should MAC treatment be continued according to the clinical practice guideline of the American Thoracic Society (ATS), European Respiratory Society (ERS), European Society of Clinical Microbiology and Infectious Diseases (ESCMID), and Infectious Diseases Society of America (IDSA)?
a. For 7 days after symptoms resolve
b. For 1 month after culture results are negative
c. For 6 months after symptoms resolve
d. For 12 months after diagnosis
e. For 12 months after culture results are negative

Case Follow-up and Outcome

The smear and culture of the sample from bronchoscopy were positive for MAC. Susceptibility testing demonstrated macrolide resistance. The patient had been treated empirically with macrolide-based triple-drug mycobacterial therapy. The use of macrolides was discontinued, and therapy was begun with a combination of antibiotics, including nebulized amikacin. Bronchial hygiene included the use of an oscillating positive expiratory pressure device, 3% hypertonic saline, and a high-frequency chest wall oscillation vest. The patient was enrolled for medication monitoring, including audiometry and liver function tests. He completed approximately 15 months of mycobacterial therapy and had sputum conversion with complete resolution of symptoms.

Discussion

Bronchiectasis is a pathologic, irreversible dilatation of bronchi. This bronchial dilatation usually results from chronic or recurrent damage to the bronchi, most commonly from infection. Patients can have an increased risk for bronchiectasis if they have certain conditions, such as cystic fibrosis (CF), acquired or inherited immune deficiency syndromes, chronic inflammatory lung disease, and chronic lung infections, especially mycobacterial infections (both tuberculous and nontuberculous mycobacteria [NTM]).

The most common chronic infections that cause bronchiectasis are fungal (eg, bronchopulmonary aspergillosis) and mycobacterial infections. Although the most common form of mycobacterial lung infection worldwide is tuberculosis, NTM infection is more prevalent in the US, and the main NTM is MAC. Bronchiectasis and MAC have a complex relationship because bronchiectasis can be both a risk factor for NTM infection and a complication of NTM infection.

Chronic airway disease, such as chronic obstructive pulmonary disease and bronchial asthma, can increase the risk for NTM infection.

Clinically, patients with MAC infection present with a history of symptoms that have persisted for weeks to months and include cough (usually productive but may be dry), fatigue, weight loss, fever, and night sweats. Two types of MAC infection are evident radiologically: the nodular-bronchiectatic form (with peribronchial tree-in-bud nodules) and cylindrical bronchiectasis, which affects the lingula and the right middle lobe. The other radiologic form of MAC infection is the cavitary form, which has an upper lobe predilection. Mixed patterns have been reported as well. This distinction is important since it helps in guiding the treatment of the MAC infection.

Before the patient begins a lengthy and risky treatment, the diagnosis should be confirmed by the presence of all the following: 1) typical pulmonary symptoms of mycobacterial infection, 2) presence of cavitary or nodular lesions on CT with or without bronchiectasis, and 3) exclusion of other diagnoses. Since radiologic findings are not specific, the 2020 clinical practice guideline of the ATS, ERS, ESCMID, and IDSA requires a microbiologic diagnosis (1). Criteria for microbiologic diagnosis of MAC infection are 1) presence of positive mycobacterial culture from at least 2 separate sputum specimens (preferably collected in early morning) or 2) at least 1 bronchial washing with positive results from a sputum culture. Hypertonic saline can be used to induce sputum. Antibiotic sensitivity should always be evaluated.

The recommended first-line treatment of MAC infection is azithromycin, rifampin, and ethambutol used in combination (Figure 3.1) (2). The frequency of treatment depends on the type of MAC infection. The cavitary type requires daily administration of antibiotics, but 3 times weekly is sufficient for the nodular-bronchiectatic type. If antibiotic sensitivity results indicate macrolide resistance, acceptable alternatives include moxifloxacin, clofazimine, bedaquiline, or inhaled liposomal amikacin. Antibiotics should be continued for at least 12 months after culture results are negative.

Figure 3.1   Treatment Algorithm for MAC Infection

Choice of antimicrobial

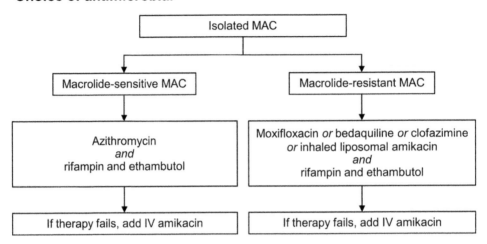

Frequency of administration

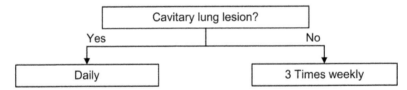

Duration of treatment

Continue antimicrobial therapy for 12 mo after culture negativity

Treatment recommendations reflect the 2020 clinical practice guidelines developed by the ATS, ERS, ESCMID, and IDSA. IV indicates intravenous.

Summary

Bronchiectasis is a pathologic, irreversible dilatation of bronchi resulting from chronic damage to the bronchi (eg, from infection). Risk factors for bronchiectasis include CF, immune deficiency syndromes, chronic inflammatory lung disease, and chronic lung infections. MAC is a common cause of bronchiectasis in the US. The diagnosis of either of the 2 types of MAC infection, cavitary and nodular-bronchiectatic, requires 2 sputum cultures positive for MAC or 1 bronchial washing culture positive for MAC. Treatment is with combination antibiotic therapy (azithromycin, rifampin, and ethambutol) that should be continued for at least 12 months after culture results are negative.

Answers

3.1. Answer c.

Evaluation of a patient with bronchiectasis should include identification of potential causes of the bronchiectasis and the presence of respiratory pathogens, including testing for infection (bacterial, fungal, and mycobacterial cultures). Testing for genetic disorders such as CF (sweat chloride testing with or without *CFTR* gene sequence variation screening) and for the AAT serum level is generally recommended. For younger patients who have bronchiectasis and sinopulmonary disease with or without infertility, consideration should be given for screening for primary cilia dyskinesia with nasal nitric oxide, and genetic screening may also be appropriate. Immunoglobulins should be checked to evaluate for hypogammaglobulinemia, which can occur with common variable immunodeficiency. Testing for rheumatologic and connective tissue disease with rheumatoid factor and antinuclear antibody titers may be warranted in select patients. If patients have chronic asthma and bronchiectasis, *Aspergillus*-specific IgE and IgG serum levels should be checked because ABPA is a common cause of bronchiectasis in patients with asthma. The association between AAT and bronchiectasis is controversial, so checking the AAT serum level should not be the first test to order. Additional information is available in the medical literature (3).

3.2. Answer b.

The distribution of bronchiectasis varies according to the cause. Bronchiectasis involving upper lung zones is more commonly associated with CF or tuberculosis, while the middle lobe and lingula are typical locations of cylindrical bronchiectasis associated with NTM lung disease, including MAC lung disease. Causes of lower lobe bronchiectasis include foreign body aspiration, hypogammaglobulinemia, gastroesophageal reflux or aspiration, and primary ciliary dyskinesia. Additional information is available in the medical literature (4).

3.3. Answer c.

For patients who have MAC lung disease without macrolide resistance, the preferred first-line antibiotics for combination therapy are a macrolide (usually azithromycin) with rifampin and ethambutol. However, if macrolide resistance is present, alternatives are amikacin and clofazimine. The CONVERT (Amikacin Liposome Inhalation Suspension for Treatment-Refractory Lung Disease Caused by MAC) trial found that adding amikacin liposomal inhalation solution to the guideline-based therapy resulted in higher rates of culture conversion but was limited to patients who had refractory MAC lung disease (positive results from sputum culture after >6 months of guideline-based therapy). Additional information is available in the medical literature (5).

3.4. Answer a.

When MAC lung disease is diagnosed, the decision to initiate antibiotic treatment should be based on clinical, microbiologic, and radiologic features in addition to shared decision making. The presence of cavitation, with or without a sputum smear that is positive for acid-fast bacilli, warrants the initiation of treatment given the increased likelihood of progressive disease. The presence of cavitary lung disease also affects the frequency of medication administration: Triple-drug mycobaterial therapy should be given daily rather than 3 times weekly. Intravenous amikacin should also be considered for patients who have cavitary MAC lung disease. An important point is that treatment of bronchiectasis with or without MAC lung disease warrants aggressive airway clearance (regular aerobic activity, active cycle breathing, use of a positive expiratory pressure valve, nebulized hypertonic saline, and a high-frequency chest wall oscillation vest) and treatment of comorbidities, including gastroesophageal reflux disease, sinus disease, chronic obstructive pulmonary disease, and asthma. Additional information is available in the medical literature (6).

3.5. Answer e.

The clinical practice guideline of the ATS, ERS, ESCMID, and IDSA recommends that in patients with macrolide-susceptible MAC lung infection, treatment should continue for at least 12 months after culture results are negative. Additional information is available in the medical literature (1).

References

1. Daley CL, Iaccarino JM, Lange C, Cambau E, Wallace RJ Jr, Andrejak C, et al. Treatment of nontuberculous mycobacterial pulmonary disease: an official ATS/ERS/ESCMID/IDSA clinical practice guideline. Clin Infect Dis. 2020;71(4):e1–e36.

2. Daley CL, Iaccarino JM, Lange C, Cambau E, Wallace RJ Jr, Andrejak C, et al. Treatment of nontuberculous mycobacterial pulmonary disease: an official ATS/ERS/ESCMID/IDSA clinical practice guideline. Eur Respir J. 2020;56(1).

3. Carreto L, Morrison M, Donovan J, Finch S, Tan GL, Fardon T, et al. Utility of routine screening for alpha-1 antitrypsin deficiency in patients with bronchiectasis. Thorax. 2020;75(7):592–3.

4. Shoemark A, Ozerovitch L, Wilson R. Aetiology in adult patients with bronchiectasis. Respir Med. 2007;101(6):1163–70.

5. Griffith DE, Eagle G, Thomson R, Aksamit TR, Hasegawa N, Morimoto K, et al. Amikacin liposome inhalation suspension for treatment-refractory lung disease caused by *Mycobacterium avium* complex (CONVERT): a prospective, open-label, randomized study. Am J Respir Crit Care Med. 2018;198(12):1559–69.

6. Munoz G, de Gracia J, Buxo M, Alvarez A, Vendrell M. Long-term benefits of airway clearance in bronchiectasis: a randomised placebo-controlled trial. Eur Respir J. 2018;51(1):1701926.

A 63-Year-Old Woman With Recurrent Exacerbations of Chronic Obstructive Pulmonary Disease

4

Amjad N. Kanj, MD, MPH, and Darlene R. Nelson, MD, MHPE

Case Presentation

A 63-year-old woman with severe chronic obstructive pulmonary disease (COPD) was seen at the pulmonary clinic for recurrent exacerbations. In the past year, she had 3 exacerbations, 1 of which required admission to the intensive care unit. She reported having shortness of breath with minimal activity (modified Medical Research Council dyspnea scale, grade 3), and she was a former smoker with a 40-pack-year history. Her treatment included continuous oxygen therapy (2-4 L/min) and nebulized albuterol, tiotropium, mometasone-formoterol, roflumilast, azithromycin, and prednisone. She recently completed pulmonary rehabilitation.

On physical examination, the patient had diffuse expiratory wheezes with a prolonged expiratory phase. Her body mass index was 23 (calculated as weight in kilograms divided by height in meters squared). Results of pulmonary function tests (PFTs) (with percentage of the predicted value) were as follows: total lung capacity (TLC), 7.3 L (151%); residual volume (RV), 6.1 L (303%); ratio of forced expiratory volume in the first second of expiration (FEV_1) to forced vital capacity (FVC), 28.5%; FEV_1, 0.44 L (19%); and diffusing capacity of lung for carbon monoxide ($DLCO$), 5.2 mL/min/mm Hg (24%). The most recent chest radiograph showed hyperinflation and emphysema with no infiltrates. The 6-minute walk distance (6MWD) was 301 m. A dobutamine stress echocardiogram was negative for ischemia. Left ventricular ejection fraction was 65%. While she was receiving oxygen (2 L/min), arterial blood gas results were the following: pH, 7.40; PCO_2, 41 mm Hg; PO_2, 68 mm Hg; and bicarbonate, 26 mmol/L.

On evaluation, the patient met the eligibility criteria for bronchoscopic lung volume reduction (BLVR). After the risks and benefits of BLVR were discussed, the patient agreed to the procedure. Results of high-resolution computed tomography (CT) of the thorax and a ventilation-perfusion lung study were carefully reviewed. A quantitative analysis of fissure completeness was performed, and the density of emphysema and the lung volumes were determined. The left lower lobe (LLL) was identified as the potential target for BLVR. The patient then underwent bronchoscopy, and the Chartis Pulmonary Assessment System (Pulmonx Corp) was used to evaluate for collateral ventilation. No collateral ventilation was identified. Four endobronchial valves were strategically placed to completely occlude all segments of the LLL.

Questions

Multiple Choice (choose the best answer)

4.1. Which statement correctly describes the use of BLVR in patients with COPD?
   a. BLVR should be considered for symptomatic patients with COPD who are receiving suboptimal medical therapy
   b. Endobronchial valves deployed during BLVR prohibit airflow into and out of the targeted lobe
   c. BLVR is associated with increased exercise capacity and decreased work of breathing
   d. BLVR is reserved for patients with upper lobe–predominant emphysema
   e. BLVR and lung volume reduction surgery have similar costs and mortality rates

4.2. Which of the following is a potential contraindication for BLVR in patients with severe COPD?
   a. Large bullae adjacent to the target lobe
   b. Heterogeneous emphysema with RV more than 175% of the predicted value on PFTs
   c. Daily use of a low dose of prednisone (<20 mg)
   d. Life expectancy of less than 5 years
   e. Consideration for lung transplant

4.3. During selection of the target lobe, which of the following lobe characteristics would not predict success with BLVR?
   a. Large volume
   b. Low perfusion
   c. Absent collateral ventilation
   d. High emphysematous destruction
   e. High collateral ventilation

4.4. Which of the following is an expected outcome from successful BLVR?
   a. Improvement of more than 50% in FEV_1
   b. Increase in RV of 10% to 15%
   c. Improvement in 6MWD and health-related quality of life
   d. Mortality benefit for most patients
   e. Greater clinical improvement with homogeneous distribution of emphysema rather than heterogenous distribution

4.5. In the first week after BLVR, what is the greatest risk for patients?
   a. Pneumonia
   b. Pneumothorax
   c. Respiratory failure
   d. COPD exacerbation
   e. Death

Case Follow-up and Outcome

After she underwent BLVR, the patient was admitted to the hospital for observation. Four hours later, chest radiography showed LLL atelectasis and a new left pneumothorax, which was managed with CT-guided insertion of a pigtail catheter. The patient was discharged on hospital day 5 after the pneumothorax resolved and the pigtail catheter was removed (Figure 4.1).

Six weeks after BLVR, CT of the lungs showed complete lobar atelectasis of the LLL (Figure 4.2). The patient's shortness of breath and work of breathing had improved, but a persistent dry cough had developed. Results of PFTs (percentage of predicted value; change from baseline value) were as follows: TLC, 6.35 L (133%; −0.91 L); RV, 4.00 L (210%; −2.35 L); FEV_1, 1.00 L (43%; + 0.56 L); and DLco, 7.1 mL/min/mm Hg (34%). Her 6MWD was 356 m (+54 m).

Discussion

BLVR is part of the treatment guidelines for patients who have severe emphysema and continue to have symptoms despite optimal standard of care medical therapy (1). The best candidates are patients with dyspnea that is mostly attributable to hyperinflation and air trapping (2).

BLVR involves the use of bronchoscopy for deployment of multiple 1-way valves into segments or subsegments of a targeted lobe. The objective is to prevent air from flowing into a hyperinflated emphysematous lobe and thereby achieve complete lobar atelectasis and allow expansion of the remaining lung (2). This leads to overall improvement in lung mechanics, which in turn reduces the work of breathing and increases exercise tolerance (3).

In eligible patients (Box 4.1), careful selection of the target lobe is essential for predicting BLVR success (4). A quantitative lung CT analysis provides data on the severity and distribution of emphysema, lobar volume, and fissure integrity. The interlobar fissure should be at least 80% complete for successful endobronchial valve (EBV) placement (2). Perfusion scintigraphy may help guide the selection of the lobe for treatment, especially in patients with homogeneous disease (3).

Characteristics of a good target lobe for BLVR are listed in Box 4.2 (1). *Interlobar collateral ventilation*, which refers to ventilation between adjacent lung lobes due to incomplete fissures, may not allow for complete lobar atelectasis. Collateral ventilation can be assessed with the use of fissure integrity on high-resolution CT and with the Chartis System, which consists of a console and a single-use catheter with a balloon at the tip. The balloon is inflated to block the airway supplying the target lobe. Air can flow only out of the target lobe, and real-time assessment of collateral ventilation is achieved (5).

Data from major trials (STELVIO, IMPACT, TRANSFORM, and LIBERATE) have shown favorable results for the BLVR groups, with improvements in lung function, exercise tolerance, severity of dyspnea, and quality of life. By 3 to 12 months after BLVR, the following had improved: FEV_1 (by 17% to 29%); RV (by −0.52 L to −0.83 L); 6MWD (by 39 m to 79 m); and the St George's Respiratory Questionnaire score (by −6.5 points to −14.7 points) (1).

These trials also identified important adverse events related to BLVR. Pneumothorax was the most commonly reported adverse event in the first 45 days after BLVR; it occurred in 27% of patients, and 76% of the occurrences were in the first 3 days after the procedure (6). Revision bronchoscopy was also required in the 12 months after BLVR for 19% to 35% of the patients for adjustment or removal of valves. Complications that required valve removal included pneumothorax, respiratory failure, and valve dislocation or migration. The dislocation or migration of only 1 valve may prevent complete lobar occlusion because of intersegmental collateral ventilation (1). Other potential adverse events include exacerbation of COPD, pneumonia, and death.

Figure 4.1 Chest Radiographs

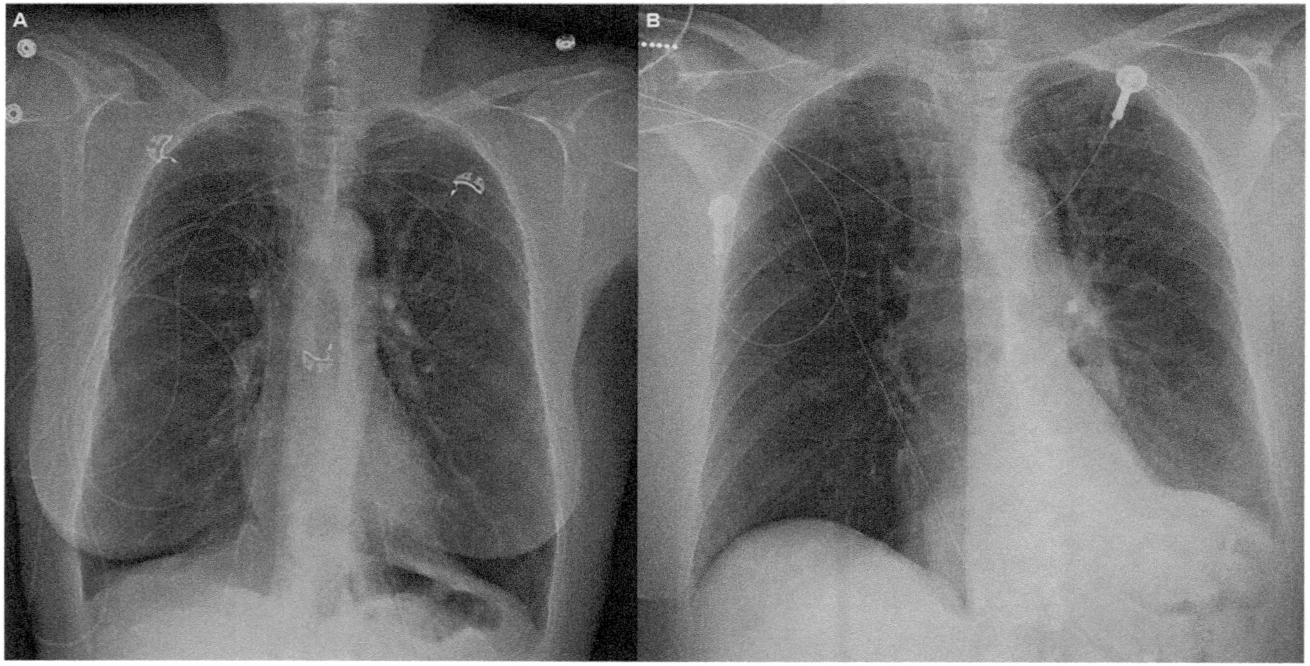

A, Anteroposterior view before BLVR shows hyperinflated lungs with emphysema. B, Anteroposterior view on day 5 after BLVR shows atelectasis of the LLL.

Figure 4.2   CT of the Chest

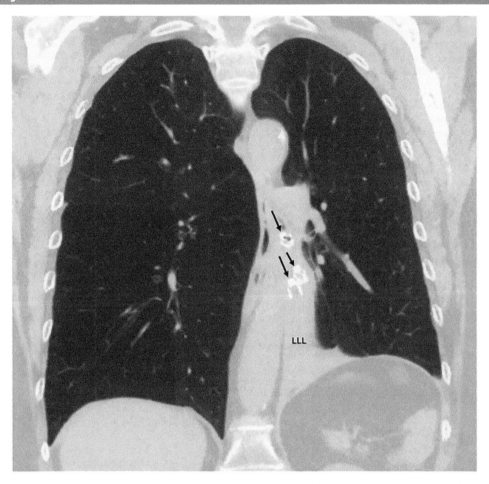

Coronal section 6 weeks after BLVR shows complete lobar atelectasis of the LLL. Arrows indicate EBVs within segmental bronchi.

Box 4.1

Eligibility Criteria for BLVR

Indications

Heterogeneous or homogeneous emphysema

Symptoms despite optimal medical therapy

FEV_1 ≥15% but <50% of the predicted value

RV >175% of the predicted value and TLC >100% of the predicted value

6MWD >100 m but <500 m after pulmonary rehabilitation

Pao_2 >45 mm Hg and $Paco_2$ <60 mm Hg while breathing room air

Contraindications

Active smoking or vaping

Active pulmonary infection

LVEF <35% or sPAP >45 mm Hg

Previous lung transplant, LVRS, or major lung surgery

Severe fibrosis or bronchiectasis or a potentially malignant nodule

Large bullae adjacent to target lobe

Abbreviations: LVEF, left ventricular ejection fraction; LVRS, lung volume reduction surgery; sPAP, systolic pulmonary artery pressure.

Box 4.2

Good Target Lobe Characteristics

Complete fissure

High emphysematous destruction

Large volume

Little interlobar collateral ventilation

Low perfusion

Low intralobar heterogeneity

Summary

BLVR benefits a subset of patients who have severe emphysema and are still symptomatic after receiving optimal medical therapy. Target lobe selection and careful assessment of collateral ventilation are important for successful BLVR. An important risk for patients undergoing BLVR is pneumothorax.

Answers

4.1. Answer c.

BLVR is associated with increased exercise capacity and decreased work of breathing. The procedure should be considered for patients who have COPD but are still symptomatic despite having received optimal medical therapy and pulmonary rehabilitation. In BLVR, 1-way valves are strategically deployed in the targeted lobe. The valves allow air to only exit; the result is lobar atelectasis and collapse. Favorable results have been shown for patients who have homogeneous emphysema or heterogeneous emphysema, although the benefit may be greater with heterogeneous emphysema. BLVR is generally less expensive and less invasive than lung volume reduction surgery, and it has lower mortality rates. Additional information is available in the medical literature (1,2).

4.2. Answer a.

When BLVR is performed in patients who have large bullae (usually larger than one-third the size of the lung) or severe bullous emphysema adjacent to the target lobe, the procedure is associated with a higher rate of pneumothorax and, in some instances, marked hypoxemia. BLVR should be a consideration for patients who have heterogeneous emphysema and high RV (>175% of the predicted value) and for patients who are receiving long-term corticosteroids for management. Life expectancy from other comorbidities of less than 12 months is a relative contraindication to BLVR. Most importantly, undergoing BLVR does not preclude patients from being considered for lung transplant at any time. Additional information is available in the medical literature (2).

4.3. Answer e.

Target lobe selection is crucial to the success of BLVR. Before valve placement, collateral ventilation must be carefully evaluated because its absence is critical for the attainment of lobar atelectasis and collapse. Lobes with the largest volume are ideal targets because large volumes indicate hyperinflation and air trapping. If multiple target lobes are available for BLVR, the lobe with the lowest perfusion may be chosen. Another key determinant in target lobe selection for BLVR is a high degree of emphysematous destruction, which is a reflection of disease in the lobe. Additional information is available in the medical literature (4).

4.4. Answer c.

Although dramatic clinical improvement has been reported, patients undergoing BLVR should be educated about outcomes and counseled to expect more modest improvement. This includes an increase of 22% to 28% in 6MWD and an improvement in health-related quality of life. It also includes an increase of 12% to 15% in FEV_1 and a decrease in RV of 10% to 15%. Clinical improvement is likely greater in patients with heterogeneous distribution of emphysema. Robust evidence on the mortality benefit is still lacking, although improved survival has been shown for certain patients when complete lobar atelectasis was achieved. Additional information is available in the medical literature (2).

4.5. Answer b.

In the LIBERATE trial, pneumothorax occurred in up to 27% of patients in the first 45 days after BLVR. Most pneumothoraces occurred in the first 3 to 5 days after the procedure. Other less common complications included exacerbation of COPD (in 8% of patients), death (3%), respiratory failure (2%), and pneumonia (1%). Additional information is available in the medical literature (6).

References

1. Hartman JE, Vanfleteren L, van Rikxoort EM, Klooster K, Slebos DJ. Endobronchial valves for severe emphysema. Eur Respir Rev. 2019;28(152):1801–21.
2. Abia-Trujillo D, Johnson MM, Patel NM, Hazelett B, Edell ES, Kern RM, et al. Bronchoscopic Lung Volume Reduction: A New Hope for Patients With Severe Emphysema and Air Trapping. Mayo Clin Proc. 2021;96(2):464–72.
3. Valipour A. Valve therapy in patients with emphysematous type of chronic obstructive pulmonary disease (COPD): from randomized trials to patient selection in clinical practice. J Thorac Dis. 2018;10(Suppl 23):S2780–S96.
4. Slebos DJ, Shah PL, Herth FJ, Valipour A. Endobronchial Valves for Endoscopic Lung Volume Reduction: Best Practice Recommendations from Expert Panel on Endoscopic Lung Volume Reduction. Respiration. 2017;93(2):138–50.
5. Koster TD, Slebos DJ. The fissure: interlobar collateral ventilation and implications for endoscopic therapy in emphysema. Int J Chron Obstruct Pulmon Dis. 2016;11: 765–73.
6. Criner GJ, Sue R, Wright S, Dransfield M, Rivas-Perez H, Wiese T, et al. A Multicenter Randomized Controlled Trial of Zephyr Endobronchial Valve Treatment in Heterogeneous Emphysema (LIBERATE). Am J Respir Crit Care Med. 2018;198(9): 1151–64.

A 28-Year-Old Woman With Worsening Cough and Hemoptysis

5

Daniel O. Pfeifle, MD, and Sarah J. Chalmers, MD

Case Presentation

A 28-year-old woman presented for evaluation of worsening pulmonary symptoms. She described having a progressively worse productive cough with green sputum, chest pain, dyspnea, fatigue, and associated weight loss for the past several years. In the past several months, she had recurrent spontaneous hemoptysis with 60 to 120 mL of bright red blood or blood-tinged sputum. During 2 episodes she sought evaluation in an emergency department, where she was given a diagnosis of pneumonia and was treated with oral antibiotics, but she had little improvement. In the past year she had not required other emergency department visits or hospitalizations for respiratory symptoms, and no other antibiotics had been prescribed.

Her medical history included chronic rhinitis, asthma, and cystic fibrosis (CF), which was diagnosed when she was 8 years old. Sweat chloride test results at that time were positive for CF (98 and 86 mmol/L), and subsequent genetic testing identified 2 sequence variations in the gene for CF transmembrane conductance regulator (CFTR) (508_1655delCTT). However, at the age of 13 years, the patient was lost to pulmonary follow-up.

When she presented at age 28 years, her medications included benzonatate 100 mg as needed for cough, albuterol-ipratropium inhalation solution 2.5 to 5.0 mg/mL as needed for cough and dyspnea, and intranasal fluticasone 50 mcg/spray in each naris daily. She had recently been prescribed prednisone 10 mg daily for presumed pleuritis and cough-associated chest pain. She had not used airway clearance therapies since she was 13 years old. Her family history was pertinent for having an identical twin sister who also had received a diagnosis of CF. The patient was estranged from her father, but no other family members were known to have respiratory disease. She lived in a rural environment with her husband and 2 children. She worked as a telemarketer, was a never-smoker, and did not drink alcohol.

On physical examination, the patient was not in acute distress, but she had an intermittent, productive cough throughout the visit. Her temperature was 36.3 °C; body mass index, 24.5 (calculated as weight in kilograms divided by height in meters squared); heart rate, 87 beats/min; blood pressure, 101/67 mm Hg; respiratory rate, 22 breaths per minute; and oxygen saturation as measured by pulse oximetry, 95% while breathing room air. Her conjunctivae were clear. The appearance of her nasal turbinates and posterior pharynx was normal, and no nasal polyps were seen. Her respiratory effort was normal. The anteroposterior chest diameter was increased. A diffuse end-expiratory wheeze was heard, but there were no rhonchi or rales. She had mild clubbing of her fingers.

The complete blood cell count results included a hemoglobin level of 15.3 g/dL and a high eosinophil count of 0.8×10^9/L. The international normalized ratio was 1.0; levels for liver enzymes, electrolytes, and vitamins A, D, and E were within the reference ranges. Hemoglobin A_{1c} was 5.0%, and confirmatory fasting blood glucose levels (86 mg/dL and 85 mg/dL) were within the reference range. A sputum culture was positive for methicillin-sensitive *Staphylococcus aureus*, *Haemophilus influenzae*, and *Pseudomonas aeruginosa* (nonmucoid).

Pulmonary function test results indicated moderate obstruction with a ratio of forced expiratory volume in the first second of expiration (FEV_1) to forced vital capacity of 55.2 (64% of the predicted value); FEV_1 was 2.08 L (66% of the predicted value). Computed tomographic (CT) angiography of the chest showed bronchiectasis predominantly in the upper lobe with evidence of mucoid compaction, patchy nodular infiltrates, and tortuous and prominent bronchial arteries.

Questions

Multiple Choice (choose the best answer)

5.1. What is the most appropriate next step in management for the patient described above?
a. Continue observation
b. Start home airway clearance therapy with observation only
c. Initiate therapy with appropriate inhaled antibiotics only
d. Initiate therapy with appropriate intravenous (IV) antibiotics on an outpatient basis
e. Admit the patient for administration of IV antibiotics

5.2. Which of the following is *not* part of an appropriate empirical treatment regimen for CF pulmonary exacerbation?
a. Routine use of corticosteroids
b. Continued use of long-term therapies
c. Increased frequency and intensity of airway clearance therapy
d. Continued use of inhaled antibiotics for long-term therapy
e. Antibiotic therapy selected according to the latest sputum culture results

5.3. For a patient with CF and scant hemoptysis, what is the best management strategy for long-term treatment, such as airway clearance and aerosol therapies?
a. Withhold all long-term airway clearance and aerosol therapies
b. Withhold long-term airway clearance therapies, and continue aerosol therapies
c. Withhold aerosol therapies, and continue long-term airway clearance therapies
d. Continue long-term airway clearance and aerosol therapies
e. Decrease the frequency of long-term airway clearance therapies

5.4. Which of the following patients with CF and hemoptysis has a definite indication for bronchial artery embolization (BAE)?
a. Patient with massive hemoptysis and unstable vital signs
b. Patient with moderate hemoptysis who is admitted to the hospital for observation
c. Patient with hemoptysis and normal vasculature
d. Patient with scant hemoptysis
e. Patient with recurrent episodes of hemoptysis

5.5. In addition to other guideline-directed therapies, which of the following therapies should be initiated to decrease pulmonary exacerbations and hospitalizations?
a. Oseltamivir 75 mg every 12 hours for 5 days
b. Prednisone 10 mg daily
c. Rotating long-term oral antibiotic therapy
d. Ivacaftor alone
e. Elexacaftor-tezacaftor-ivacaftor combination therapy

Case Follow-up and Outcome

The patient was admitted to the hospital, and therapy was begun with IV cefepime and oral trimethoprim-sulfamethoxazole. Airway clearance therapy was provided 4 times daily with bronchodilators, nebulized hypertonic saline, and chest physiotherapy. Given the patient's previous hemoptysis and tortuous vessels on CT angiography of the chest, she underwent prophylactic BAE. On hospital day 6, after she showed symptomatic and spirometric improvement, she was discharged to her home with continuation of outpatient antibiotic therapy for a planned 21-day course.

Discussion

This patient presented with signs and symptoms concerning for pulmonary exacerbation of CF, a multiorgan disease characterized by progressively worse lung function due to mucociliary dysfunction with mucus plugging, microbe colonization, chronic inflammation, bronchiectasis, and recurrent pulmonary exacerbations. When patients have acute worsening of respiratory signs and symptoms, or pulmonary exacerbations, they typically have increased cough, increased sputum production, dyspnea, decreased lung function, and worsening of other signs and symptoms (1). Frequency and severity of exacerbations have been shown to be correlated with progressive and irreversible worsening in lung function, decreased quality of life, increased mortality, and increased health care costs (2).

Factors that should be considered for treatment of pulmonary exacerbation include antibiotic selection, dose and duration, and mode of administration (IV or oral) and the treatment setting (inpatient or outpatient). Current guidelines for treatment of CF pulmonary exacerbations recommend prescribing systemic antibiotics, continuing long-term therapies, and increasing

airway clearance therapy (ie, increasing the duration of each treatment and the frequency of treatments) (1). In an initial trial that compared administration of IV antibiotic therapy at home with administration of IV antibiotic therapy in the hospital, many outcome measures had similar results (3). A more recent retrospective observational study confirmed that there was no difference in baseline FEV_1 with home treatment compared to in-hospital treatment; among the patients who received inpatient treatment in combination with home treatment (ie, therapy was started in the hospital, and the patients finished their antibiotics at home), a longer course of treatment in the hospital was associated with a longer duration before their next pulmonary exacerbation (4). Administration of IV antibiotics in the inpatient setting is probably more appropriate than administration on a solely outpatient basis, especially if the patient has comorbidities that may complicate care or has too much distress to self-administer appropriate therapies (1). Inpatient therapy could include additional nutritional support, closely monitored insulin therapy for CF-related diabetes, or monitoring of patients who have kidney dysfunction.

The selection of antimicrobial therapy during pulmonary exacerbations should be guided by the most recent results from sputum culture. Additional sputum cultures are useful when exacerbations occur, and antibiotic therapy should be changed as appropriate according to the most recent culture results. In many patients with CF, *P aeruginosa* is the most common pathogen and is the one most often associated with a risk of exacerbation and worsening of pulmonary function. Previously, some patients were treated with 2 antipseudomonal drugs to enhance activity and decrease the risk of resistance (5). However, in a large observational study from the Cystic Fibrosis Foundation Patient Registry, treatment with a single antipseudomonal agent was equivalent to dual coverage (6). Optimal duration of antibiotic therapy is unclear but typically ranges from 10 to 28 days (7).

During pulmonary exacerbations, patients with CF should continue therapy with their long-term medications. In previous studies of patients with acute exacerbations, long-term therapies were continued, and no other evidence has refuted this strategy. Individual considerations should be made for the specific clinical scenario. For instance, continuing the use of high doses of nonsteroidal anti-inflammatory agents (NSAIDs) while IV aminoglycosides are being administered may increase the risk of nephrotoxicity (1).

Airway clearance therapy has long been a standard and crucial aspect of therapy for maintenance and for pulmonary exacerbations in CF. During a pulmonary exacerbation, patients have more airway inflammation and mucus production, which further limit mucociliary clearance, worsen airway obstruction, and render maintenance airway clearance therapies insufficient. Thus, patients usually need intensified therapy, which can be individualized but usually requires more frequent and intensive treatments (1).

Patients with CF can also present with other respiratory complications, including hemoptysis or pneumothorax, that occur separately or as part of pulmonary exacerbations. Hemoptysis is common in these patients; approximately 9.1% of patients have hemoptysis over a 5-year period, and the average annual incidence is 1 in 115 patients (8). Hemoptysis occurs when the pulmonary vasculature is disrupted because of chronic inflammation, and the severity ranges from scant (<5 mL) to massive (>240 mL). Because hemoptysis may be a sign of pulmonary exacerbation, patients with hemoptysis that is more than scant (ie, ≥5 mL) should receive antibiotic treatment even if hemoptysis is the only symptom of exacerbation or infection (8). Therapy for many patients with CF includes long-term therapy with NSAIDs, which should be withheld during episodes with at least mild hemoptysis. Patients who have scant hemoptysis can continue airway clearance and aerosol therapies. However, those therapies may need to be withheld if patients have more severe hemoptysis because treatments such as hypertonic saline may exacerbate cough and worsen hemoptysis (8).

Patients with massive hemoptysis have a high risk of death and should therefore be hospitalized for further care. If patients have massive hemoptysis and hemodynamic instability, BAE is first-line treatment, and lung resection should be considered as a last resort. Although some episodes of massive hemoptysis stop spontaneously, the risk of recurrence is high. Therefore, BAE of all abnormal vessels should be considered even in patients who are hemodynamically stable (8).

Summary

CF is a multiorgan disease process characterized by progressive worsening in lung function due to chronic inflammation and impaired mucociliary clearance. Pulmonary exacerbations are associated with worsening lung function, and patients typically have symptoms such as increased cough, increased sputum production, and dyspnea. Typical treatment of a CF exacerbation includes admission to the hospital, administration of IV antibiotics targeted to culture-specific microbes, continuation of long-term therapies with intensification of airway clearance therapies, and initiation of CFTR modulator therapy.

Hemoptysis can occur as an independent pulmonary complication of CF, or it may indicate acute pulmonary exacerbation. The amount of hemoptysis can range from scant, which can be managed in the outpatient setting, to massive, which requires hospitalization. BAE is first-line therapy for patients with massive hemoptysis, particularly if they have hemodynamic instability.

Answers

5.1. Answer e.

Although CF pulmonary exacerbation has not been clearly defined, typical symptoms include increased cough and sputum production, fatigue, dyspnea, anorexia, and hemoptysis. Patients with CF who have signs and symptoms of pulmonary exacerbation, such as the patient described in this case, should be treated and not simply observed. Treatment of pulmonary exacerbations includes airway clearance therapy, but airway clearance therapy alone is insufficient. Inhaled antibiotics are used predominantly for eradication of new infection or treatment of chronic infection, particularly if sputum cultures are positive for *P aeruginosa*. Inhaled antibiotics alone are insufficient antimicrobial treatment for pulmonary exacerbations.

When outpatient therapy for pulmonary exacerbations is compared with inpatient therapy, the evidence is conflicting. However, current guidelines, which are based on available evidence and expert opinion, recommend administration of IV antibiotic therapy in the inpatient setting only. Inpatient administration of IV antibiotics may be more appropriate for patients who have comorbidities that complicate care and for patients who have more severe exacerbations and may not be able to administer therapy appropriately at home. Additional information is available in the medical literature (1,3,5).

5.2. Answer a.

Treatment of pulmonary exacerbation includes systemic antibiotics chosen on the basis of the most recent sputum culture results, increased frequency and intensity of airway clearance therapies, and continuation of long-term therapies at home. Limited evidence is available on the use of corticosteroids in CF pulmonary exacerbations, and current guidelines do not recommend their routine use in pulmonary exacerbations. This recommendation is based on 2 small trials that did not show a significant difference in FEV_1 with the use of corticosteroids. Although the use of corticosteroids may be appropriate in certain circumstances (eg, a patient with CF and concurrent asthma), there is insufficient evidence to recommend their routine use. Additional information is available in the medical literature (1,3,5).

5.3. Answer d.

If patients have massive hemoptysis, all long-term therapies should be stopped and the hemoptysis should be treated promptly. However, if patients have scant hemoptysis, expert opinion recommends the continuation of long-term airway clearance therapies and aerosol therapies. Many aerosolized medications (eg, inhaled tobramycin) and medications used in airway clearance therapy (eg, hypertonic saline) can irritate the lungs and cause bronchospasm and increased cough. Therefore, concern has been expressed for continuing these medications if hemoptysis develops. For patients with CF and scant hemoptysis, the current guidelines, based on expert consensus, recommend that all airway clearance therapies and aerosolized medications should be continued. The use of these therapies for patients who have mild to moderate hemoptysis is not clear. For patients with scant hemoptysis, the frequency of airway clearance therapies does not need to be decreased. Additional information is available in the medical literature (8).

5.4. Answer a.

In most patients who have CF and hemoptysis, the bleeding will stop spontaneously. Therefore, not every patient who presents with hemoptysis requires intervention. However, in select patients, BAE is appropriate. The consensus reflected in the current guidelines is to proceed with embolization in patients who have massive hemoptysis and are clinically unstable.

Other scenarios, which did not meet sufficient consensus for the guidelines but may be considered for embolization, include patients who have massive hemoptysis and are clinically stable but still bleeding and patients who have abnormal vessels, defined as dilated and tortuous vessels, because of the possibility of future bleeding episodes. Additional information is available in the medical literature (8).

5.5. Answer e.

CFTR modulators are a relatively new drug class approved for the treatment of patients who have CF and a qualifying genetic mutation. These drugs modify or potentiate the CFTR protein (the abnormal protein in CF) and thereby improve protein production, processing, or function. The US Food and Drug Administration has approved 3 CFTR modulators for use (elexacaftor, tezacaftor, and ivacaftor), and they have been studied in combination. The use of elexacaftor-tezacaftor-ivacaftor combination therapy, when used with other guideline-based therapies, has been shown to decrease the rate of pulmonary exacerbations by 63% and improve FEV_1 by up to 14 percentage points at 6 months. The use of this combination therapy (elexacaftor-tezacaftor-ivacaftor) has shown more benefit than the use of ivacaftor alone. Oseltamivir may be appropriate therapy for patients who have CF and infection with influenza virus, but the drug should not be used in patients who have a pulmonary exacerbation not due to influenza virus. Long-term therapy with prednisone should be avoided in patients who have CF but not asthma or allergic bronchopulmonary aspergillosis because of the risk of adverse effects such as hyperglycemia and cataracts. The use of long-term rotating oral antibiotic therapy is not recommended. Additional information is available in the medical literature (9,10).

References

1. Flume PA, Mogayzel PJ, Jr., Robinson KA, Goss CH, Rosenblatt RL, Kuhn RJ, et al. Cystic fibrosis pulmonary guidelines: treatment of pulmonary exacerbations. Am J Respir Crit Care Med. 2009;180(9):802–8.

2. Sanders DB, Bittner RC, Rosenfeld M, Redding GJ, Goss CH. Pulmonary exacerbations are associated with subsequent FEV1 decline in both adults and children with cystic fibrosis. Pediatr Pulmonol. 2011;46(4):393–400.

3. Thornton J, Elliott R, Tully MP, Dodd M, Webb AK. Long term clinical outcome of home and hospital intravenous antibiotic treatment in adults with cystic fibrosis. Thorax. 2004;59(3):242–6.

4. Collaco JM, Green DM, Cutting GR, Naughton KM, Mogayzel PJ, Jr. Location and duration of treatment of cystic fibrosis respiratory exacerbations do not affect outcomes. Am J Respir Crit Care Med. 2010;182(9):1137–43.

5. Regelmann WE, Elliott GR, Warwick WJ, Clawson CC. Reduction of sputum Pseudomonas aeruginosa density by antibiotics improves lung function in cystic fibrosis more than do bronchodilators and chest physiotherapy alone. Am Rev Respir Dis. 1990;141(4 Pt 1):914–21.

6. Cogen JD, Faino AV, Onchiri F, Hoffman LR, Kronman MP, Nichols DP, et al. Association between number of intravenous antipseudomonal antibiotics and clinical outcomes of pediatric cystic fibrosis pulmonary exacerbations. Clin Infect Dis. 2021;73(9):1589–96.

7. West NE, Beckett VV, Jain R, Sanders DB, Nick JA, Heltshe SL, et al. Standardized Treatment of Pulmonary Exacerbations (STOP) study: physician treatment practices and outcomes for individuals with cystic fibrosis with pulmonary Exacerbations. J Cyst Fibros. 2017;16(5):600–6.

8. Flume PA, Mogayzel PJ, Jr., Robinson KA, Rosenblatt RL, Quittell L, Marshall BC, et al. Cystic fibrosis pulmonary guidelines: pulmonary complications: hemoptysis and pneumothorax. Am J Respir Crit Care Med. 2010;182(3):298–306.

9. Middleton PG, Mall MA, Drevinek P, Lands LC, McKone EF, Polineni D, et al. Elexacaftor-tezacaftor-ivacaftor for cystic fibrosis with a single Phe508del allele. N Engl J Med. 2019;381(19):1809–19.

10. Mogayzel PJ, Jr, Naureckas ET, Robinson KA, Mueller G, Hadjiliadis D, Hoag JB, et al. Cystic fibrosis pulmonary guideline: chronic medications for maintenance of lung health. Am J Respir Crit Care Med. 2013;187(7):680–9.

An 84-Year-Old Man With Chronic Obstructive Pulmonary Disease and Cirrhosis

Kirtivardhan Vashistha, Rahul Kashyap, MBBS, MBA, and Ashokakumar M. Patel, MD

Case Presentation

An 84-year-old man with a past medical history of cirrhosis and chronic obstructive pulmonary disease (COPD) presented for evaluation of the COPD. His shortness of breath was severe enough to limit his daily activities, such as getting dressed in the morning, and he had a productive cough that persisted through the day along with mild intermittent wheezing. He used an albuterol inhaler once a month and regularly scheduled budensonide-formoterol and tiotropium. He did not have chest pain, palpitations, orthopnea, paroxysmal nocturnal dyspnea, or fever. In the past year, he had not required any antibiotic or oral corticosteroid therapy for exacerbations. He had leg edema bilaterally for the previous 4 years, which is when cirrhosis was diagnosed incidentally on computed tomography (CT) of the chest for evaluation of emphysema. He smoked for 16 years and quit at age 30 years. He drank alcohol only socially, 1 or 2 times per week, and he had not used substances. He did not have a history of any other environmental or occupational exposure. His family history was notable for a sister having COPD.

The patient received a diagnosis of COPD 20 years ago, and results of pulmonary function tests (PFTs) showed a decrease of 30% in pulmonary function. He was treated with fluticasone and an albuterol inhaler when needed. A few years later, when he had increasing dyspnea on mild exertion, he was prescribed ipratropium bromide–albuterol, but when he felt better a few months later, he stopped taking all his medication. However, results of PFTs showed a slight decrease in forced expiratory volume in the first second of expiration (FEV_1) (1.93 L) and forced vital capacity (FVC) (4.74 L) and no response to bronchodilator. Total lung capacity (TLC) was 9.02 L, diffusing capacity of lung for carbon monoxide (D_{LCO}) was 17.1 mL/min/mm Hg, oxygen saturation as measured by pulse oximetry (Spo_2) at rest was 95%, and a chest radiograph showed bilateral alveolar opacities. He was advised to resume taking ipratropium bromide–albuterol. Eight years after COPD was diagnosed, results of PFTs showed the following: FEV_1, 1.80 L; FEV_1/FVC, 40%; TLC, 9.05 L; and D_{LCO}, 59% of the predicted value. He was prescribed tiotropium for treatment of COPD symptoms.

His past medical history included ascites due to cirrhosis. At that time, therapeutic and diagnostic paracentesis was used to remove 2.5 L of fluid, which was a transudate. At presentation, management of ascites was with salt restriction, paracentesis as needed, furosemide 20 mg daily, and spironolactone 50 mg daily.

Physical examination findings included the following: blood pressure, 110/63 mm Hg;

heart rate, 84 beats/min; temperature, 35.6 °C; Spo$_2$, 90%; height, 1.74 m; weight, 63.3 kg; and body mass index, 21 (calculated as weight in kilograms divided by height in meters squared). On lung auscultation, the patient had a prolonged expiratory phase, mild expiratory wheezes, diminished breath sounds throughout the lung fields, and no crackles. On heart auscultation, the rate and rhythm were regular and an S$_4$ was audible. Radial pulses were equal and palpable bilaterally, extremities were warm, and the patient wore compression stockings on the lower portion of his legs, which were not edematous. He did not have abdominal distention or hepatosplenomegaly.

The latest CT of the chest without an intravenous (IV) contrast agent showed increased cylindrical and cystic bronchiectasis with associated bronchial inflammatory changes, mucoid impactions, and fluid levels consistent with infection. He also had persistent mild to moderate increases in transaminase levels: alanine aminotransferase, 56 uL; aspartate aminotransferase, 72 uL.

Questions

Multiple Choice (choose the best answer)

6.1. Which of the following would be the most likely diagnosis?
  a. Hypersensitivity pneumonitis
  b. Hemochromatosis
  c. Amyloidosis
  d. Cor pulmonale
  e. Deficiency of α_1-antitrypsin (AAT)

6.2. Which of the following is correct for the suspected disease?
  a. Serial CT scanning of the chest should be done to monitor progression of the disease
  b. Annual monitoring of liver disease is not recommended
  c. Manifestations of AAT deficiency include emphysema-predominant COPD, bronchiectasis, panniculitis, or chronic liver disease
  d. Lung volume reduction surgery is recommended for patients with COPD related to AAT deficiency

6.3. Which of the following alleles is associated with liver disease in AAT deficiency?
  a. Null
  b. SS
  c. ZZ
  d. MM
  e. MZ

6.4. Which of the following diseases is associated with AAT deficiency?
  a. Hashimoto thyroiditis
  b. Polyarteritis nodosa
  c. Cryoglobulinemia
  d. Antineutrophil cytoplasmic autoantibody (ANCA)-associated vasculitis
  e. Ankylosing spondylitis

6.5. Which of the following is an exclusion criterion for augmentation therapy with pooled human AAT?
  a. Age older than 60 years
  b. AAT level less than 57 mg/dL
  c. Current smoker
  d. FEV_1 less than 30% of the predicted value
  e. Evidence of emphysema on CT of the chest

e. PFTs would show low lung volumes and normal D_{LCO}

Case Follow-up and Outcome

Results of the patient's iron studies were normal, and results of hepatitis A serology were negative. The patient's serum AAT level was 31 mg/dL, and his genotype was ZZ. Results of PFTs were as follows: FEV_1/FVC, 38%; increased FVC (4.73 L); decreased FEV_1 (1.80 L; 63% of the predicted value); and DLco, 38.5% of the predicted value. He was given a diagnosis of AAT deficiency associated with COPD and cirrhosis. He was advised to use nebulized hypertonic saline (3%) twice daily for clearance of mucus, to use supplemental oxygen as needed (to maintain arterial oxygen saturation at 88% or more) and with exercise to improve shortness of breath, and to continue use of corticosteroid, long-acting β_2-agonist, and long-acting muscarinic antagonist inhalers.

Discussion

AAT deficiency is among the most common genetic disorders inherited in a codominant fashion. It is caused by a deficiency or an absence of the enzyme AAT, which is in the superfamily of proteins called serpins (ie, serine protease inhibitors), and causes a wide spectrum of diseases. Most commonly AAT deficiency causes panlobular emphysema in lungs from unchecked activity of elastase and liver disorders due to accumulation of an abnormal AAT protein (1-3). Other clinical manifestations include panniculitis, bronchiectasis, glomerulonephritis, and ANCA-associated vasculitis (4-6). The estimated prevalence in the US is 70,000 to 100,000 persons, but it is thought that the disease is undiagnosed in many instances. A population-based study in Europe estimated that the prevalence of various types of genotypes affecting the functioning of AAT is close to 40 million. Patients often present in the later stages of the disease and so have increased morbidity and a poor prognosis (7,8).

Clinical practice guidelines published in the *Journal of the COPD Foundation* (9) state that the following individuals should be tested for AAT deficiency: 1) those with COPD regardless of age or ethnicity; 2) those with unexplained chronic liver disease; and 3) those with necrotizing panniculitis, granulomatosis with polyangiitis, or unexplained bronchiectasis (8).

Clinical clues that suggest AAT deficiency include a family history of a COPD-related disorder, liver disorder, panniculitis, emphysema in a person 45 years or younger or without risk factors, predominant bibasilar changes on chest radiography, neonatal hepatitis, hepatocellular carcinoma, cirrhosis, or any unexplained liver disease (6,10).

Diagnosis involves measuring serum levels of AAT (by nephelometry or equivalent tests) with isoelectric focusing or genotype testing (11). An algorithm for the diagnosis of AAT deficiency is shown in Figure 6.1 (12).

For patients with COPD or emphysema due to AAT deficiency, treatment is similar to that for patients with COPD or emphysema not due to AAT deficiency with additional recommendations (Table 6.1). Patients should stop smoking because smoking hastens the lung parenchymal insult. Follow-up of adult patients should occur annually and include spirometry. IV augmentation therapy with pooled human AAT is known to decrease the progression of emphysema (20,21). However, patients who meet any of the following exclusion criteria should not be considered for augmentation therapy: current smoker, younger than 18 years, allergic reaction to AAT formulation, liver transplant patient, and presence of volume overload (22). Moreover, this therapy is recommended only for patients with lung disease; the therapy is not known to work for patients with liver disease (22). There is strong evidence for clinical efficacy in patients with an FEV_1 that is no more than 65% of the predicted value, but before initiation of therapy, patients should be involved in a discussion of the risks and benefits and the cost-effectiveness of therapy (23).

Figure 6.1 Algorithm for Diagnosis of AAT Deficiency

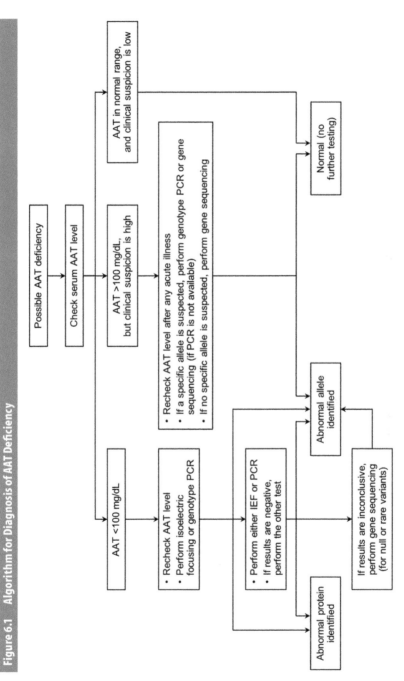

IEF indicates isoelectric focusing; PCR, polymerase chain reaction.

Table 6.1	Therapy for AAT Deficiency		
Therapy		**Route**	**Frequency**
Plasma-derived IV augmentation		IV	Weekly
Plasma-derived inhaled augmentation		Inhalational	100 mg twice daily (13)
Recombinant or transgenic augmentation (14)		Inhalational	Investigational
Recombinant AAT (15)		IV	60 mg/kg weekly
Hormonal derivative (eg, danazol, tamoxifen, and progesterone) (16,17)		Oral	Danazol, 200 mg 3 times daily Tamoxifen, 10 mg twice daily
Gene therapy (18,19)		IV	Once?

Summary

AAT deficiency is an underdiagnosed, widely prevalent systemic disease, and clinicians should maintain a high degree of awareness during evaluation of patients with COPD, unexplained liver disease, or specific skin manifestations. Early identification of the disease helps to provide specific therapy for patients, improve the prognosis, and decrease the associated morbidity and mortality. The choice of therapy should be based on the patient's candidacy and comorbidities and on the risks, benefits, and cost of treatment. Family members should be involved in medical genetics counseling and evaluation for the presence of the abnormal gene for AAT, and family members who have symptoms should undergo genotyping for early detection.

Answers

6.1. Answer e.

The most likely diagnosis is AAT deficiency, which is supported by the patient's low serum AAT level and his ZZ genotype. AAT deficiency is among the most common genetic disorders inherited in a codominant fashion. Typically, AAT deficiency causes panlobular pulmonary emphysema from unchecked activity of elastase and liver disorders due to accumulation of an abnormal AAT protein. Additional information is available in the medical literature (1-3,24).

6.2. Answer c.

Besides pulmonary emphysema, other clinical manifestations of AAT deficiency include panniculitis, bronchiectasis, glomerulonephritis, and ANCA-associated vasculitis. Additional information is available in the medical literature (6).

6.3. Answer c.

Homozygosity of the Z allele is the most common cause of AAT, and the Z allele is most commonly associated with liver disease. Additional information is available in the medical literature (22).

6.4. Answer d.

Other clinical manifestations of AAT deficiency besides panlobular pulmonary emphysema are panniculitis, bronchiectasis, glomerulonephritis, and ANCA-associated vasculitis. Additional information is available in the medical literature (4).

6.5. Answer c.

IV augmentation therapy with pooled human AAT decreases the progression of emphysema, but patients who meet any of the following exclusion criteria should not be considered for augmentation therapy: current smoker, age younger than 18 years, allergic reaction to AAT formulation, liver transplant recipient, and presence of volume overload. Additional information is available in the medical literature (16,25).

References

1. Kohnlein T, Welte T. Alpha-1 antitrypsin deficiency: pathogenesis, clinical presentation, diagnosis, and treatment. Am J Med. 2008;121(1):3–9.
2. Brantly ML, Paul LD, Miller BH, Falk RT, Wu M, Crystal RG. Clinical features and history of the destructive lung disease associated with alpha-1-antitrypsin deficiency of adults with pulmonary symptoms. Am Rev Respir Dis. 1988;138(2):327–36.
3. Sandhaus RA, Knebel AR. Might your respiratory patient have alpha-1 antitrypsin deficiency? Heart Lung. 2015;44(6):463–4.
4. Morris H, Morgan MD, Wood AM, Smith SW, Ekeowa UI, Herrmann K, et al. ANCA-associated vasculitis is linked to carriage of the Z allele of α_1 antitrypsin and its polymers. Ann Rheum Dis. 2011;70(10):1851–6.
5. Davis ID, Burke B, Freese D, Sharp HL, Kim Y. The pathologic spectrum of the nephropathy associated with alpha 1-antitrypsin deficiency. Hum Pathol. 1992;23(1):57–62.
6. American Thoracic Society; European Respiratory Society. American Thoracic Society/European Respiratory Society statement: standards for the diagnosis and management of individuals with alpha-1 antitrypsin deficiency. Am J Respir Crit Care Med. 2003;168(7):818–900.
7. de Serres FJ. Worldwide racial and ethnic distribution of alpha1-antitrypsin deficiency: summary of an analysis of published genetic epidemiologic surveys. Chest. 2002;122(5):1818–29.
8. Blanco I, de Serres FJ, Fernandez-Bustillo E, Lara B, Miravitlles M. Estimated numbers and prevalence of PI*S and PI*Z alleles of alpha1-antitrypsin deficiency in European countries. Eur Respir J. 2006;27(1):77–84.
9. Yawn BB, Thomashaw B, Mannino DM, Han MK, Kalhan R, Rennard S, et al. The 2017 Update to the COPD Foundation COPD Pocket Consultant Guide. Chronic Obstr Pulm Dis. 2017;4(3):177–85.
10. Miravitlles M, Dirksen A, Ferrarotti I, Koblizek V, Lange P, Mahadeva R, et al. European Respiratory Society statement: diagnosis and treatment of pulmonary disease in α_1-antitrypsin deficiency. Eur Respir J. 2017;50(5):1700610.
11. Stoller JK, Hupertz V, Aboussouan LS. Alpha-1 antitrypsin deficiency. 2006 Oct 27 [Updated 2020 May 21]. In: Adam MP, Ardinger HH, Pagon RA, Wallace SE, Bean LJH, Stephens K, et al., editors. GeneReviews® [Internet]. Seattle (WA): University of Washington, Seattle; 1993-2020. Available from: https://www.ncbi.nlm.nih.gov/books/NBK1519/.
12. Snyder MR, Katzmann JA, Butz ML, Wiley C, Yang P, Dawson DB, et al. Diagnosis of alpha-1-antitrypsin deficiency: an algorithm of quantification, genotyping, and phenotyping [published correction appears in Clin Chem. 2007 Sep;53(9):1724. Wiley, Carmen (added)]. Clin Chem. 2006;52(12):2236–42.
13. Griese M, Scheuch G. Delivery of alpha-1 antitrypsin to airways. Ann Am Thorac Soc. 2016;13 Suppl 4:S346–51.
14. Arjmand S, Bidram E, Lotfi AS, Shamsara M, Mowla SJ. Expression and purification of functionally active recombinant human alpha 1-antitrypsin in methylotrophic yeast pichia pastoris. Avicenna J Med Biotechnol. 2011;3(3):127–34.
15. Pirooznia N, Hasannia S, Arab SS, Lotfi AS, Ghanei M, Shali A. The design of a new truncated and engineered alpha1-antitrypsin based on theoretical studies: an antiprotease therapeutics for pulmonary diseases. Theor Biol Med Model. 2013;10:36.
16. Tonelli AR, Brantly ML. Augmentation therapy in alpha-1 antitrypsin deficiency: advances and controversies. Ther Adv Respir Dis. 2010;4(5):289–312.
17. Wewers MD, Brantly ML, Casolaro MA, Crystal RG. Evaluation of tamoxifen as a therapy to augment alpha-1-antitrypsin concentrations in Z homozygous alpha-1-antitrypsin-deficient subjects. Am Rev Respir Dis. 1987;135(2):401–2.
18. Wilson AA, Kwok LW, Hovav AH, Ohle SJ, Little FF, Fine A, et al. Sustained expression of alpha1-antitrypsin after transplantation of manipulated hematopoietic stem cells. Am J Respir Cell Mol Biol. 2008;39(2):133–41.
19. Chiuchiolo MJ, Crystal RG. Gene therapy for alpha-1 antitrypsin deficiency lung disease. Ann Am Thorac Soc. 2016;13 Suppl 4(Suppl 4):S352–69.
20. Sandhaus RA. alpha1-Antitrypsin deficiency: new and emerging treatments for alpha1-antitrypsin deficiency. Thorax. 2004;59(10):904–9.
21. Stoller JK, Aboussouan LS. alpha1-Antitrypsin deficiency. 5: intravenous augmentation therapy: current understanding. Thorax. 2004;59(8):708–12.
22. Mitchell EL, Khan Z. Liver disease in alpha-1 antitrypsin deficiency: current approaches and future directions [published correction appears in Curr Pathobiol Rep. 2018;6(1):97]. Curr Pathobiol Rep. 2017;5(3):243–52.
23. Sandhaus RA, Turino G, Brantly ML, Campos M, Cross CE, Goodman K, et al. The diagnosis and management of alpha-1 antitrypsin deficiency in the adult. Chronic Obstr Pulm Dis. 2016;3(3):668–82.
24. Strnad P, McElvaney NG, Lomas DA. Alpha$_1$-antitrypsin deficiency. N Engl J Med. 2020 Apr 9;382(15):1443–55.
25. Rahaghi FF. Alpha-1 antitrypsin deficiency research and emerging treatment strategies: what's down the road? Ther Adv Chronic Dis. 2021 Jul 29;12 suppl:20406223211014025.

Critical Care Medicine

A 67-Year-Old Woman With Hyperglycemia

Yosuf W. Subat, MD, Kianna M. Nguyen,
and Richard A. Oeckler, MD, PhD

Case Presentation

A 67-year-old woman presented to the emergency department with hyperglycemia. Her past medical history was notable for widely metastatic small cell lung cancer (SCLC), hypertension, type 2 diabetes, and atrial fibrillation, for which she received apixaban. She was in her usual state of health until earlier in the day, when her blood glucose level was 540 mg/dL at home. The diabetes had been controlled relatively well, with blood glucose levels typically less than 200 mg/dL and a hemoglobin A_{1c} level of 6.8%. However, she had noticed that her blood glucose levels were increasing over the previous several weeks, often with values exceeding 350 mg/dL. She also described polyuria and a feeling of unsteadiness.

In the emergency department, the patient was hypertensive (blood pressure, 162/88 mm Hg), but her other vital signs were normal. On physical examination she had a cushingoid habitus, but other findings were unremarkable. Point-of-care ultrasonography showed a collapsible inferior vena cava and a hyperdynamic left ventricle. A metabolic panel showed the following notable results: sodium, 146 mmol/L; potassium, 2.3 mmol/L; chloride, 97 mmol/L; bicarbonate, 29 mmol/L; serum urea nitrogen, 36.4 mg/dL; creatinine, 0.7 mg/dL; and glucose, 371 mg/dL. The lactate level was high (4.1 mmol/L). The other laboratory findings were normal and included results for additional electrolytes, β-hydroxybutyrate, and arterial blood gases. The urinalysis showed severe glucosuria. Blood and urine culture results were negative. The patient was admitted to the hospital for rehydration, electrolyte repletion, and blood glucose control. However, hypokalemia persisted despite aggressive potassium supplementation.

Concern for Cushing syndrome increased because of the cushingoid body habitus and persistent electrolyte disturbances. The morning cortisol level was 46 µg/dL (reference range, 7-25 µg/dL), the corticotropin level was 148 pg/mL (reference range, 7.2-63 pg/mL), and the aldosterone level was low (<4.0 ng/dL). The 24-hour urine free cortisol result was extremely high (3,157 µg; reference range, 3-45 µg). The patient received a diagnosis of Cushing syndrome secondary to corticotropin-releasing SCLC. After she began treatment with ketoconazole 200 mg 3 times daily, the potassium and cortisol levels were in the reference ranges. She was discharged from the hospital with a plan for close outpatient follow-up.

The patient underwent fluorodeoxyglucose F 18–positron emission tomography, which showed considerable worsening of the metastatic SCLC. One week later, she was readmitted to the hospital with severe, recurrent hyperglycemia. The potassium level was 3.3 mmol/L, and the cortisol level was elevated (51 µg/dL) despite treatment with ketoconazole. She was admitted to the intensive care unit for the initiation of etomidate infusion for severe Cushing syndrome and a plan for bilateral adrenalectomy.

Questions

Multiple Choice (choose the best answer)

7.1. Which combination of abnormal laboratory test results is most likely present when a patient has severe Cushing syndrome?
   a. Hyponatremia, hyperkalemia, and non–anion gap metabolic acidosis
   b. Hypokalemia, hypophosphatemia, and hypomagnesemia
   c. Hyperkalemia, hyperphosphatemia, hyperuricemia, and hypocalcemia
   d. Hypokalemia, hypernatremia, and metabolic alkalosis
   e. Hypokalemia, hypochloremia, and metabolic alkalosis

7.2. A 52-year-old man presents with fatigue, easy bruising, muscle atrophy and weakness, and severely abnormal electrolyte levels. He has a cushingoid body habitus. Laboratory test results (with reference ranges) are as follows: morning cortisol, 57 µg/dL (5-25 µg/dL); corticotropin, 2 pg/mL (10-60 pg/mL); and 24-hour urine free cortisol, 1,270 µg (3-45 µg).
   What is the most likely source of the high cortisol level?
   a. Exogenous corticosteroids
   b. Adrenal adenoma
   c. Pituitary adenoma
   d. SCLC

   e. Physiologic hypercortisolism

7.3. Which of the following will decrease cortisol levels most effectively and rapidly in patients with severe Cushing syndrome?
   a. Ketoconazole
   b. Metyrapone
   c. Mitotane
   d. Etomidate
   e. Hemodialysis

7.4. In addition to corticotropin, which hormone is most commonly released ectopically in SCLC?
   a. Antidiuretic hormone
   b. Gastrin
   c. Aldosterone
   d. Parathyroid hormone–related peptide
   e. Glucagon

7.5. Which of the following correctly describes the use of etomidate for induction of anesthesia during intubation of critically ill patients?
   a. For patients with septic shock, etomidate is associated with increased risk of death compared to other induction agents
   b. Glucocorticoids should be used prophylactically with etomidate to prevent adrenal insufficiency
   c. Etomidate increases the risk of post-intubation seizure
   d. Etomidate provides analgesic effects
   e. A single dose of etomidate has been shown to decrease cortisol levels

Case Follow-up and Outcome

Etomidate infusion was initiated at 0.04 mg/kg/h and was increased to 0.06 mg/kg/h. Cortisol levels were checked every 6 hours with a target range of 18 to 29 µg/dL. Sedation scoring was conducted every 2 hours for the first 24 hours and then every 6 hours thereafter. Within 36 hours after the etomidate infusion had been initiated, the patient's cortisol levels were in the reference range. The patient did not have any sedative effects from the low-dose infusion of etomidate. Bilateral adrenalectomy was delayed because of anticoagulation with apixaban, and the etomidate infusion was continued until surgical intervention. The etomidate infusion was stopped while the patient was transported to the operating room, where she underwent uncomplicated bilateral adrenalectomy. She was discharged 3 days later, and her therapy included hydrocortisone 50 mg twice daily. Although she did not have a recurrence of hypercortisolemia, she began receiving palliative care 4 months later and died shortly thereafter.

Discussion

Cushing syndrome has a wide spectrum of clinical manifestations and can be caused by several conditions, including exogenous corticosteroid use, corticotropin-releasing pituitary adenomas (Cushing disease), ectopic corticotropin syndrome, and excessive cortisol production from adrenal tumors or hyperplasia. Clinical manifestations of Cushing syndrome can include alterations in body habitus and skin, such as dorsocervical fat pad (or buffalo hump), rounded (or moonlike) face, central obesity, muscle wasting, skin thinning, abdominal striae, and easy bruising (1). Additionally, chronically high cortisol levels in patients with Cushing syndrome can increase the risk of several conditions, including obesity, hypertension, glucose intolerance, obstructive sleep apnea, osteoporosis, and mood disturbances. In patients with rapidly progressive Cushing syndrome and ectopic corticotropin syndrome, severe electrolyte disturbances and infections are potentially life-threatening complications.

Ectopic corticotropin syndrome can be caused by various tumors, but the most common are thymic, pancreatic, and pulmonary neuroendocrine tumors (2). SCLC has neuroendocrine markers, which may suggest a neuroendocrine origin. SCLC is responsible for 8% to 20% of cases of ectopic corticotropin syndrome, and corticotropin production is associated with a worse prognosis (3,4). The patient described above in the Case Presentation had a short life expectancy (probably weeks to months) because of the underlying metastatic SCLC. However, after hypercortisolemia rapidly progressed, her life expectancy was drastically shortened—to days without urgent intervention. Patients in similar situations require rapid control of cortisol levels, thus prompting admission to the intensive care unit for etomidate infusion and ultimately bilateral adrenalectomy.

Several medications are available for medical management of Cushing syndrome, and they are classified according to their mechanism of action. The most commonly used medications are adrenal steroidogenesis inhibitors (eg, ketoconazole, metyrapone, mitotane, and etomidate). All these agents inhibit at least 1 enzyme involved in steroid biosynthesis in the adrenal cortex (5). Drugs targeting the pituitary, such as pasireotide, cabergoline, and temozolomide, are not used as commonly as adrenal steroidogenesis inhibitors, which can inhibit cortisol production regardless of the source (6). Because ketoconazole, metyrapone, and mitotane act more slowly in the short-term reduction of cortisol levels, their effectiveness (49%-85%) is less than that of etomidate (100%). Etomidate inhibits steroidogenesis at multiple levels, particularly at the enzyme 11β-hydroxylase (7). Several studies have shown that etomidate infusion can rapidly decrease cortisol levels within hours and serve as a bridge to surgical intervention (eg, resection of local SCLC or bilateral adrenalectomy in metastatic SCLC) (8-11).

The current recommendation for etomidate infusion is to begin with a low dose (0.02 mg/kg/h) and increase it by 0.01 to 0.02 mg/kg/h to a cortisol level of about 10 to 20 μg/dL or slightly higher if the patient is physiologically stressed (12). This recommendation is in contrast to the larger bolus dosing of 0.2 to 0.3 mg/kg that is commonly given during endotracheal intubation. The use of a low dose for etomidate infusion is unlikely to cause sedation that would require endotracheal intubation and appears to be safe and effective for use even outside the intensive care unit (13). The fact that etomidate is formulated in propylene glycol should be considered when patients have metabolic acidosis with an elevated osmolar gap.

One controversial consideration is whether etomidate can cause clinically relevant adrenal suppression when used for induction of anesthesia in critically ill patients. Transient decreases in adrenal steroidogenesis have been identified, but this effect lasts less than 24 hours whether patients are healthy or critically ill (14).

The majority of evidence suggests that in most clinical situations the temporary adrenal suppression is not likely to lead to worse outcomes (14-19). However, some intensivists avoid the use of etomidate in patients who have severe septic shock.

Summary

SCLC can cause ectopic corticotropin release and development of Cushing syndrome. Life-threatening complications of rapidly progressive hypercortisolemia include severe electrolyte abnormalities and infections. Etomidate is a highly effective inhibitor of adrenal steroidogenesis and should be considered in patients who require urgent correction of cortisol levels. A low-dose infusion of etomidate is unlikely to cause sedation and may serve as a bridge to surgical intervention in patients with refractory hypercortisolemia.

Answers

7.1. Answer d.

Although not always present, hypokalemia, hypernatremia, and metabolic alkalosis are most likely to occur in severe Cushing syndrome. They result from the mineralocorticoid effect of cortisol, leading to sodium retention, potassium wasting, and proton loss in the kidneys. The opposite effect could be seen in patients with adrenal insufficiency, which can cause hyponatremia, hyperkalemia, and non–anion gap metabolic acidosis. Low serum levels of potassium, phosphate, and magnesium can occur in refeeding syndrome. Tumor lysis syndrome can cause hyperkalemia, hyperphosphatemia, hyperuricemia, and hypocalcemia from widespread cellular lysis and the release of intracellular contents. Gastric acid loss, such as from vomiting or high output from a gastric tube, could lead to hypochloremia, hypokalemia, and metabolic alkalosis. Additional information is available in the medical literature (20).

7.2. Answer b.

Adrenal adenoma is the source of increased cortisol production in nearly 10% of patients who have Cushing syndrome. Adrenal adenomas are most likely to cause corticotropin-independent cortisol secretion (an increased level of cortisol with a low level of corticotropin). Exogenous corticosteroids would lead to decreased levels of morning cortisol and corticotropin. Corticotropin-secreting pituitary adenoma (Cushing disease) and ectopic corticotropin release by SCLC would increase morning cortisol levels and corticotropin levels. Physiologic (ie, nonneoplastic) hypercortisolism can be caused by several conditions, including pregnancy, severe obesity, obstructive sleep apnea, severe psychological stress or major depressive disorder, and, rarely, chronic alcoholism. However, they would be unlikely to cause the cutaneous and muscle signs of Cushing syndrome and the extremely high levels of plasma and urinary cortisol. Additional information is available in the medical literature (21).

7.3. Answer d.

Etomidate is most effective in rapidly decreasing cortisol levels in patients who have severe Cushing syndrome. Ketoconazole, metyrapone, mitotane, and etomidate are classified as steroidogenesis inhibitors because they each inhibit 1 or more enzymes in cortisol biosynthesis. Ketoconazole, metyrapone, and mitotane can decrease cortisol levels, but they act more slowly and less effectively than etomidate. Hemodialysis is not an effective method of decreasing blood cortisol levels. Additional information is available in the medical literature (6).

7.4. Answer a.

In addition to causing ectopic corticotropin release, SCLC can also cause the syndrome of inappropriate antidiuretic hormone secretion in 7% to 16% of patients, which is important to recognize because the syndrome is associated with poor outcomes and can lead to severe hyponatremia. Gastrin can be released ectopically by small-bowel or pancreatic neuroendocrine tumors (gastrinomas), leading to Zollinger-Ellison syndrome. Ectopic aldosterone-secreting tumors are extremely rare and can arise from aberrant adrenocortical tissue outside the adrenal gland, but they do not occur in patients with SCLC. Parathyroid hormone–related peptide can be released by several different cancers, including breast cancer, kidney cancer, lymphoma, and leukemia, but it is much more likely to be released by squamous cell lung cancer than by SCLC. A glucagonoma is a pancreatic neuroendocrine tumor that can cause glucose intolerance and necrotizing migratory erythema. Additional information is available in the medical literature (22,23).

7.5. Answer e.

A single dose of etomidate has been shown to decrease cortisol levels temporarily within the first 24 hours after intubation in critically ill patients. However, the majority of evidence suggests that this is not likely to lead to worse outcomes in most clinical situations. In a systematic review of 8 clinical trials, the use of etomidate in critically ill patients undergoing endotracheal intubation was not associated with an increased risk of mortality. There is no evidence that glucocorticoids should be used prophylactically in conjunction with etomidate. However, it would be reasonable to administer stress doses of corticosteroids in patients if refractory hypotension develops after they receive etomidate. Myoclonic movements can occur after the use of etomidate (in a dose-dependent manner), but they are not related to seizure activity. Etomidate does have some anticonvulsant properties, including decreasing cerebral oxygen consumption and intracranial pressure. Etomidate does not have any important analgesic effects. Additional information is available in the medical literature (14-18).

References

1. Loriaux DL. Diagnosis and differential diagnosis of Cushing's syndrome. N Engl J Med. 2017;376(15):1451–9.

2. Ilias I, Torpy DJ, Pacak K, Mullen N, Wesley RA, Nieman LK. Cushing's syndrome due to ectopic corticotropin secretion: twenty years' experience at the National Institutes of Health. J Clin Endocrinol Metab. 2005;90(8):4955–62.

3. Aniszewski JP, Young WF Jr, Thompson GB, Grant CS, van Heerden JA. Cushing syndrome due to ectopic adrenocorticotropic hormone secretion. World J Surg. 2001;25(7):934–40.

4. Isidori AM, Kaltsas GA, Pozza C, Frajese V, Newell-Price J, Reznek RH, et al. The ectopic adrenocorticotropin syndrome: clinical features, diagnosis, management, and long-term follow-up. J Clin Endocrinol Metab. 2006;91(2):371–7.

5. Broersen LHA, Jha M, Biermasz NR, Pereira AM, Dekkers OM. Effectiveness of medical treatment for Cushing's syndrome: a systematic review and meta-analysis. Pituitary. 2018;21(6):631–41.

6. Hinojosa-Amaya JM, Cuevas-Ramos D, Fleseriu M. Medical management of Cushing's syndrome: current and emerging treatments. Drugs. 2019;79(9):935–56.

7. Tritos NA, Biller BMK. Current management of Cushing's disease. J Intern Med. 2019;286(5):526–41.

8. Preda VA, Sen J, Karavitaki N, Grossman AB. Etomidate in the management of hypercortisolaemia in Cushing's syndrome: a review. Eur J Endocrinol. 2012;167(2):137–43.

9. Heyn J, Geiger C, Hinske CL, Briegel J, Weis F. Medical suppression of hypercortisolemia in Cushing's syndrome with particular consideration of etomidate. Pituitary. 2012;15(2):117–25.

10. Allolio B, Schulte HM, Kaulen D, Reincke M, Jaursch-Hancke C, Winkelmann W. Nonhypnotic low-dose etomidate for rapid correction of hypercortisolaemia in Cushing's syndrome. Klin Wochenschr. 1988;66(8):361–4.

11. Schulte HM, Benker G, Reinwein D, Sippell WG, Allolio B. Infusion of low dose etomidate: correction of hypercortisolemia in patients with Cushing's syndrome and dose-response relationship in normal subjects. J Clin Endocrinol Metab. 1990;70(5):1426–30.

12. Carroll TB, Peppard WJ, Herrmann DJ, Javorsky BR, Wang TS, Patel H, et al. Continuous etomidate infusion for the management of severe cushing syndrome: validation of a standard protocol. J Endocr Soc. 2019;3(1):1–12.

13. Constantinescu SM, Driessens N, Lefebvre A, Furnica RM, Corvilain B, Maiter D. Etomidate infusion at low doses is an effective and safe treatment for severe Cushing's syndrome outside intensive care. Eur J Endocrinol. 2020;183(2):161–7.

14. Bruder EA, Ball IM, Ridi S, Pickett W, Hohl C. Single induction dose of etomidate versus other induction agents for endotracheal intubation in critically ill patients. Cochrane Database Syst Rev. 2015;1:CD010225.

15. Cohan P, Wang C, McArthur DL, Cook SW, Dusick JR, Armin B, et al. Acute secondary adrenal insufficiency after traumatic brain injury: a prospective study. Crit Care Med. 2005;33(10):2358–66.

16. den Brinker M, Joosten KF, Liem O, de Jong FH, Hop WC, Hazelzet JA, et al. Adrenal insufficiency in meningococcal sepsis: bioavailable cortisol levels and impact of interleukin-6 levels and intubation with etomidate on adrenal function and mortality. J Clin Endocrinol Metab. 2005;90(9):5110–7.

17. Jackson WL Jr. Should we use etomidate as an induction agent for endotracheal intubation in patients with septic shock?: a critical appraisal. Chest. 2005;127(3):1031–8.

18. Schenarts CL, Burton JH, Riker RR. Adrenocortical dysfunction following etomidate induction in emergency department patients. Acad Emerg Med. 2001;8(1):1–7.

19. Basciani RM, Rindlisbacher A, Begert E, Brander L, Jakob SM, Etter R, et al. Anaesthetic induction with etomidate in cardiac surgery: a randomised controlled trial. Eur J Anaesthesiol. 2016;33(6):417–24.

20. Lobo Ferreira T, Nunes da Silva T, Canario D, Francisca Delerue M. Hypertension and severe hypokalaemia associated with ectopic ACTH production. BMJ Case Rep. 2018;2018:bcr2017223406.

21. Invitti C, Pecori Giraldi F, de Martin M, Cavagnini F; Study Group of the Italian Society of Endocrinology on the Pathophysiology of the Hypothalamic-Pituitary-Adrenal Axis. Diagnosis and management of Cushing's syndrome: results of an Italian multicentre study. J Clin Endocrinol Metab. 1999;84(2):440–8.

22. Lokich JJ. The frequency and clinical biology of the ectopic hormone syndromes of small cell carcinoma. Cancer. 1982;50(10):2111–4.

23. Gross AJ, Steinberg SM, Reilly JG, Bliss DP Jr, Brennan J, Le PT, et al. Atrial natriuretic factor and arginine vasopressin production in tumor cell lines from patients with lung cancer and their relationship to serum sodium. Cancer Res. 1993;53(1):67–74.

A 52-Year-Old Man With Suicidal Ideation and Bipolar Disorder

Kavitha Gopalratnam, MBBS, and Sara E. Hocker, MD

Case Presentation

A 52-year-old man with a history of suicide attempts and bipolar disorder who had been prescribed various medications was brought to the hospital after he was found unresponsive on the floor with multiple empty medication bottles nearby. At presentation he was lethargic but arousable. Laboratory test results were negative for a toxicology screen and normal for a complete blood cell count and electrolytes.

The patient's wife said that recently he had received lithium treatment for several weeks and that his test results had shown elevated blood levels of lithium for which he had undergone 2 sessions of hemodialysis until his lithium levels normalized. According to her description, however, he continued to express suicidal ideation and had pressured speech and mild agitation.

Over the next day in the hospital, his clinical condition continued to deteriorate, and he had febrile episodes (41 °C), severe agitation, diaphoresis, and increased tremulousness. He was given an intravenous dexmedetomidine infusion, but he had minimal response. On clinical examination, he had flushed, diaphoretic skin, and he was agitated and unable to follow commands. On neurologic examination, he had a bilateral, equal and reactive pupillary response with slow, continuous horizontal eye movements; he could not follow commands for assessment of motor strength; and he had symmetric hypertonicity, inducible clonus, and hyperreflexia in all extremities (more prominent in the legs than the arms).

Questions

Multiple Choice (choose the best answer)

8.1. The patient's clinical signs are most consistent with which of the following diagnoses?
    a. Neuroleptic malignant syndrome (NMS)
    b. Malignant hyperthermia
    c. Serotonin syndrome
    d. Anticholinergic overdose
    e. Agitated delirium

8.2. Which of the following statements describes a useful distinction between serotonin syndrome and NMS?
    a. Serotonin syndrome causes hyperthermia
    b. Serotonin syndrome causes autonomic dysfunction
    c. NMS causes hyporeflexia
    d. NMS causes altered mental status
    e. Serotonin syndrome causes lead pipe rigidity

8.3. In addition to aggressive cooling measures, which of the following is the most appropriate next step in management of this patient's condition?
    a. Intubation and sedation with fentanyl and propofol
    b. Intubation, sedation with midazolam infusion, and paralysis with cisatracurium
    c. Intubation and sedation with dexmedetomidine and fentanyl
    d. Intubation, sedation with dexmedetomidine, and intravenous haloperidol as needed
    e. Intubation, sedation with propofol, and initiation of hemodialysis

8.4. Despite the above measures, this patient continues to have increased hypertonicity without much improvement neurologically. Which of the following medications would be indicated at this time?
    a. Dantrolene
    b. Cyproheptadine
    c. Bromocriptine
    d. Haloperidol
    e. Dexmedetomidine

8.5. After the patient's home medications are reviewed, which of the following combinations could be implicated in the patient's current condition?
    a. Tramadol and ondansetron
    b. Acetaminophen and haloperidol
    c. Ibuprofen and aspirin
    d. Haloperidol and ibuprofen
    e. Ibuprofen and doxycycline

Case Follow-up and Outcome

Further evaluation of the home medications showed that the patient had consumed unknown quantities of sertraline and citalopram in addition to lithium, so a diagnosis of serotonin syndrome was confirmed. His agitation and mental status continued to worsen, and he was intubated for airway protection. A midazolam infusion was started, and, given the severity of his symptoms, cyproheptadine was also begun. His clinical condition improved gradually over the next few days, and he was successfully extubated. He was weaned from cyproheptadine therapy over the next week.

Discussion

Serotonin syndrome is associated with a constellation of clinical signs and symptoms that result from increased serotonergic stimulation of the central and peripheral serotonergic receptors in response to medications. The signs can range from very mild neurologic derangements to life-threatening conditions. Although serotonin syndrome has been difficult to assess epidemiologically, Ibister et al [1] reported a 14% to 16% incidence among patients who have had an overdose of selective serotonin reuptake inhibitors (SSRIs). Early recognition of toxicity or adverse reaction to these medications and management can prevent the life-threatening complications of serotonin syndrome.

Serotonin, a neurotransmitter produced by the decarboxylation of L-tryptophan, acts on serotonin-1A and possibly serotonin-2A receptors in the central nervous system, which are located in the raphe nuclei in the midbrain, pons, and medulla. Serotonin assists with thermoregulation, sleep and wakefulness, attention, behavior, and motor tone. In the peripheral nervous system, serotonin helps regulate vascular tone and gastrointestinal motility.

Overstimulation of these receptors results in serotonin syndrome [2].

Medications such as SSRIs (eg, sertraline, fluoxetine, and citalopram), monoamine oxidase inhibitors (MAOIs), tricyclic antidepressants, antiemetics (ondansetron, granisetron, and metoclopramide), opiates (fentanyl and tramadol), antibiotics (linezolid), lithium, and recreational drugs such as methylenedioxymethamphetamine (MDMA or "ecstasy") are the more commonly implicated causes of serotonin syndrome [3]. Often a combination of those medications potentiates a more severe form of the disease such as in the patient described in this case.

Serotonin syndrome is characterized by a wide spectrum of changes in mental status, neuromuscular hyperactivity, and symptoms of autonomic dysfunction. A patient with a mild to moderate case of serotonin syndrome can present with vital sign abnormalities (eg, hypertension, tachycardia, and hyperthermia) that are associated with diaphoresis, mydriasis, and occasionally increased tone and hyperreflexia that are more apparent in the lower extremities than the upper extremities. Patients with more severe disease may have encephalopathy, spontaneous or inducible clonus, ocular clonus, and severe agitation. In life-threatening disease, the core body temperature may increase to more than 41.1 °C mainly because of increased muscle hyperactivity. Uncontrolled hyperthermia in combination with severe hypertension and tachycardia can lead to severe metabolic acidosis, rhabdomyolysis, renal failure, seizures, and death.

Given the variable symptoms and presentations associated with serotonin syndrome, multiple diagnostic criteria have been proposed over the years. The Hunter Serotonin Toxicity Criteria [4], developed after a retrospective evaluation of over 2,000 patients, have been shown to be both sensitive (about 84%) and specific (about 97%) for the diagnosis of serotonin syndrome.

To fulfill the criteria, a patient must have a known exposure to a serotonergic agent within the previous 5 weeks and meet 1 of the following conditions: 1) spontaneous clonus; 2) inducible clonus and either agitation or diaphoresis;

3) ocular clonus and either agitation or diaphoresis; 4) tremor and hyperreflexia; or 5) muscle rigidity, core body temperature higher than 38 °C, and either ocular clonus or inducible clonus.

The differential diagnosis includes malignant hyperthermia, NMS, autoimmune encephalitis, nonconvulsive status epilepticus, and anticholinergic poisoning. These conditions can be differentiated from serotonin syndrome on the basis of the history and clinical examination findings.

For example, patients with malignant hyperthermia, which occurs after exposure to inhalational anesthetic agents, may have hyporeflexia, mottled and cyanotic skin, and rigidity that resembles rigor mortis. In contrast, patients with NMS, which occurs after exposure to dopamine antagonists, is characterized by a slow onset of bradykinesia or akinesia, lead pipe rigidity, and hyporeflexia (which is the main feature that helps to differentiate serotonin syndrome from NMS).

For patients with serotonin syndrome, symptom duration and rate of improvement largely depend on the combination of medications ingested and the half-lives of those medications. MAOIs, which inhibit monoamine oxidase A, are associated with a more severe form of the disease, especially when used in combination with SSRIs or MDMA.

The mainstay of management of serotonin syndrome is to discontinue use of the triggering agent in addition to providing supportive care, which centers on controlling agitation and managing autonomic instability and hyperthermia (2). Mild to moderate cases of serotonin syndrome can usually be managed with removal of the offending agent, supportive care with oral or intravenous benzodiazepines, and aggressive temperature control to prevent hyperthermia. In severe cases or if the patient's temperature exceeds 41.1 °C, the patient should be intubated and supported with mechanical ventilation and receive nondepolarizing agents for neuromuscular blockade, which helps to eliminate excessive muscle activity and thereby prevent the life-threatening complications of rhabdomyolysis and hyperkalemia. Benzodiazepines

are also recommended for the management of agitation associated with serotonin syndrome; in animal models, benzodiazepines have been shown to blunt the hyperadrenergic component of the syndrome. Autonomic instability is a key component that requires stabilization of the heart rate and blood pressure in severe cases. For example, to treat hypotension that results from MAOI interactions, sympathomimetic agents are recommended (eg, norepinephrine, phenylephrine, and epinephrine). Hypertension that results from the poisoning itself is treated with esmolol or nitroprusside, which have a short duration of action.

The use of cyproheptadine is strongly recommended for treatment of severe serotonin syndrome when vital signs and agitation do not improve with supportive care and benzodiazepines, but its efficacy has not been clearly established (5). Cyproheptadine is a histamine$_1$ receptor antagonist and a nonspecific antagonist to serotonin-1A and serotonin-2A receptors. The recommended treatment is to begin with a loading dose of 12 mg and use a maintenance dose of 8 mg every 6 hours orally or by nasogastric tube especially in patients with severe disease. When symptoms subside, the dose can be tapered gradually over a few days.

The use of medications such a bromocriptine, dantrolene, and propranolol is not recommended in serotonin syndrome.

Summary

Patients with serotonin syndrome present with the triad of mental status changes, neuromuscular abnormalities, and autonomic dysfunction after exposure to a serotonergic drug. A high degree of awareness is required for an accurate diagnosis. Prompt discontinuation of the drug and symptom management are the mainstays of therapy.

Answers

8.1. Answer c.

The timeline of clinical signs and constellation of neurologic signs for this patient are consistent with serotonin syndrome. The patient has ocular clonus, hyperreflexia, hypertonicity of muscles, and inducible clonus along with a fever. These findings fulfill the Hunter Serotonin Toxicity Criteria, which are used in the diagnosis of serotonin syndrome. Agitated delirium can be excluded because patients do not present with neurologic manifestations of hyperreflexia and inducible and ocular clonus. Additional information is available in the medical literature (4).

8.2. Answer c.

These signs are not particularly diagnostic when the details about the ingested medications are unknown. The main distinction between serotonin syndrome and NMS is that serotonin syndrome is associated with hyperreflexia and hypertonicity, whereas NMS occurs with hyporeflexia and lead pipe ridigity. Additional information is available in the medical literature (2).

8.3. Answer b.

In patients with severe serotonin syndrome, as described above, the mainstay of management (in addition to aggressive cooling measures to prevent hyperthermia) is supportive care in combination with nondepolarizing paralytic agents, which can reduce muscle hyperactivity and thereby prevent adverse events such as rhabdomyolysis. Benzodiazepines not only help to decrease the patient's agitation but also help to blunt the hyperadrenergic drive and improve autonomic instability. The use of dexmedetomidine and haloperidol have not been shown to have a direct role in the management of serotonin syndrome. In addition, this patient had already undergone hemodialysis with normalization of lithium levels, so those drugs would provide no benefit at this stage. Additional information is available in the medical literature (2).

8.4. Answer b.

Cyproheptadine is a histamine$_1$ receptor antagonist and a nonspecific antagonist of serotonin-1A and serotonin-2A receptors. Addition of cyproheptadine is recommended when appropriate supportive measures do not result in improvements in agitation and vital signs. The drug is available as an oral formulation only and should be administered by the nasogastric or orogastric route if needed. After an initial loading dose of 12 mg is administered, 8 mg is given every 6 hours until a response is evident, and then the dose is tapered over a few days. Additional information is available in the medical literature (5).

8.5. Answer a.

Analgesics such as tramadol, fentanyl, methadone, meperidine, and remifentanil have been implicated in serotonin syndrome. Antiemetic agents such as ondansetron, granisetron, and metoclopramide have also been identified as causes. Besides tramadol and ondansetron, none of the other listed combinations have been implicated in serotonin syndrome. An important reminder is that a patient taking a combination of medications often presents with a more severe form of the disease. Additional information is available in the medical literature (2).

References

1. Isbister GK, Bowe SJ, Dawson A, Whyte IM. Relative toxicity of selective serotonin reuptake inhibitors (SSRIs) in overdose. J Toxicol Clin Toxicol. 2004;42(3):277–85.
2. Boyer EW, Shannon M. The serotonin syndrome [published correction appears in N Engl J Med. 2007 Jun 7;356(23):2437] [published correction appears in N Engl J Med. 2009 Oct 22;361(17):1714]. N Engl J Med. 2005;352(11):1112–20.
3. Birmes P, Coppin D, Schmitt L, Lauque D. Serotonin syndrome: a brief review. CMAJ. 2003;168(11):1439–42.
4. Dunkley EJ, Isbister GK, Sibbritt D, Dawson AH, Whyte IM. The Hunter Serotonin Toxicity Criteria: simple and accurate diagnostic decision rules for serotonin toxicity. QJM. 2003;96(9):635–42.
5. Graudins A, Stearman A, Chan B. Treatment of the serotonin syndrome with cyproheptadine. J Emerg Med. 1998;16(4):615–9.

A 66-Year-Old Man With Fatigue, Dyspnea, and Hypoxemia

Michael Bourne, MD, and Daniel A. Diedrich, MD

Case Presentation

A 66-year-old man presented to the hospital with a 3-day history of worsening fatigue, dyspnea, and weakness. His past medical history included chronic lymphocytic leukemia with splenectomy and allogeneic bone marrow transplant 5 years previously that was complicated by graft-vs-host disease of the liver and gastrointestinal tract. Other past medical history included *Pneumocystis* pneumonia (PCP) 6 years previously and necrotizing pneumonia due to *Pseudomonas aeruginosa* 2 years previously.

Before he presented to the hospital the patient had been evaluated by his primary care provider who, because the influenza season was in progress, empirically began therapy with oseltamivir. The patient's medications included prophylactic acyclovir, azathioprine, dapsone, and posaconazole in addition to diltiazem, inhaled fluticasone, gabapentin, and pantoprazole. He denied smoking, illicit drug use, or recent contact with anyone who was ill. In the past, he had an allergic reaction (rash) to sulfa.

On presentation, he was febrile, hypotensive, cyanotic, and dyspneic. Chest radiography did not show any focal infiltrate. His oxygen saturation as measured by pulse oximetry (Spo_2) was 87% while he received supplemental oxygen at 15 L/min with a nonrebreather mask. His blood pressure was 94/57 mm Hg, his respiratory rate was 14 breaths/min, and his heart rate was 70 beats/min. When intravenous fluids were administered, his blood pressure improved. Blood cultures were obtained, and therapy was initiated with broad-spectrum antibiotics (piperacillin-tazobactam and vancomycin). Pulmonary thromboembolism was ruled out with a D-dimer test. Computed tomography showed a small amount of bibasilar atelectasis and consolidation in the posterior lung fields, but these findings were not thought to fully account for the degree of hypoxemia. The patient was admitted to the intensive care unit for refractory hypoxemia.

The patient received supplemental oxygen through a high-flow nasal cannula with a fraction of inspired oxygen (Fio_2) of 100% and a flow of 55 L/min with a maximum Spo_2 of 92%. Persistent hypoxia prompted arterial blood gas (ABG) analysis with co-oximetry, which had the following results: pH 7.38, $Paco_2$ 36 mm Hg, Pao_2 212 mm Hg, bicarbonate 21 mmol/L, oxyhemoglobin 90.2%, and methemoglobin 9.4%.

Questions

Multiple Choice (choose the best answer)

9.1. Which of the following is true about the diagnosis of methemoglobinemia?
a. It can be diagnosed with standard pulse oximetry
b. SpO_2 will not normalize with supplemental oxygen
c. ABG analysis will show decreased PaO_2 despite high FIO_2
d. The arterial blood will appear brighter red than normal arterial blood
e. An arterial blood sample is required for diagnosis

9.2. Which medication is not known to cause or worsen methemoglobinemia?
a. Inhaled nitric oxide
b. Benzocaine
c. Amlodipine
d. Methylene blue
e. Nitroprusside

9.3. After the offending agent is discontinued, when should acquired methemoglobinemia be treated with additional therapies such as methylene blue?
a. Only when the patient is symptomatically dyspneic, regardless of the methemoglobin level

b. When the patient is symptomatic and methemoglobin is greater than 5% but no more than 10% on co-oximetry
c. When the patient is symptomatic and methemoglobin is greater than 10% but no more than 20% on co-oximetry
d. When the patient is symptomatic and methemoglobin is greater than 20% on co-oximetry or when methemoglobin is greater than 30% regardless of symptoms
e. Only when the patient appears cyanotic regardless of symptoms or methemoglobin level

9.4. Which is *not* an accepted therapy for methemoglobinemia?
a. *N*-acetylcysteine
b. Vitamin C
c. Methylene blue
d. Removal of oxidizing agent
e. Exchange transfusion

9.5. What would be the most effective, safest, and cost-effective option for ongoing PCP prophylaxis in this patient?
a. Another trial of dapsone
b. Monthly pentamadine
c. Sulfamethoxazole-trimethoprim desensitization
d. Atovaquone
e. Lower dose of dapsone in addition to pyrimethamine and leucovorin

Case Follow-up and Outcome

This patient received a diagnosis of methemoglobinemia, and the use of dapsone was discontinued. Reverse transcriptase–polymerase chain reaction results were positive for Influenzavirus A, and treatment with oseltamivir was continued. Because co-oximetry showed that methemoglobin was only 9.4% of the total hemoglobin and because the patient's acute dyspnea was largely attributed to influenza, treatment with methylene blue was deferred in favor of continued oxygen, dapsone avoidance, and oseltamivir therapy. The patient's condition improved, so he was weaned from supplemental oxygen over the next few days, and he successfully underwent sulfamethoxazole-trimethoprim desensitization for further PCP prophylaxis.

Discussion

Methemoglobin is defined as a hemoglobin molecule with the central iron atom oxidized from ferrous iron (Fe^{2+}) to ferric iron (Fe^{3+}), which cannot bind oxygen. An abnormally high concentration of methemoglobin results in a functional anemia and lower oxygen-carrying capacity of the blood. About 1% to 3% of total body hemoglobin is oxidized to methemoglobin every hour, but this is easily reduced by cytochrome $b5$ reductase (1).

Methemoglobinemia can be congenital or acquired. Congenital methemoglobinemia is secondary to enzymatic deficiencies that result in decreased reduction of methemoglobin. Acquired methemoglobinemia is most commonly caused by drugs, but other sources of oxidative stress, such as surgical procedures, have been implicated (2,3).

The diagnosis of methemoglobinemia requires a high degree of clinical awareness and corresponding ABG and co-oximetry results. ABG testing shows low arterial oxygen saturation (Sao_2) with a normal or high Pao_2, and co-oximetry is diagnostic because percentages of oxyhemoglobin, carboxyhemoglobin, and methemoglobin can be quantified. Another helpful diagnostic feature for methemoglobinemia is the abnormal color of arterial blood (Figure 9.1), which is often described as brown or chocolate, and the color does not change to bright red when exposed to oxygen (1).

Methemoglobinemia should be suspected when a patient has cyanosis with a normal PaO_2. Pulse oximeters with multiple wavelengths are reported to be useful for identifying multiple types of human hemoglobin, including methemoglobin; however, those pulse oximeters are not reliable when SpO_2 is less than 95% (4). Methemoglobinemia should be a consideration if a patient has a low pulse oximetry reading in spite of adequate oxygen supplementation and normal PaO_2. At higher methemoglobin levels, the pulse oximetry reading tends to stabilize at about 85% regardless of the actual oxyhemoglobin percentage.

Treatment depends on the percentage of methemoglobin and the degree of symptoms attributable to the methemoglobinemia. Should treatment be indicated, methylene blue is administered at a dose of 1 to 2 mg/kg. Methylene blue is generally not administered unless the methemoglobin percentage is greater than 30% regardless of symptoms or if the patient has a methemoglobin level that is greater than 20% and the patient is symptomatic or has cardiopulmonary comorbidities. With this therapy, methemoglobin is reduced to oxyhemoglobin, and the carrying capacity of blood oxygen is quickly restored (5). In patients with glucose-6-phosphate dehydrogenase (G6PD) deficiency, methylene blue can paradoxically increase methemoglobin levels. In this scenario vitamin C can be administered instead, but effective reduction of methemoglobin with vitamin C takes much longer (6).

Figure 9.1   Blood Sample From a Patient With Methemoglobinemia

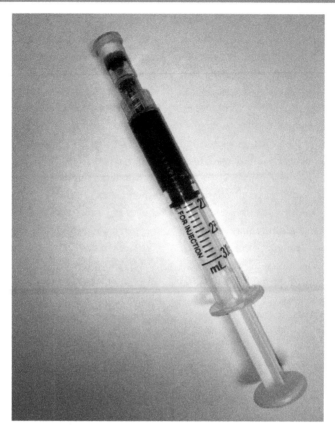

The color is often described as brown or chocolate, and it does not change to bright red when exposed to oxygen.

Summary

Acquired methemoglobinemia occurs when oxidative stress oxidizes hemoglobin-bound Fe^{2+} to Fe^{3+}, producing methemoglobin, a state of hemoglobin that cannot bind oxygen. The result is a functional anemia and decreased blood oxygen content. Commonly implicated oxidative stressors include drugs such as dapsone and benzocaine. A high degree of clinical awareness with corresponding ABG testing and co-oximetry should allow for confirmation of the diagnosis. Treatment depends on the percentage of methemoglobin and the presence of symptoms. Most patients who require treatment beyond removal of the offending agent and supportive care can be treated with methylene blue.

Answers

9.1. Answer b.

Increased methemoglobin levels interfere with normal pulse oximetry. Abnormally low SpO_2 on pulse oximetry can be a clue that a hemoglobinopathy is present but is not diagnostic. Even with an increased FIO_2, the measured SpO_2 will not improve because of the inability of methemoglobin to appropriately bind oxygen despite a high PaO_2. ABG samples will appear brown or chocolate (Figure 9.1) as opposed to the normal bright red. Methemoglobinemia may be diagnosed from an arterial or venous blood sample, although an arterial blood sample may be useful because it allows for a stark comparison between the high PaO_2 and the low saturation of hemoglobin. Additional information is available in the medical literature (1,4).

9.2. Answer c.

All medications listed are known to trigger or worsen methemoglobinemia except amlodipine. Curiously, even methylene blue has been known to trigger or worsen methemoglobinemia in certain patients, such as those with G6PD deficiency. Baseline and periodic methemoglobin levels must be checked when inhaled nitric oxide is used in the intensive care unit. Additional information is available in the medical literature (1-3).

9.3. Answer d.

Most patients with methemoglobinemia can be treated with supportive care and withdrawal of the offending agent (as in the patient described in this case). It is generally accepted that when a patient is symptomatic or has cardiopulmonary comorbidities and methemoglobin is greater than 20% on co-oximetry, or when methemoglobin is greater than 30% regardless of symptoms, treatment with methylene blue is indicated. Treatment consists of methylene blue 1 to 2 mg/kg given intravenously over 5 minutes. Dosing may be repeated after 1 hour if the methemoglobin level remains elevated or is increasing. Caution must be exercised when methylene blue is used in patients with G6PD deficiency. Additional information is available in the medical literature (1,5).

9.4. Answer a.

All the listed therapies except *N*-acetylcysteine are known treatments for methemoglobinemia. *N*-acetylcysteine has shown some efficacy in reducing methemoglobin in vitro, but is not used clinically. Vitamin C is used in treating patients with G6PD deficiency. Methylene blue requires the reduced form of nicotinamide adenine dinucleotide phosphate (NADPH) to reduce methemoglobin to hemoglobin (vitamin C reduces methemoglobin in an NADPH-independent pathway). G6PD causes a scarcity of NADPH, and methylene blue decreases stores of NADPH further, possibly resulting in hemolysis. Offending agents should be removed for all patients who have methemoglobinemia. Exchange transfusion can be considered if methemoglobinemia is refractory to other treatments. Additional information is available in the medical literature (5,6).

9.5. Answer c.

All listed options are acceptable forms of PCP prophylaxis; however, sulfamethoxazole-trimethoprim is considered first-line therapy in terms of efficacy and cost. It is generally well tolerated, and patients with sulfa allergies can be desensitized. Data are less robust for other regimens such as atovaquone. Trials have shown the superiority of sulfamethoxazole-trimethoprim over dapsone and pentamidine. Therefore, if patients can tolerate desensitization, sulfamethoxazole-trimethoprim is generally accepted as a superior regimen. Additional information is available in the medical literature (7).

References

1. Ash-Bernal R, Wise R, Wright SM. Acquired methemoglobinemia: a retrospective series of 138 cases at 2 teaching hospitals. Medicine (Baltimore). 2004;83(5):265–73.
2. Kane GC, Hoehn SM, Behrenbeck TR, Mulvagh SL. Benzocaine-induced methemoglobinemia based on the Mayo Clinic experience from 28 478 transesophageal echocardiograms: incidence, outcomes, and predisposing factors. Arch Intern Med. 2007;167(18):1977–82.
3. Esbenshade AJ, Ho RH, Shintani A, Zhao Z, Smith LA, Friedman DL. Dapsone-induced methemoglobinemia: a dose-related occurrence? Cancer. 2011;117(15):3485–92.
4. Feiner JR, Bickler PE, Mannheimer PD. Accuracy of methemoglobin detection by pulse CO-oximetry during hypoxia. Anesth Analg. 2010;111(1):143–8.
5. Modarai B, Kapadia YK, Kerins M, Terris J. Methylene blue: a treatment for severe methaemoglobinaemia secondary to misuse of amyl nitrite. Emerg Med J 2002;19: 270–1.
6. Rino PB, Scolnik D, Fustinana A, Mitelpunkt A, Glatstein M. Ascorbic acid for the treatment of methemoglobinemia: the experience of a large tertiary care pediatric hospital. Am J Ther. 2014;21(4):240–3.
7. Ioannidis JP, Cappelleri JC, Skolnik PR, Lau J, Sacks HS. A meta-analysis of the relative efficacy and toxicity of Pneumocystis carinii prophylactic regimens. Arch Intern Med. 1996 Jan 22;156(2): 177–88.

A 51-Year-Old Man With Fever, Dyspnea, and Productive Cough

10

Tyler L. Herzog, MD, Bryan T. Kelly, MD, and Diana J. Kelm, MD

Case Presentation

A 51-year-old man with a history of hypertension and obesity presented to the emergency department (ED) with a 6-day history of fever, dyspnea, chills, productive cough, anosmia, ageusia, and diarrhea. His wife was concurrently being evaluated for similar symptoms. He had no other known sick contacts and no recent travel. In the ED, he was hypoxemic (a nonrebreather mask was required), tachypneic, and febrile (39.2 °C). Portable radiography of the chest (CXR) showed bilateral patchy alveolar and interstitial opacities. The clinical diagnosis was COVID-19, which was subsequently confirmed with nasopharyngeal polymerase chain reaction testing. With an increasing oxygen requirement, the patient was transferred to the medical intensive care unit (MICU) for management of acute hypoxemic respiratory failure.

In the MICU, the patient was treated with a high-flow nasal cannula (HFNC) with settings for 90% fraction of inspired oxygen (FIO_2) at 50 L/min. Over the next several days, bilevel positive airway pressure was used and then changed to continuous positive airway pressure (CPAP) to maintain his oxygenation because he did not tolerate the HFNC. CPAP settings were 15 cm H_2O and 80% FIO_2 after his respiratory status stabilized. The patient received best practice medications and trial medications that were deemed appropriate during the COVID-19 pandemic. His treatment included remdesivir for 5 days, dexamethasone for 10 days, enoxaparin, ceftriaxone, and azithromycin and involvement in a clinical trial that used merimepodib. CPAP settings were maintained at 15 cm H_2O as his oxygen requirement slowly decreased over the course of a week to an FIO_2 of 45%. However, the patient's oxygen requirement then abruptly increased over a few hours to an FIO_2 of 60%. He did not have any new symptoms or complaints. CXR showed pneumomediastinum (Figure 10.1).

Figure 10.1   Portable CXR Showing Pneumomediastinum (Anteroposterior View)

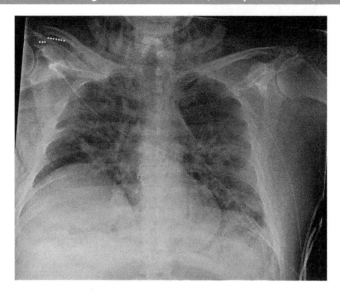

Questions

Multiple Choice (choose the best answer)

10.1. Which of the following patients, if their other characteristics are similar, would have the greatest risk of pneumomediastinum?

a. A patient receiving a tidal volume of 7 mL/kg

b. A patient with a plateau pressure of 23 cm H$_2$O

c. A patient undergoing neuromuscular blockade to maintain ventilator synchrony

d. A patient with high auto positive end-expiratory pressure (PEEP)

e. A patient whose use of mechanical ventilation is discontinued as soon as parameters allow

10.2. Compared to no therapy, which of the following may hasten the resolution of pneumomediastinum?

a. Analgesics

b. Use of 100% oxygen

c. Exercise

d. Antibiotics

e. No oral nutrition

10.3. If each of the following patients has pneumomediastinum, for which patient would mediastinotomy be most appropriate?

a. A 45-year-old woman with crepitus after repeated vomiting

b. A 54-year-old man who is asymptomatic but has pneumomediastinum that was incidentally seen on CXR

c. A 23-year-old man who has a history of asthma and presents with acute neck discomfort

d. A 31-year-old woman with mild dyspnea after childbirth

e. A 56-year-old man who has been intubated and whose blood pressure is decreasing rapidly

10.4. What is the most common mechanism for development of pneumoperitoneum in patients with coexisting pneumomediastinum from barotrauma?

a. Air tracks through the esophageal hiatus entering the abdominal wall and then the peritoneal space

b. Visceral perforation from extensive aerophagia

c. Diaphragmatic rupture

d. Formation of a mediastinal-peritoneal fistula

e. Air movement through microscopic diaphragmatic defects

10.5. For patients with pneumoperitoneum from pneumomediastinal extension, which of the following would be an indication for abdominal decompression?

a. Urinary bladder with intravesical pressure of 9 mm Hg

b. Severe nausea with intermittent vomiting

c. New kidney dysfunction with oliguria progressing to anuria

d. Abdominal distention with a girth increase of 5 cm

e. Worsening abdominal pain with stable vital signs

Case Follow-up and Outcome

After pneumomediastinum was identified, the use of a HFNC was resumed. When desaturation developed despite high levels of F_{IO_2}, the use of CPAP was resumed at a decreased pressure (10 cm H_2O). The next day, the pneumomediastinum had nearly completely resolved (Figure 10.2), but on the day after that, the patient reported abdominal bloating without pain. On physical examination he had an obese abdomen with mild distention but no tenderness, rebound, or guarding. An upright abdominal radiograph showed the double-wall sign, which suggested the possibility of pneumoperitoneum (Figure 10.3) that was confirmed from a lateral decubitus radiograph. Follow-up abdominal computed tomography (CT) was negative for visceral perforation, and pneumoperitoneum was presumed to have developed from the migration of air from the pneumomediastinum. The patient was monitored with serial examinations and chest radiographs. The F_{IO_2} was increased to

100% for nitrogen washout and to facilitate resorption. The patient's therapy was transitioned to bilevel positive airway pressure and then to a nonrebreather mask to minimize the positive-pressure contribution. His condition continued to improve slowly, and he was discharged after 2 weeks in the hospital without having to undergo intervention for pneumomediastinum or pneumoperitoneum. Pneumomediastinum was not visible on CXR at discharge.

Discussion

The *mediastinum* is the area within the thoracic cavity between the right and left parietal pleurae. *Pneumomediastinum* refers to air within the mediastinum. Air can be introduced into the mediastinum from various sources, including the lungs, airways, and esophagus and from external trauma. When the lungs are the source of air, barotrauma causes alveolar overdistention

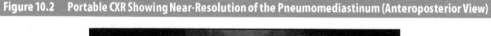

Figure 10.2   Portable CXR Showing Near-Resolution of the Pneumomediastinum (Anteroposterior View)

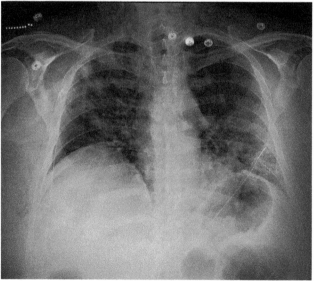

Figure 10.3   Portable Radiography of the Abdomen Showing Pneumoperitoneum

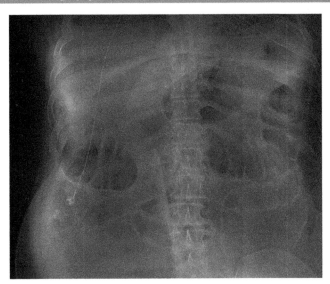

This anteroposterior view shows the double-wall sign.

and rupture. Free air then tracks along the bronchovascular sheaths to the mediastinum (Figure 10.4). Within the mediastinum, air can travel along fascial planes and, for instance, cause subcutaneous emphysema in the neck.

Patients with pneumomediastinum typically present with dyspnea and retrosternal chest pain, which can radiate to the neck or back. Additional symptoms may include dysphagia, neck swelling, and neck pain (1). Some patients are asymptomatic. The most common physical examination finding is subcutaneous emphysema, which is present in about 56% of patients who have pneumomediastinum (1,2). About 18% of patients have the Hamman sign, which is a crunching sound synchronous with the heartbeat (2,3).

The diagnosis of pneumomediastinum is usually determined with CXR. However, CXR may not show spontaneous pneumomediastinum in up to 30% of cases (4). When CXR is inconclusive, CT can be used for confirmation of smaller amounts of air causing pneumomediastinum and to differentiate pneumomediastinum and pneumoperitoneum. Bedside ultrasonography

has been used for the rapid diagnosis of pneumomediastinum in more urgent situations. On bedside ultrasonography, parasternal and apical views are obstructed because of air artifact, but subxiphoid views are unobstructed because the pericardium is in direct contact with the diaphragm, so that pneumomediastinum can be differentiated from pneumopericardium. However, this finding alone cannot differentiate pneumomediastinum from other causes of air artifact on parasternal and apical views (eg, pneumothorax) (5). Pneumomediastinum is classified as spontaneous or secondary, which includes iatrogenic and traumatic causes.

Spontaneous pneumomediastinum occurs without an obvious precipitating event or identifiable cause. Risk factors for spontaneous pneumomediastinum include smoking, underlying lung disorders (eg, asthma, interstitial lung disease, and chronic obstructive pulmonary disease), and substance use (2). Spontaneous pneumomediastinum occurs most often in younger adult patients and pediatric patients. However, case reports also describe spontaneous pneumomediastinum arising from infectious

Figure 10.4   CT of the Chest

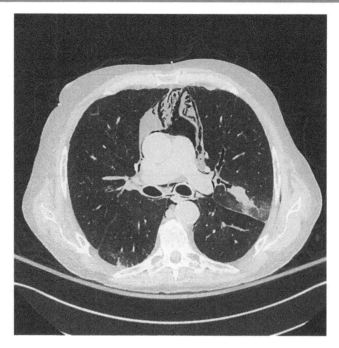

This axial view shows that free air has tracked along bronchovascular structures to the mediastinum.

causes (6), such as during the COVID-19 pandemic (7,8). The incidence in a recent case series is approximately 1 in 30,000 ED presentations (1). For most patients with spontaneous pneumomediastinum, the course is benign. Although no guidelines exist, management includes observation, rest, oxygen therapy, and pain management (1). Use of high-concentration oxygen may help to increase the absorption of free air through increases in the diffusion pressure of nitrogen in the interstitium (9).

Secondary pneumomediastinum refers to pneumomediastinum for which an underlying cause can be found. Most frequently secondary pneumomediastinum results from iatrogenic and traumatic causes. Iatrogenic causes include invasive and noninvasive ventilation, procedures such as central line placement and intubation, and endoscopic procedures. Traumatic causes include penetrating injuries (eg, stab or gunshot wound) and blunt force trauma (eg, motor vehicle accident) to either the airway or the esophagus. Additional considerations include other causes of increased thoracic pressure, including Boerhaave syndrome and childbirth. In a study conducted at a single center where a large cohort of patients with pneumomediastinum was evaluated, approximately 90% of patients were admitted with secondary pneumomediastinum that was due to trauma (90% of patients), esophageal injury (5.5%), or pneumothorax or airway injury (3.5%) (10).

Patients with pneumomediastinum due to trauma require targeted surgical management to repair any underlying injuries contributing to the pneumomediastinum. Patients with esophageal injury should be evaluated to identify any esophageal tears that require surgical repair. After the underlying injuries are repaired, the mainstay of therapy is observation, rest, oxygen therapy, and pain management.

For secondary pneumomediastinum due to barotrauma, the primary goal is prevention with lung-protective ventilation. The clinician should also take steps to eliminate or minimize the development of auto-PEEP, which, if untreated, may lead to alveolar overdistention and precipitate alveolar rupture. If pneumomediastinum develops from barotrauma, measures should be taken to decrease the risk of further trauma and air leak. These measures include decreasing the pressures by maintaining a goal plateau pressure of less than 30 cm H_2O, ventilating with a tidal volume less than 6 to 8 mL/kg ideal body weight, and decreasing PEEP (11). Another consideration is to increase the level of sedation or perform neuromuscular blockade in mechanically ventilated patients to reduce asynchrony and patient distress. Ideally, mechanical or noninvasive ventilation should be discontinued as soon as possible. As in spontaneous pneumothorax, a high concentration of oxygen may help increase the resorption of free air, so an increase in F_{IO_2} should be considered.

A rare complication of pneumomediastinum is tension pneumomediastinum, which was first demonstrated in laboratory studies that showed that pneumomediastinum could lead to compression of the heart and its vessels and thereby lead to cardiac tamponade (9). If the situation is not recognized, hypotension and shock can develop from decreased venous return to the heart causing low cardiac output. An early case report described a 23-year-old man who required cardiopulmonary resuscitation because of tension pneumomediastinum that had been managed with needle decompression (12). The mainstay of therapy for tension pneumomediastinum is mediastinal drainage in addition to conservative management and correction of the underlying cause.

Pneumoperitoneum is defined as free air within the peritoneal cavity. In most cases (about 90%), it results from a perforated abdominal viscus. However, pneumoperitoneum can also have a thoracic cause (13). Pneumoperitoneum resulting from mechanical ventilation is rare; only 40 cases were described in a literature review published in 2000 (14). Pneumoperitoneum from noninvasive ventilation is very rare but has been described (15). In ventilated patients, pneumoperitoneum may occur as free air from an alveolar rupture passes from the mediastinum through the esophageal hiatus into the anterior abdominal wall and then into the peritoneum. Diagnosis is often made with identification of free air on chest or abdominal radiographs that show the free air under the diaphragm on upright radiographs or the double-wall sign (eponym, Rigler sign), which describes visualization of both the outer and the inner walls of the bowel (16). Even when free air is recognized on plain radiographs, CT should be pursued to rule out rupture of an abdominal viscus.

Conservative management is appropriate in most cases of pneumoperitoneum related to ventilation. Patients should be monitored closely because abdominal compartment syndrome can occur. Manifestations of abdominal compartment syndrome include hepatic, mesenteric, or kidney dysfunction from direct compression and cardiac or respiratory compromise from diaphragm elevation. Monitoring of intravesical (bladder) pressures is a common screening tool for abdominal compartment syndrome; if it is identified, the patient should undergo decompression (17).

Summary

Pneumomediastinum and pneumoperitoneum are rare pulmonary disorders. They can occur spontaneously or result from medical treatment (iatrogenic causes), underlying disorders, or trauma. In patients receiving ventilation, pneumomediastinum and pneumoperitoneum result from barotrauma and alveolar rupture. Currently, no guidelines exist to guide evaluation and management of either disorder. Most patients present with mild, self-limited disease that resolves with conservative treatment. Administration of high concentrations of oxygen may help speed resorption of the free air. An underlying cause should be sought and treated as necessary. Rarely, patients may have a more serious complication, such as tension pneumomediastinum or abdominal compartment syndrome, that necessitates emergent treatment with decompression.

Answers

10.1. Answer d.

Increasing auto-PEEP may lead to alveolar overdistention and precipitation of alveolar rupture, causing pneumomediastinum. The other answer choices are all consistent with lung-protective ventilation, which is intended to prevent alveolar rupture and includes delivering a tidal volume less than 6 to 8 mL/kg ideal body weight, maintaining a plateau pressure less than 30 cm H_2O, improving patient-ventilator synchrony, and discontinuing use of mechanical ventilation as soon as possible. Additional information is available in the medical literature (11).

10.2. Answer b.

A patient breathing 100% oxygen may have faster resorption of free air and faster resolution of pneumomediastinum than a patient who is not receiving oxygen therapy. No other definitive management strategies have been studied to help resolve pneumomediastinum more quickly. The mainstay of therapy is observation and supportive care, which can include analgesics, but those measures will not resolve the underlying pneumomediastinum. The use of antibiotics and no oral nutrition may be indicated for specific causes of pneumomediastinum but would not be expected to improve resolution of free air alone.

Additional information is available in the medical literature (1,9).

10.3. Answer e.

A patient whose blood pressure is decreasing rapidly may have potentially life-threatening tension pneumomediastinum, which requires intervention. The patients in the other answer choices have mild cases that most likely will follow a benign, self-limited course. Additional information is available in the medical literature (12).

10.4. Answer a.

Although all the answer choices pose reasonable consideration for the development of pneumoperitoneum, early studies indicated that the most common mechanism is air tracking along the esophagus through the esophageal hiatus. Additional information is available in the medical literature (13).

10.5. Answer c.

The patient's new kidney dysfunction is indicative of organ dysfunction related to abdominal compartment syndrome, which requires intervention. The other findings listed can occur in pneumoperitoneum, but they do not indicate abdominal compartment syndrome. A bladder with an intravesical pressure greater than 25 mm Hg is typically associated with abdominal compartment syndrome, but that value is not an absolute cutoff. Additional information is available in the medical literature (17).

References

1. Newcomb AE, Clarke CP. Spontaneous pneumomediastinum: a benign curiosity or a significant problem? Chest. 2005;128(5):3298–302.

2. Sahni S, Verma S, Grullon J, Esquire A, Patel P, Talwar A. Spontaneous pneumomediastinum: time for consensus. N Am J Med Sci. 2013;5(8):460–4.

3. Hamman L. Spontaneous mediastinal emphysema. Bull Johns Hopkins Hosp. 1939;64:1–21.

4. Kaneki T, Kubo K, Kawashima A, Koizumi T, Sekiguchi M, Sone S. Spontaneous pneumomediastinum in 33 patients: yield of chest computed tomography for the diagnosis of the mild type. Respiration. 2000;67(4):408–11.

5. Zachariah S, Gharahbaghian L, Perera P, Joshi N. Spontaneous pneumomediastinum on bedside ultrasound: case report and review of the literature. West J Emerg Med. 2015;16(2):321–4.

6. Chekkoth SM, Supreeth RN, Valsala N, Kumar P, Raja RS. Spontaneous pneumomediastinum in H1N1 infection: uncommon complication of a common infection. J R Coll Physicians Edinb. 2019;49(4):298–300.

7. Romano N, Fischetti A, Melani EF. Pneumomediastinum related to Covid-19 pneumonia. Am J Med Sci. 2020;360(6):e19–e20.

8. Volpi S, Ali JM, Suleman A, Ahmed RN. Pneumomediastinum in COVID-19 patients: a case series of a rare complication. Eur J Cardiothorac Surg. 2020;58(3):646–7.

9. Macklin MT, Macklin, C.C. Malignant interstitial emphysema of the lungs and mediastinum as an important occult complication in many respiratory diseases and other conditions: interpretation of the clinical literature in the light of laboratory experiment. Medicine. 1944;23:281–358.

10. Banki F, Estrera AL, Harrison RG, Miller CC, 3rd, Leake SS, Mitchell KG, et al. Pneumomediastinum: etiology and a guide to diagnosis and treatment. Am J Surg. 2013;206(6):1001–6; discussion 6.

11. Ioannidis G, Lazaridis G, Baka S, Mpoukovinas I, Karavasilis V, Lampaki S, et al. Barotrauma and pneumothorax. J Thorac Dis. 2015;7(Suppl 1):S38–43.

12. Shennib HF, Barkun AN, Matouk E, Blundell PE. Surgical decompression of a tension pneumomediastinum. A ventilatory complication of status asthmaticus. Chest. 1988;93(6):1301–2.

13. Williams NM, Watkin DF. Spontaneous pneumoperitoneum and other nonsurgical causes of intraperitoneal free gas. Postgrad Med J. 1997;73(863):531–7.

14. Mularski RA, Sippel JM, Osborne ML. Pneumoperitoneum: a review of nonsurgical causes. Crit Care Med. 2000;28(7):2638–44.

15. Planchard D, Verdaguer M, Levrat V, Caron F, Adoun M, Meurice JC. [Pneumoperitoneum and pneumomediastinum complicating non-invasive ventilation]. Rev Mal Respir. 2005;22(1 Pt 1):147–50.

16. Rigler LG. Spontaneous pneumoperitoneum: a roentgenologic sign found in the supine position. 1941;37(November):604–7.

17. Chang MC, Miller PR, D'Agostino R, Jr, Meredith JW. Effects of abdominal decompression on cardiopulmonary function and visceral perfusion in patients with intra-abdominal hypertension. J Trauma. 1998;44(3):440–5.

A 49-Year-Old Man With Massive Upper Gastrointestinal Tract Bleeding

Kelly M. Pennington, MD, and Michael E. Wilson, MD

Case Presentation

A 49-year-old man with a past medical history of gallstone pancreatitis complicated by chronic superior mesenteric vein thrombosis and an unprovoked pulmonary embolism (PE) 10 years previously was admitted to the intensive care unit (ICU) with massive bleeding in the upper gastrointestinal tract. Two weeks previously, deep vein thrombosis (DVT) in the proximal right lower extremity was diagnosed, and therapy was initiated with warfarin and an enoxaparin bridge to achieve a therapeutic international normalized ratio. Subsequently the patient had melenic stools and a decrease of 8 g/dL in the hemoglobin level, which prompted esophagogastroduodenoscopy (EGD). During EGD, large duodenal varices were punctured and resulted in massive bleeding in the upper gastrointestinal tract. Massive blood transfusion protocols were initiated, and endoscopic control of the bleeding was attempted with balloon tamponade.

The patient was subsequently transferred to the ICU. Upon arrival in the ICU, he was normotensive and mildly tachycardic. He continued to have bloody emesis around his endotracheal tube. He subsequently underwent transhepatic and portal venography, during which no active blood loss was visualized. Since the patient had an ongoing bleeding risk and a high risk for thromboembolic disease, an inferior vena cava filter (IVCF) was placed. Two days later, EGD was repeated with gluing of his duodenal varices. After that procedure, the patient had a sudden cardiac arrest characterized by pulseless, monomorphic ventricular tachycardia. With resuscitation, spontaneous circulation returned and he could follow commands. Point-of-care ultrasonography showed a mobile echodense mass within the right atrium and right ventricle. Computed tomography with angiography showed an acute saddle PE with leftward deviation of the intraventricular septum, and the IVCF was located in the right ventricle (Figure 11.1).

Presented in part at the CHEST annual meeting, San Antonio, Texas, October 6-10, 2018.

Figure 11.1   Computed Tomography of the Chest, Axial Views

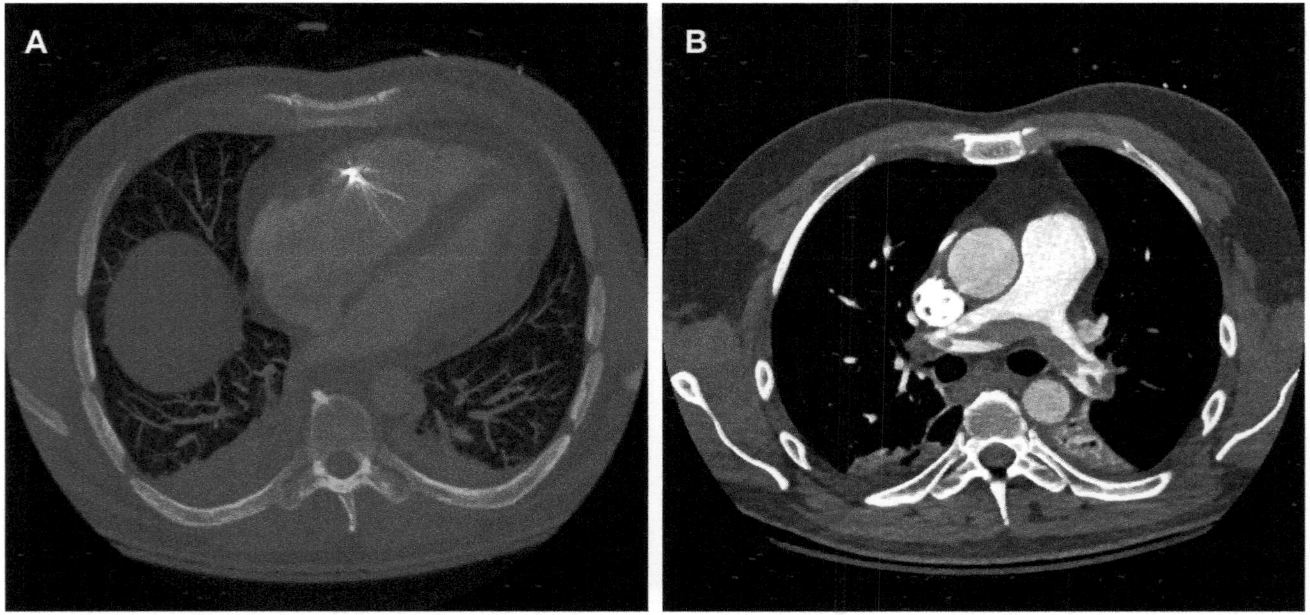

A, Minimal-intensity projection shows an inferior vena cava filter in the right ventricle. B, On angiography, a bilateral pulmonary artery filling defect is consistent with a saddle pulmonary embolism.

Multiple Choice (choose the best answer)

11.1. What is the only indication for placement of an IVCF that is agreed upon by all societal guidelines?
   a. Acute venothromboembolic disease in a patient who cannot receive anticoagulant therapy
   b. Anticoagulation failure
   c. Massive PE with evidence of thrombosis in a lower extremity
   d. Prophylaxis in high-risk populations
   e. Postoperative patients at high risk for VTE

11.2. When placed in appropriate patients, IVCFs can decrease the risk of which of the following?
   a. DVT
   b. Mortality
   c. PE
   d. Symptomatic PE
   e. Thrombophlebitis

11.3. What is the most common device-related complication of an IVCF?
   a. Filter embolization
   b. Filter fracture
   c. Occlusion of the IVCF
   d. Recurrent PE
   e. No known complications exist

11.4. In what clinical setting should mechanical clot evacuation be considered?
   a. Mechanical clot evacuation should never be considered
   b. Submassive PE in an adult with chronic debilitation
   c. Massive PE without active bleeding or a high risk for bleeding
   d. Massive PE with active bleeding or a high risk for bleeding
   e. Low-risk PE

11.5. In what clinical setting is systemic thrombolysis the treatment of choice?
   a. Massive PE without active bleeding or a high risk for bleeding
   b. Massive PE with massive, uncontrolled bleeding
   c. Submassive PE in a patient on postoperative day 2 after repair of a ruptured abdominal aortic aneurysm
   d. Submassive PE in a patient after recent intracranial surgery for cortical abscess
   e. Low-risk PE

Case Follow-up and Outcome

The patient underwent emergent sternotomy with thromboembolectomy and retrieval of the embolized IVCF. Another IVCF was placed intraoperatively because he continued to have a high risk for bleeding. Acute kidney failure developed postoperatively and required renal replacement therapy for several days. Otherwise, the postoperative course was uncomplicated. The patient made a complete recovery and was discharged to independent living.

Discussion

IVCFs were developed in 1967 as a mechanism to prevent PE in patients with DVT. Since that time, the reasons for IVCF placement have evolved. Currently, IVCFs are placed in patients for acute thromboembolic disease with active bleeding or a high risk for bleeding, anticoagulation failure, massive or submassive PE with ongoing DVT in a lower extremity, prophylaxis (in patients at high risk for PE), mobile thrombus, or ileocaval DVT (1-5). Societal guidelines support the use of IVCFs for acute thromboembolic disease in a patient who cannot receive anticoagulant therapy (1-5), and many support the use of IVCFs if anticoagulation has failed (3-5). The data supporting IVCF placement, however, are limited. Only 2 randomized trials have evaluated the efficacy of IVCFs. Both studies examined the use of anticoagulation compared to IVCF in combination with anticoagulation in patients with acute venothromboembolic disease (6,7). Both studies showed a reduction in PE with IVCF placement compared with anticoagulation alone; however, neither study showed an improvement in mortality with IVCF placement (6-8). Data for other indications of IVCF placement are limited to retrospective studies and expert opinion.

Although complication rates with IVCFs are relatively low, the complications can be severe. The most common postprocedural IVCF complications are DVT and caval thrombosis (9). Filter fracture and inferior vena cava perforation are uncommon and are usually of no clinical consequence (9). Embolization of an IVCF to an intracardiac location occurs in less than 1% of all IVCF placements but can lead to cardiac arrhythmias and sudden death (10). Intracardiac embolization occurs most often at device deployment as an intraprocedural deployment malfunction. Less frequently, IVCFs embolize after the procedure, and the usual cause is an enlarged vena cava ("mega cava"), filter fracture, or mobilization of the filter with a surrounding clot (10). When IVCFs embolize, treatment is endovascular or surgical retrieval of the embolized filter (10).

For massive PE, catheter-directed or systemic thrombolysis is indicated (1). Catheter-directed thrombolysis, systemic thrombolysis, or embolectomy can also be considered in otherwise healthy patients with submassive PE to prevent chronic thromboembolic pulmonary hypertension (1,4). When a massive PE results in sudden cardiac arrest, systemic thrombolysis is indicated unless contraindications exist. The 2016 American College of Chest Physicians guidelines for venous thromboembolic disease list structural intracranial disease, previous intracranial hemorrhage, ischemic stroke within 3 months, active bleeding, recent neurosurgery, and recent head trauma with brain injury as major contraindications for systemic or catheter-directed thrombolytic therapy (1).

Embolectomy or clot evacuation may be indicated in a patient with a massive PE when systemic or catheter-directed thrombolysis is otherwise contraindicated (1).

Summary

IVCFs are indicated in patients with acute venothrombembolic disease and in patients with active bleeding or a high risk for bleeding. Complications associated with IVCFs are rare but can be associated with morbidity and mortality. Massive PE requires treatment with systemic or catheter-directed thrombolysis or mechanical clot evacuation.

Answers

11.1. Answer a.

Acute venothromboembolic disease in a patient who cannot receive anticoagulant therapy is the only indication for IVCF placement that is agreed upon by all societal guidelines. IVCF can be considered in patients who have massive PE with evidence of lower extremity DVT, but this is controversial. Anticoagulation failure and prophylaxis are not indications for IVCF placement. Additional information is available in the medical literature (1-5).

11.2. Answer c.

An IVCF reduces the risk of PE but may increase the risk of DVT because of slowed venous return from the extremities due to partial occlusion of the inferior vena cava (IVC) by the IVCF. Another reason for increased risk of DVT is that the thrombogenic effects of the filter in the IVC can result in IVC thrombus formation. An IVCF does not reduce mortality or the rate of symptomatic PE. Additional information is available in the medical literature (6-8).

11.3. Answer c.

Occlusion of the IVCF due to clot extension or thrombus formation is the most common complication. For this reason, anticoagulation should be initiated as soon as possible. In addition, the IVCF should be removed when it is no longer required. Filter embolization is a very rare complication of an IVCF. While filter fracture occurs more frequently, it is still a rare complication. Additional information is available in the medical literature (9).

11.4. Answer d.

Thrombolysis is the favored treatment for massive PE, but mechanical clot evacuation is required in patients who have active bleeding or a high risk for bleeding. Mechanical clot evacuation or thrombolysis can be considered for otherwise healthy patients with submassive PE but not for chronically debilitated patients with submassive PE. Additional information is available in the medical literature (1).

11.5. Answer a.

Systemic thrombolysis is the treatment of choice for massive PE unless the patient has active bleeding or a high risk for bleeding. Systemic thrombolysis should not be considered in patients who have active bleeding or a high risk for bleeding. Thrombolysis is not used in patients with low-risk PE. Additional information is available in the medical literature (1).

References

1. Kearon C, Akl EA, Ornelas J, Blaivas A, Jimenez D, Bounameaux H, et al. Antithrombotic therapy for VTE disease: CHEST Guideline and Expert Panel Report [published correction appears in Chest. 2016 Oct;150(4):988]. Chest. 2016;149(2):315–52.
2. Kearon C, Akl EA, Comerota AJ, Prandoni P, Bounameaux H, Goldhaber SZ, et al. Antithrombotic therapy for VTE disease: Antithrombotic therapy and prevention of thrombosis, 9th ed: American College of Chest Physicians Evidence-Based Clinical Practice Guidelines [published correction appears in Chest. 2012 Dec;142(6):1698-704]. Chest. 2012;141(2 Suppl):e419S–96S.
3. Kaufman JA, Kinney TB, Streiff MB, Sing RF, Proctor MC, Becker D, et al. Guidelines for the use of retrievable and convertible vena cava filters: report from the Society of Interventional Radiology multidisciplinary consensus conference. Surg Obes Relat Dis. 2006;2(2):200–12.
4. Jaff MR, McMurtry MS, Archer SL, Cushman M, Goldenberg N, Goldhaber SZ, et al, American Heart Association Council on Cardiopulmonary, Critical Care, Perioperative and Resuscitation; American Heart Association Council on Peripheral Vascular Disease; American Heart Association Council on Arteriosclerosis, Thrombosis and Vascular Biology. Management of massive and submassive pulmonary embolism, iliofemoral deep vein thrombosis, and chronic thromboembolic pulmonary hypertension: a scientific statement from the American Heart Association [published correction appears in Circulation. 2012 Aug 14;126(7):e104] [published correction appears in Circulation. 2012 Mar 20;125(11):e495]. Circulation. 2011;123(16):1788–830.
5. Caplin DM, Nikolic B, Kalva SP, Ganguli S, Saad WEA, Zuckerman DA, Society of Interventional Radiology Standards of Practice Committee. Quality improvement guidelines for the performance of inferior vena cava filter placement for the prevention of pulmonary embolism. J Vasc Interv Radiol. 2011;22(11):1499–506.
6. Mismetti P, Laporte S, Pellerin O, Ennezat P-V, Couturaud F, Elias A, et al, PREPIC2 Study Group. Effect of a retrievable inferior vena cava filter plus anticoagulation vs anticoagulation alone on risk of recurrent pulmonary embolism: a randomized clinical trial. JAMA. 2015;313(16):1627–35.
7. Decousus H, Leizorovicz A, Parent F, Page Y, Tardy B, Girard P, et al. A clinical trial of vena caval filters in the prevention of pulmonary embolism in patients with proximal deep-vein thrombosis. Prévention du Risque d'Embolie Pulmonaire par Interruption Cave Study Group. N Engl J Med. 1998;338(7):409–15.
8. PREPIC Study Group. Eight-year follow-up of patients with permanent vena cava filters in the prevention of pulmonary embolism: the PREPIC (Prevention du Risque d'Embolie Pulmonaire par Interruption Cave) randomized study. Circulation. 2005;112(3):416–22.
9. Van Ha TG. Complications of inferior vena caval filters. Semin Intervent Radiol. 2006;23(2):150–5.
10. Owens CA, Bui JT, Knuttinen MG, Gaba RC, Carrillo TC, Hoefling N, et al. Intracardiac migration of inferior vena cava filters: review of published data. Chest. 2009;136(3):877–87.

A 74-Year-Old Man With Shortness of Breath, Cough, Rigors, and Malaise

12

Gautam Raju Mehta, MBBS, and Craig E. Daniels, MD

Case Presentation

A 74-year-old man with a previous 75-pack-year smoking history and moderate chronic obstructive pulmonary disease (forced expiratory volume in the first second of expiration, 1.48 L; 50% predicted with reversible component) presented at the hospital with shortness of breath. His symptoms included productive cough, rigors, and malaise. He was recently hospitalized for community-acquired pneumonia and type 2 non–ST-segment elevation myocardial infarction and discharged with a short course of oral antibiotics. Two days later he returned with worsening symptoms, and he was admitted to the medical unit for supplemental oxygen therapy, bronchodilators, and intravenous antibiotics. Further medical history included coronary artery disease, chronic congestive heart failure with a decreased ejection fraction of 34%, deep vein thrombosis while he was receiving warfarin, and squamous cell carcinoma of the left lung (treated with left upper lobe resection and locoregional radiotherapy).

On chest radiography the patient had diffuse interstitial and airspace opacities throughout the right lung that had progressed since his previous admission. Transthoracic echocardiography, performed to further evaluate the cause of the patient's dyspnea, showed that overall left ventricular function was stable compared with previous echocardiographic results; however, a new finding was a 3×1.5-cm apical left ventricular thrombus. The patient continued use of warfarin,

and, with antibiotic treatment, the international normalized ratio (INR) ranged from therapeutic to supratherapeutic throughout his hospital stay.

Acute respiratory failure developed, however, and was accompanied by large-volume hemoptysis and increased oxygen requirements. The patient was subsequently transferred to the medical intensive care unit for further care. After a brief trial of noninvasive positive pressure ventilation, he was intubated and given mechanical ventilation.

Physical examination findings were blood pressure 104/66 mm Hg, heart rate 104 beats/min, respiratory rate 18 breaths/min, and oxygen saturation as measured by pulse oximetry of 91% at 80% fraction of inspired oxygen. Breath sounds were diminished bilaterally, with scattered end-expiratory wheezes and no crackles. Laboratory test results showed that hemoglobin had decreased from 13.4 g/dL to 11.0 g/dL and the INR was 4.8. The lactate level was normal. The INR decreased with parenteral vitamin K administration. Given the concern for active bronchial bleeding and the history of lung malignancy, emergent bronchoscopy was performed. The right tracheobronchial tree had a large amount of bloody secretions with no active source of bleeding, and the left upper lobe had a visible and intact upper lobectomy staple line. The left lower lobe was difficult to enter because of architectural distortion, but there was no evidence of bleeding.

Chest radiography was performed later that evening because oxygen saturation had worsened and peak airway pressures were elevated. Radiography showed complete collapse of the left lower lobe with a leftward mediastinal shift. Urgent bronchoscopy showed a large, obstructing clot in the left mainstem bronchus emanating from the left lower lobe bronchus. The clot was removed with a cryotherapy probe, but bleeding continued at the site despite multiple instillations of cold saline lavage. Topical epinephrine was not used because of the patient's recent history of active coronary artery disease and the concern for increased myocardial oxygen demand or arrhythmia. Instead, tranexamic acid (TXA) was instilled twice in aliquots of 500 mg mixed with 20 mL of saline, and the bleeding eventually abated.

Questions

Multiple Choice (choose the best answer)

12.1. In relatively affluent countries, hemoptysis is most commonly caused by bronchitis, bronchogenic carcinoma, or bronchiectasis. Conversely, which of the following is the most common cause of hemoptysis in low-income countries?
   a. Trauma
   b. *Mycobacterium tuberculosis*
   c. Bronchogenic carcinoma
   d. Cystic fibrosis
   e. Pulmonary embolism

12.2. To clinically stabilize a patient who has massive hemoptysis, which of the following should *not* be performed initially?
   a. Secure the airway with an endotracheal tube
   b. Position the patient so that the presumed bleeding lung is in the dependent position
   c. Attempt bronchoscopy
   d. Reverse any suspected coagulopathy
   e. Check the serum hemoglobin level and administer a transfusion if necessary

12.3. A 65-year-old man with a history of coronary artery disease and supraventricular tachycarida presents with hemoptysis of unknown origin. Which endobronchial therapy should be used with caution?
   a. Epinephrine
   b. Vasopressin
   c. Cold saline
   d. TXA
   e. Naloxone

12.4. A 44-year-old patient has massive hemoptysis that is presumed to be secondary to a large mass in the left lung. Which of the following may be protective?
   a. Placement of an endotracheal tube 3 to 5 cm above the carina
   b. Selective left mainstem bronchus intubation
   c. Selective right mainstem bronchus intubation
   d. Emergent cricothyroidotomy
   e. Urgent radiotherapy

12.5. TXA is useful in controlling bleeding by which of the following mechanisms?
   a. Preventing fibrinolysis by inhibiting plasmin formation
   b. Activating platelets
   c. Augmenting vitamin K activity
   d. Increasing factor X activity
   e. Replacing coagulation factors

After the bleeding abated, the patient had no further episodes of hemoptysis, and chest imaging showed gradual improvement of the left-sided opacification with improved oxygenation and ventilation. When bronchoscopy was performed 24 hours later, there was no active bleeding and only a trace of residual nonobstructing clot. Subsequently, systemic anticoagulation was reintroduced cautiously because of the known intraventricular thrombus.

Discussion

Massive hemoptysis is a medical emergency requiring urgent identification of the cause and prompt intervention. There are many causes of hemoptysis, and the differential diagnosis includes disorders directly related to airway diseases, pulmonary parenchymal diseases, vascular disorders, coagulopathies, iatrogenic causes, and various adverse effects of drugs. *Massive hemoptysis*, commonly described as more than 500 mL of blood expectorated over 24 hours, is most often associated with bronchiectasis, bronchogenic carcinoma, tuberculosis, and iatrogenic causes (1,2).

The source of bleeding in massive hemoptysis is frequently identified with bronchoscopy, which should be performed early in the evaluation (3). In a 2001 study, the site of bleeding was identified through bronchoscopy in 26 of 28 patients (92.9%) (4).

Early management of massive hemoptysis involves positioning the patient so that the suspected bleeding lung is down (to protect the nonbleeding lung from spillage of blood) and selectively intubating the nonbleeding lung. Bronchoscopic interventions may include placement of a balloon tamponade with a Fogarty catheter or an Arndt endobronchial blocker as a temporizing measure. Topical therapy may be a useful adjunct.

The source of bleeding can be lavaged directly with iced saline in 50-mL aliquots. Iced saline is thought to act through local vasoconstriction, hemostasis, and reduction of blood flow (2). Other topical treatments may include the use of endobronchially administered epinephrine or vasopressin. Systemic effects of endobronchial epinephrine are well-known but unpredictable. Cardiac dysrhythmias have occurred in addition to blood pressure variations (5). Epinephrine administration should be used with caution in patients who are elderly or who have underlying arrhythmias and coronary artery disease because of the risk of coronary vasospasm, increased myocardial oxygen demand, and worsening dysrhythmias (5). Potentially fatal ventricular fibrillation has occurred in patients with no underlying risk factors after the use of endobronchial epinephrine (6).

TXA is a synthetic amino acid derivative that reversibly binds to plasminogen and prevents plasmin formation, which results in the inhibition of fibrinolysis. Systemic TXA is commonly used to control bleeding during surgery and in cardiopulmonary bypass procedures. Endobronchial instillation of TXA to control pulmonary bleeding has not been widely adopted. A 2010 prospective study evaluated the effect of TXA on pulmonary bleeding in 48 patients who did not respond to the traditional use of cold saline lavage or endobronchial epinephrine (7). In 39 of those 48 patients (81%), TXA successfully controlled bleeding without additional adverse events (7). Another randomized control trial, which included 50 patients, evaluated the effectiveness of epinephrine compared with TXA in controlling bronchial bleeding that did not initially respond to cold saline lavage; between the 2 groups there was no significant difference in the ability to control bleeding or the time to control bleeding (8). In a 2018 study of patients admitted with nonmassive hemoptysis, 47 patients were randomly assigned to receive nebulized TXA instead of saline; the patients who received TXA had a smaller volume of expectorated blood, earlier resolution of hemoptysis, shorter length of stay, and fewer requirements for invasive procedures (9). Other endoscopic interventions may include laser therapy, electrocautery, argon plasma coagulation, or cryotherapy. Arteriographic embolization is sometimes necessary, and surgery is rarely performed.

Summary

Hemoptysis is a commonly encountered symptom in patients needing intensive care. Life-threatening hemoptysis is a medical emergency requiring prompt evaluation and treatment. Bronchoscopy is both diagnostic and therapeutic in many patients. Traditionally, cold saline lavage is attempted first to control bleeding. Epinephrine is also commonly used for its local vasoconstrictive effects, yet its use carries the risk of cardiac dysrhythmias and hemodynamic instability. TXA is an antifibrinolytic agent that has been shown to be effective in controlling pulmonary bleeding when administered by the endobronchial route. Its use should be considered especially in patients with cardiac instability who have ongoing pulmonary bleeding. Laser therapy, electrocautery, argon plasma coagulation, or cryotherapy may be needed. Arteriographic embolization is sometimes necessary, and surgery is rarely performed.

12.1. Answer b.

In retrospective analyses of the underlying causes of hemoptysis in patients undergoing diagnostic bronchoscopy in the US, the most common causes were bronchitis, bronchogenic carcinoma, and bronchiectasis. In contrast, similar studies performed in Southeast Asia found that pulmonary infection with *Mycobacterium tuberculosis* was overwhelmingly the leading cause of hemoptysis (accounting for >75% of cases in 1 study). Additional information is available in the medical literature (1,10).

12.2. Answer e.

Initial management of a patient with massive hemoptysis should focus on stabilization of the airway, breathing, and circulation. This may involve securing the airway with an endotracheal tube. The nonbleeding lung may be protected by turning the patient so the bleeding side is down. Knowledge of the patient's clinical status, medications (including anticoagulant or antiplatelet agents), and the presence of thrombocytopenia or uremia may aid in determining whether rapid reversal of a suspected coagulopathy is warranted. Flexible bronchoscopy may be used for clearing the airway of blood products to ensure adequate oxygenation and ventilation and for localizing the source of bleeding to administer endobronchial therapies. Further laboratory evaluation should be considered, but it is not the first priority. Additional information is available in the medical literature (11).

12.3. Answer a.

Epinephrine, a vasopressor that acts on α_1-adrenergic receptors and causes vasoconstriction, has been useful when administered endobronchially in patients who have hemoptysis. However, because epinephrine also acts on β_1 and β_2 receptors, it may induce inotropic and chronotropic effects and thereby increase myocardial oxygen demand, which may precipitate cardiac ischemia or induce arrhythmias in a patient with a history of cardiac disease. Vasopressin, cold saline, and TXA all have utility in hemoptysis without the potential adverse effects of epinephrine. Additional information is available in the medical literature (6).

12.4. Answer c.

In this patient who has massive hemoptysis, and given that the source of bleeding is likely secondary to a large mass in the left lung, selective right mainstem intubation may be protective. In a patient with uncontrolled bleeding, selective intubation of the nonbleeding lung with a single-lumen endotracheal tube may be performed quickly and easily. Even though single-lung ventilation will not allow for immediate intervention, oxygenation and ventilation may be maintained. Double-lumen endotracheal intubation is also possible; however, placement requires experience, bronchoscopic confirmation, and often more time. Selective placement of the endotracheal tube in the left lung would impair oxygenation and ventilation in the nonbleeding lung. Cricothyroidotomy would not be indicated at this time unless a definitive airway cannot be established. Urgent radiotherapy would not be indicated for a patient who has active hemorrhage and a risk of decompensation. Additional information is available in the medical literature (11).

12.5. Answer a.

TXA, a derivative of lysine, inhibits fibrinolysis by inhibiting the formation of plasmin from plasminogen. TXA does not activate platelets, augment vitamin K activity, increase factor X activity, or replace depleted coagulation factors. Additional information is available in the medical literature (7).

References

1. Hirshberg B, Biran I, Glazer M, Kramer MR. Hemoptysis: etiology, evaluation, and outcome in a tertiary referral hospital. Chest. 1997;112(2):440–4.
2. Cahill BC, Ingbar DH. Massive hemoptysis: assessment and management. Clin Chest Med. 1994;15(1):147–67.
3. Sakr L, Dutau H. Massive hemoptysis: an update on the role of bronchoscopy in diagnosis and management. Respiration. 2010;80(1):38–58.
4. Hsiao EI, Kirsch CM, Kagawa FT, Wehner JH, Jensen WA, Baxter RB. Utility of fiberoptic bronchoscopy before bronchial artery embolization for massive hemoptysis. AJR Am J Roentgenol. 2001;177(4):861–7.
5. Khoo KL, Lee P, Mehta AC. Endobronchial epinephrine: confusion is in the air. Am J Respir Crit Care Med. 2013;187(10):1137–8.
6. Steinfort DP, Herth FJ, Eberhardt R, Irving LB. Potentially fatal arrhythmia complicating endobronchial epinephrine for control of iatrogenic bleeding. Am J Respir Crit Care Med. 2012;185(9):1028–30.
7. Marquez-Martin E, Vergara DG, Martin-Juan J, Flacon AR, Lopez-Campos JL, Rodriguez-Panadero F. Endobronchial administration of tranexamic acid for controlling pulmonary bleeding: a pilot study. J Bronchology Interv Pulmonol. 2010;17(2):122–5.
8. Fekri MS, Hashemi-Bajgani SM, Shafahi A, Zarshenas R. Comparing adrenaline with tranexamic acid to control acute endobronchial bleeding: a randomized controlled trial. Iran J Med Sci. 2017;42(2):129–35.
9. Wand O, Guber E, Guber A, Epstein Shochet G, Israeli-Shani L, Shitrit D. Inhaled tranexamic acid for hemoptysis treatment: a randomized controlled trial. Chest. 2018;154(6):1379–84.
10. Prasad R, Garg R, Singhal S, Srivastava P. Lessons from patients with hemoptysis attending a chest clinic in India. Ann Thorac Med. 2009 Jan;4(1):10–2.
11. Radchenko C, Alraiyes AH, Shojaee S. A systematic approach to the management of massive hemoptysis. J Thorac Dis. 2017 Sep;9(Suppl 10):S1069–86.

A 63-Year-Old Woman With Back Pain, Weakness, Tachycardia, and Hypertension

Catarina N. Aragon Pinto and Alice Gallo de Moraes, MD

Case Presentation

A 63-year-old woman presented with a 2-day history of low back pain and generalized weakness. The weakness rapidly progressed until she could not walk independently. She reported no fever, paresthesias, shortness of breath, chest pain, dysuria, fecal or urinary incontinence, or recent infection. Her past medical history included ulcerative colitis and colectomy, rheumatoid arthritis, biliary neoplasm, and prior hepaticojejunostomy with secondary complications of malnutrition while receiving total parenteral nutrition. She reported no use of tobacco, recreational drugs, or alcohol and no recent travel. Her current medications included low-dose aspirin, duloxetine, zolpidem, bupropion, aripiprazole, and atorvastatin.

On admission, the patient had tachycardia (heart rate, 110-140 beats/min) and hypertension (systolic pressure, 170-180 mm Hg; diastolic pressure, 100-110 mm Hg). Electrocardiography showed sinus tachycardia. Chest radiography showed bilateral basilar atelectasis. Computed tomography of the head was negative for an acute intracranial abnormality. After the patient had been admitted, and during a physical therapy session, she had labored breathing and gurgles, so suction was attempted. After having cardiac arrest

with pulseless electrical activity, she underwent 5 rounds of cardiopulmonary resuscitation and received 3 mg intravenous epinephrine before spontaneous circulation returned. She was intubated and transferred to the medical intensive care unit. Computed tomographic angiography of the chest was negative for pulmonary embolism but did show acute rib fractures.

Without sedation and with normal oxygenation, the patient followed commands and was temporarily extubated, but bradycardia developed (heart rate, 49 beats/min) with apnea that required bag mask ventilation. Before she was intubated again, she could not lift her extremities or her head from the bed. During a neurologic consultation and examination, she had diffuse flaccid quadriparesis with absent reflexes in the lower extremities and normal reflexes in the upper extremities. Sensation was normal. Results from nerve conduction studies (NCS) and electromyography (EMG) were consistent with an early demyelinating polyradiculoneuropathy. Cerebrospinal fluid (CSF) analysis confirmed albuminocytologic dissociation with less than 1 cell/μL and protein 62 mg/dL (reference range, 0-35 mg/dL). CSF glucose was normal. Findings from magnetic resonance imaging of the cervical spine were unremarkable.

Questions

Multiple Choice (choose the best answer)

13.1. Of the differential diagnosis for acute flaccid paralysis, which of the following is most frequently associated with respiratory failure?
    a. Botulism
    b. Guillain-Barré syndrome (GBS)
    c. Transverse myelitis
    d. Myositis
    e. Myasthenia gravis

3.2. Which of the following statements is correct for the diagnosis of this patient's condition?
    a. NCS and EMG are required for the diagnosis
    b. Respiratory failure develops in approximately one-third of patients
    c. Virtually all patients have a precipitating factor
    d. Albuminocytologic dissociation is specific for this condition
    e. Creatine kinase is always elevated

13.3. Which of the following would rule out this patient's condition?
    a. Normal muscle stretch reflexes
    b. Normal CSF protein level
    c. Unilateral weakness
    d. Abnormal mental status
    e. Ophthalmoplegia

13.4. What treatments are currently available for this condition?
    a. Corticosteroids and intravenous immunoglobulin (IVIG)
    b. IVIG and plasma exchange
    c. Corticosteroids and plasma exchange
    d. Rituximab and IVIG
    e. Rituximab and corticosteroids

13.5. Which respiratory parameters are indications for elective intubation in this condition?
    a. Forced vital capacity (FVC), 15 mL/kg; maximum inspiratory pressure, 20 cm H_2O; maximum expiratory pressure, 30 cm H_2O
    b. FVC, 30 mL/kg; maximum inspiratory pressure, 40 cm H_2O; maximum expiratory pressure, 50 cm H_2O
    c. Weak cough and tachypnea
    d. Dysphagia and tachypnea
    e. Generalized weakness

Case Follow-up and Outcome

A diagnosis of GBS was made. The patient began receiving IVIG 2 g/kg divided over 5 days. After completion of the immunotherapy trial, her maximum inspiratory pressure was 30 cm H_2O and vital capacity was more than 20 mL/kg. After an uneventful T-piece trial, extubation proceeded successfully. Length of stay was 11 days in the intensive care unit (total hospital stay, 17 days). At discharge, the patient was walking with the assistance of a walker.

Discussion

The differential diagnosis for acute flaccid paralysis is broad and includes myopathies, myasthenic syndromes, acute transverse myelitis, and peripheral neuropathies. Myopathies rarely present in an acute fashion, and the patient's creatine kinase was normal. A myasthenic syndrome is unlikely because the patient did not have eyelid ptosis, dysphagia, dysarthria, or dysphonia. A transverse myelitis is ruled out because of the absence of sphincter dysfunction or a sensory level and because findings on magnetic resonance imaging of the cervical spine were unremarkable. The ascending paralysis with respiratory failure and absent reflexes in the lower extremities are typical of GBS, but the presence of muscle stretch reflexes in the upper extremities was quite unusual for this condition. The use of NCS with EMG is the gold standard test for the diagnosis of a neuromuscular disorder, and it confirmed the clinical suspicion for this particular patient. NCS and EMG are not required for the diagnosis of GBS, which is essentially clinical. However, NCS and EMG can be used to help determine whether the patient has a classic demyelinating GBS (acute inflammatory demyelinating polyradiculoneuropathy) or axonal GBS (acute motor and sensory axonal polyradiculoneuropathy). Patients with the axonal variant tend to need more time for recovery. CSF analysis can support the diagnosis and show the classic albuminocytologic dissociation (elevated CSF protein with normal cellularity), which occurs in approximately 60% of patients at 1 week after symptom onset and in 90% of patients at 3 weeks. CSF cell counts rarely exceed 10/μL and very rarely exceed 50/μL (1,2).

GBS is the most common cause of acute flaccid paralysis. Its worldwide overall incidence is 1 to 2 cases per 100,000 per year. It usually starts in the lower extremities and ascends to the upper extremities, causing proximal and distal weakness. It affects cranial nerves, especially the facial nerves, in approximately 50% of patients and can cause respiratory failure necessitating ventilatory support in 30% of patients. Half the patients, like our patient, present with acute low back pain due to nerve root inflammation. By definition, symptoms are the worst in less than 4 weeks after their onset, and for most patients, symptoms are the worst within the first 2 weeks. Two-thirds of patients have a precipitating factor such as a gastrointestinal tract infection, upper respiratory viral syndrome, vaccination, or surgery. GBS is a symmetric polyradiculoneuropathy, so if a patient has overtly asymmetric or unilateral findings, another diagnosis should be considered (3). All patients with GBS should be hospitalized for respiratory and cardiac monitoring. As with the patient described above, neuromuscular respiratory failure can occur suddenly, and arterial blood gas analysis and pulse oximetry are not sensitive for the prediction of respiratory failure in these patients. Measurement of respiratory pressures and FVC should be done regularly. If FVC is less than 20 mL/kg, maximum inspiratory pressure is less than 30 cm H_2O, or maximum expiratory pressure is less than 40 cm H_2O, elective endotracheal intubation should be performed. This is the 20/30/40 rule for neuromuscular respiratory failure (4,5).

In the patient described above, the early cardiac arrest and subsequent bradycardia after return to spontaneous circulation were likely due to dysautonomia, which occurs in approximately 70% of patients with GBS. The most common dysautonomic features in GBS are diarrhea or constipation (15.5%), syndrome of inappropriate antidiuretic hormone secretion (4.8%), and bradycardia (4.7%). Recognition of severe autonomic dysfunction is important because it is occasionally associated with sudden death. Labile blood pressure (mean change in arterial pressure >50 mm Hg from baseline) occurs in up to 25% of patients with GBS and tends to occur in more severe cases (6). Acute weakness in combination with dysautonomia strongly suggests the diagnosis of GBS.

A patient who cannot walk 10 m without assistance should be treated with immunotherapy. The only GBS treatments that are approved by the US Food and Drug Administration are IVIG and plasma exchange. Neither affects patient survival, but they hasten recovery. The recommended dosage for IVIG is 2 g/kg divided over 5 consecutive days. Complications from this therapy are rare, but the most common are headache and a flulike syndrome. Deep vein thrombosis and acute kidney dysfunction are also associated with this therapy, so prophylaxis with low-molecular-weight heparin and avoidance of dehydration are highly recommended. Plasma exchange is recommended for 4 to 6 times, usually every other day, for the treatment of GBS. Compared with IVIG, plasma exchange has more potential adverse effects and complications because it usually requires central line placement, it increases the risk of infection, and it is challenging to use in patients who have hemodynamic instability. Both treatments are equally efficacious.

Corticosteroids can worsen the prognosis, so their use should be avoided. Supportive care is extremely important because 30% of patients need ventilator support, and dysautonomia is common in these patients. Prophylaxis for deep vein thrombosis, bladder and bowel care, physical and occupational therapy, and psychological support are essential (1,2,5).

Summary

GBS is the most common cause of acute flaccid paralysis. Attention should be given to neuromuscular respiratory failure and arrhythmias. Regular measurement of respiratory pressures and FVC and continuous cardiac monitoring are lifesaving for patients with GBS. IVIG and plasma exchange are the currently available immunotherapies. However, pharmacologic treatment does not improve survival, and supportive therapy is extremely important in the care of these patients.

Answers

13.1. Answer b.

GBS is the acute flaccid paralysis most often associated with respiratory compromise. Botulism is a rare cause, and transverse myelitis and myositis rarely cause respiratory failure. Patients with myasthenia gravis usually present with ocular and bulbar weakness and normal tendon reflexes. Additional information is available in the medical literature (4).

13.2. Answer b.

GBS causes respiratory failure in approximately one-third of patients. NCS and EMG are not mandatory for the diagnosis, but the results of those studies support the diagnosis. Two-thirds of patients have a precipitating factor, which is usually an upper respiratory infection or diarrhea. Although albuminocytologic dissociation occurs in up to 90% of patients by the third week after onset of symptoms, it is not specific for GBS and can occur in patients with type 2 diabetes, lumbar spinal stenosis, or other immune-mediated neuropathies. The creatine kinase level is usually normal in GBS. Additional information is available in the medical literature (1).

13.3. Answer c.

Unilateral weakness does not occur in GBS and rules out its diagnosis. GBS usually presents as a rapidly ascending symmetric weakness with areflexia and elevated CSF protein. However, rarely patients do have normal reflexes or CSF protein levels. A variant called Bickerstaff brainstem encephalitis causes altered mental status, ataxia, and external ophthalmoplegia. Additional information is available in the medical literature (2,3).

13.4. Answer b.

Only IVIG and plasma exchange are approved by the US Food and Drug Administration for the treatment of GBS. Corticosteroids may worsen outcomes. Additional information is available in the medical literature (2).

13.5. Answer a.

Patients with GBS can have respiratory failure, so monitoring their respiratory status regularly with FVC and respiratory pressures is extremely important in their care. Patients should undergo elective endotracheal intubation if FVC is less than 20 mL/kg, maximum inspiratory pressure is greater than 30 cm H_2O, or maximum expiratory pressure is less than 40 cm H_2O. Clinical findings do not accurately predict the risk of respiratory failure. Additional information is available in the medical literature (4).

References

1. Donofrio PD. Guillain-Barré syndrome. Continuum (Minneap Minn). 2017;23(5, Peripheral Nerve and Motor Neuron Disorders):1295–1309.
2. Wijdicks EF, Klein CJ. Guillain-Barré syndrome. Mayo Clin Proc. 2017;92(3):467–79.
3. Hughes RA, Cornblath DR. Guillain-Barré syndrome. Lancet. 2005;366(9497):1653–66.
4. Rabinstein AA. Acute neuromuscular respiratory failure. Continuum (Minneap Minn). 2015;21(5 Neurocritical Care):1324–45.
5. Willison HJ, Jacobs BC, van Doorn PA. Guillain-Barré syndrome. Lancet. 2016;388(10045):717–27.
6. Anandan C, Khuder SA, Koffman BM. Prevalence of autonomic dysfunction in hospitalized patients with Guillain-Barré syndrome. Muscle Nerve. 2017; 56(2):331–3.

Diffuse Parenchymal Lung Disease

A 45-Year-Old Man With Worsening Dyspnea and Hypoxemia

Melissa K. Myers, MD, Mark E. Wylam, MD, and Muhammad A. Rishi, MBBS

Case Presentation

A 45-year-old man who had never smoked was transferred from another hospital with a 2-week history of worsening dyspnea and hypoxemia. His medical history included hypertension, obesity, and alcohol abuse. For the past year he has had chronic hypoxemia that began after an initial episode of respiratory failure with diffuse interstitial and alveolar infiltrates bilaterally. At that time, bronchoscopic and transbronchial biopsy findings were nondiagnostic. He was presumed to have hypersensitivity pneumonitis due to occupational exposure to organic dust in a furniture factory. Corticosteroids were prescribed, but his condition did not improve, and his respiratory symptoms gradually worsened.

An acute exacerbation of dyspnea prompted his current episode of care. At the referring hospital he had bilateral pulmonary infiltrates, and he was treated with levofloxacin and corticosteroids, but he showed no improvement. When transferred, he required supplemental oxygen (5 L/min by nasal cannula) to maintain oxygen saturation as measured by pulse oximetry (Spo_2) higher than 90%.

On physical examination he had tachypnea, increased work of breathing, and only a few crackles with good air movement. Laboratory evaluation showed polycythemia, a mildly elevated white blood cell count, a brain-type natriuretic peptide value of 461 pg/mL, and normal values for creatinine, sedimentation rate, and C-reactive protein. Procalcitonin was undetectable. A rheumatologic evaluation was also unremarkable with a normal level of serum creatine kinase and negative results for anti–cyclic citrullinated peptide antibodies, double-stranded DNA antibodies, and rheumatoid factor. Results of tuberculosis and HIV screening were negative.

Computed tomography (CT) of the chest (Figure 14.1) showed diffuse, patchy ground-glass opacities with interlobular septal thickening and consolidative opacities that were worse in the upper lobes and had progressed when compared to findings from 1 year before.

Figure 14.1   CT of the Chest

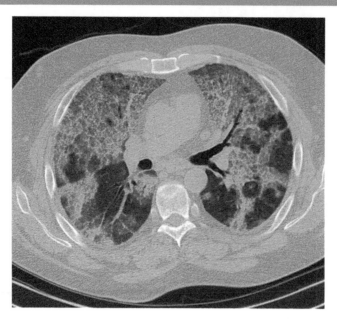

This image shows diffuse, patchy ground-glass opacities bilaterally in a geographic distribution with interlobular septal thickening and consolidative opacities.

Questions

Multiple Choice (choose the best answer)

14.1. What should be the next diagnostic test?
   a. Transbronchial biopsy
   b. Sputum culture
   c. Open lung biopsy
   d. Bronchoscopy with bronchoalveolar lavage (BAL)
   e. CT-guided biopsy

14.2. Which of the following is diagnostic of pulmonary alveolar proteinosis (PAP)?
   a. Predominant lymphocytosis on BAL
   b. Positive periodic acid–Schiff (PAS) staining on BAL
   c. Rapidly progressive dyspnea
   d. "Crazy-paving" pattern on CT
   e. Lipid-laden macrophages on BAL

14.3. What is the underlying pathophysiology of PAP?
   a. Chronic infection
   b. Exposure to an allergic trigger
   c. Accumulation of alveolar surfactant
   d. Gradually progressive fibrosis
   e. Drug-related pulmonary toxicity

14.4. What are the features of PAP on pulmonary function tests (PFTs)?
   a. Obstructive pulmonary physiology with impaired diffusing capacity
   b. Obstructive pulmonary physiology with normal diffusing capacity
   c. Restrictive pulmonary physiology with normal diffusing capacity
   d. Decreased diffusing capacity out of proportion to restrictive pulmonary physiology
   e. Mixed obstructive and restrictive pulmonary physiology pattern with normal diffusing capacity

14.5. What is the traditional standard treatment of patients with PAP who have functional limitation due to their respiratory status?
   a. Whole-lung lavage
   b. Systemic corticosteroid therapy
   c. Percussion therapy
   d. Pulmonary rehabilitation
   e. Inhaled corticosteroid therapy

Case Follow-up and Outcome

When bronchoscopy was performed, BAL showed progressively turbid, opaque, white fluid. PAS staining was positive and consistent with PAP. The patient underwent whole-lung lavage with 1-L aliquots of warm (37 °C) saline into each lung (right side, 11 L; left side, 12 L). His Spo_2 improved, but he still required supplemental oxygen (3 L/min by nasal cannula), so whole-lung lavage was performed a second time 6 days later (right side, 11 L; left side, 10 L). At hospital dismissal his Spo_2 with room air was normal. Serum anti–granulocyte-macrophage colony-stimulating factor (GM-CSF) antibodies were identified, and the patient was treated with inhaled GM-CSF. More than 1 year later he was asymptomatic, and his chest radiograph was normal.

Discussion

In adults PAP most often presents in the fourth or fifth decade (1). According to estimates from insurance claim databases, the US prevalence is 6.87 per million and is similar for males and females (2). Estimates for autoimmune PAP in Japan, by comparison, are an incidence of 1.65 per million and a prevalence of 26.6 per million (3). Although the incidence is higher among smokers, 90% of adult patients have an autoimmune origin due to acquired GM-CSF autoantibody (4).

Clinical presentations typically include insidious development of dyspnea with or without cough. Fatigue is common. Lung examination findings are often unremarkable, and patients have normal breath sounds. However, faint crackles and digital clubbing may be present (5). PFT results may be normal, but patients with more severe disease may have results consistent with restrictive lung disease and a diffusing capacity that is impaired out of proportion to the reduction in lung volume.

Interstitial infiltrates are seen on plain chest radiographs. Often the patients are treated for community-acquired pneumonia initially. CT of the chest shows ground-glass opacities in the lung parenchyma in combination with interlobular septal thickening, which is recognized as the crazy-paving pattern and helps to differentiate PAP from other interstitial pulmonary processes (6). The imaging differential diagnosis includes acute respiratory distress syndrome, pneumocystis pneumonia, atypical pulmonary edema, diffuse alveolar hemorrhage, organizing pneumonia, acute interstitial pneumonia, drug-induced pneumonitis, and lipoid pneumonia. In chronic disease, CT features of diffuse alveolar damage superimposed on usual interstitial pneumonia may also resemble the crazy-paving pattern (7). In general, a clinician needs a high level of awareness for PAP because the CT findings are compatible with many clinical syndromes.

Accumulation of alveolar surfactant due to reduced clearance or abnormal production of surfactant (congenital surfactant deficiency syndromes) elicits the clinical picture of PAP. Accumulation of lipoprotein-rich surfactant material in the air spaces impairs gas exchange and may eventually lead to the development of fibrosis.

Surfactant homeostasis is the net balance between production by type II pneumocytes and alveolar macrophage clearance. Macrophage activation is regulated in part by binding of GM-CSF to receptors on the macrophage (8). Autoimmune PAP due to GM-CSF autoantibody diminishes GM-CSF activity and therefore reduces macrophage activation (9). In secondary PAP, surfactant accumulation is caused by macrophage dysfunction due to overwhelming silica or metal dust exposure, hematopoietic stem cell transplant, or lung transplant (10,11). Congenital surfactant deficiency syndromes (ie, congenital PAP) typically present in childhood and are usually due to mutations in the genes coding for surfactant apoproteins B and C or the phospholipid transporter gene *ABCA3* (12). Surfactant protein B and ABCA3 are required for the normal organization and packaging of surfactant phospholipids into specialized secretory organelles, known as lamellar bodies, while surfactant proteins B and C are important for adsorption of secreted surfactant phospholipids to the alveolar surface. Of all patients in the US who have PAP, 91.5% have autoimmune PAP; 3%, hereditary PAP caused by GM-CSF receptor mutations; 4%, secondary PAP; and 1.5%, congenital PAP (2).

The diagnostic hallmark of PAP is the finding of PAS stain–positive material in BAL or lung biopsy specimens. PAS oxidizes adjacent hydroxyl groups (vicinal diols) on surfactant glycoproteins and glycolipids to aldehydes, which stain with Schiff reagent and give a purple color to the accumulated surfactant in the air space (13). During bronchoscopy, BAL may show progressively turbid white fluid, which creates sediment that settles in the container over time. This observational feature is highly suggestive of PAP but may not be obvious in less severe cases. PAS staining is not routinely performed on BAL specimens. Moreover, BAL specimens are unremarkable with relatively few inflammatory cells unless there is concomitant infection. Although fluid from BAL with PAS staining is usually sufficient for the diagnosis (5), if results are inconclusive, surgical lung biopsy is essentially 100% sensitive and specific (14). Electron microscopy on either BAL fluid or lung tissue can show abnormal lamellar body formation and is more specific than PAS staining (15).

Testing for serum anti–GM-CSF antibodies is highly sensitive and specific for autoimmune PAP but is not performed in all medical laboratories. Evaluation for secondary causes of PAP generally relies on a thorough clinical history and evaluation for hematologic abnormalities.

When adults present with PAP, genetic testing for mutations affecting surfactant is not typically warranted. Patients with PAP are at risk for concomitant superimposed infection such as nocardiosis, and evaluation should include bacterial, mycobacterial, and fungal cultures and testing for *Pneumocystis jiroveci*.

There are no distinct guidelines for the appropriate treatment of PAP. Whole-lung lavage, a mainstay of treatment, involves intubation with a double-lumen endotracheal tube and then sequential instillation of warm saline aliquots and drainage (16). The use of chest oscillation during whole-lung lavage may improve the yield (17). GM-CSF supplemental therapy may be inhaled or subcutaneously administered and appears to be effective in many patients (18,19). Alternatives include GM-CSF antibody–reducing strategies, such as the use of rituximab or plasmapheresis (or both), although robust data to support their efficacy are lacking.

Summary

PAP is caused by excess accumulation of surfactant within alveoli and results in a crazy-paving pattern on CT. PAP may be categorized as congenital, autoimmune (most commonly), or secondary. Diagnosis is made with positive PAS staining of BAL fluid, transbronchial biopsy, or surgical lung biopsy. Whole-lung lavage improves gas exchange immediately. Established alternatives are GM-CSF supplementation or GM-CSF antibody depletion.

Answers

14.1. Answer d.

Of the listed options, bronchoscopy with BAL is the least invasive procedure and is often sufficient for diagnosis. Transbronchial biopsy and CT-guided biopsy are reasonable diagnostic options, but they are more invasive than BAL, and their yield is subject to the degree of involvement of the biopsied tissue. Sputum culture is appropriate for the diagnosis of pulmonary infections but not PAP. If other methods are inconclusive, open lung biopsy is essentially 100% sensitive and specific. However, less invasive options should be considered first. Additional information is available in the medical literature (5,14).

14.2. Answer b.

Positive PAS staining on BAL or lung tissue is the diagnostic hallmark of PAP. Lymphocytosis is not typically present on BAL for patients with PAP and should prompt consideration of a superimposed infection or alternative diagnoses. Progressive dyspnea is a nonspecific symptom and typically develops insidiously in PAP. The "crazy-paving" pattern on CT of the chest is highly suggestive of PAP but is nonspecific and insufficient for diagnosis. Lipid-laden macrophages are not a characteristic of PAP and should prompt consideration of other causes of interstitial lung disease, including lipoid pneumonia. Additional information is available in the medical literature (6,7,13).

14.3. Answer c.

Accumulation of alveolar surfactant is the underlying cause of PAP. Chronic infection and exposure to allergic triggers are not involved in the development of PAP, but they are responsible for other interstitial pulmonary diseases. Gradually progressive fibrosis may occur in advanced PAP but does not describe the pathophysiology, and drug-related pulmonary toxicity is not the cause of PAP. Additional information is available in the medical literature (12).

14.4. Answer d.

PFT results may be normal in PAP, but as surfactant accumulates, diffusing capacity gradually becomes more impaired, and the surfactant burden and development of fibrosis may ultimately result in a restrictive pattern on PFTs. However, the diffusing capacity at this point in the disease is impaired out of proportion to the degree of restriction when compared with other restrictive lung diseases. PAP does not cause an obstructive pattern on PFT. Additional information is available in the medical literature (1,5).

14.5. Answer a.

Whole-lung lavage involves instillation of large volumes of saline into the lungs to effectively remove excess surfactant that has accumulated. Although percussion therapy may improve yield when performed during whole-lung lavage, it is not used independently in the treatment of PAP. Systemic corticosteroids, pulmonary rehabilitation, and inhaled corticosteroids have not been shown to provide benefit to patients with PAP. Additional information is available in the medical literature (16,17).

References

1. Prakash UB, Barham SS, Carpenter HA, Dines DE, Marsh HM. Pulmonary alveolar phospholipoproteinosis: experience with 34 cases and a review. Mayo Clin Proc. 1987;62(6):499–518.

2. McCarthy C, Avetisyan R, Carey BC, Chalk C, Trapnell BC. Prevalence and healthcare burden of pulmonary alveolar proteinosis. Orphanet J Rare Dis. 2018;13(1):129. Published 2018 Jul 31.

3. Kitamura N, Ohkouchi S, Tazawa R, Ishii H, Takada T, Sakagami T, et al. Incidence of autoimmune pulmonary alveolar proteinosis estimated using Poisson distribution. ERJ Open Res. 2019;5(1):00190–2018. Published 2019 Mar 18.

4. Stanley E, Lieschke GJ, Grail D, Metcalf D, Hodgson G, Gall JA, et al. Granulocyte/macrophage colony-stimulating factor-deficient mice show no major perturbation of hematopoiesis but develop a characteristic pulmonary pathology. Proc Natl Acad Sci U S A. 1994;91(12):5592–6.

5. Inoue Y, Trapnell BC, Tazawa R, Arai T, Takada T, Hizawa N, et al; Japanese Center of the Rare Lung Diseases Consortium. Characteristics of a large cohort of patients with autoimmune pulmonary alveolar proteinosis in Japan. Am J Respir Crit Care Med. 2008;177(7):752–62.

6. Holbert JM, Costello P, Li W, Hoffman RM, Rogers RM. CT features of pulmonary alveolar proteinosis. AJR Am J Roentgenol. 2001;176(5):1287–94.

7. Nunomura S, Tanaka T, Nakayama T, Otani K, Ishii H, Tabata K, et al. Pulmonary alveolar proteinosis-like change: a fairly common reaction associated with the severity of idiopathic pulmonary fibrosis. Respir Investig. 2016;54(4):272–9.

8. Shibata Y, Berclaz PY, Chroneos ZC, Yoshida M, Whitsett JA, Trapnell BC. GM-CSF regulates alveolar macrophage differentiation and innate immunity in the lung through PU.1. Immunity. 2001;15(4):557–67.

9. Uchida K, Nakata K, Trapnell BC, Terakawa T, Hamano E, Mikami A, et al. High-affinity autoantibodies specifically eliminate granulocyte-macrophage colony-stimulating factor activity in the lungs of patients with idiopathic pulmonary alveolar proteinosis. Blood. 2004;103(3):1089–98.

10. Buechner HA, Ansari A. Acute silico-proteinosis: a new pathologic variant of acute silicosis in sandblasters, characterized by histologic features resembling alveolar proteinosis. Dis Chest. 1969;55(4):274–8.

11. Chaulagain CP, Pilichowska M, Brinckerhoff L, Tabba M, Erban JK. Secondary pulmonary alveolar proteinosis in hematologic malignancies. Hematol Oncol Stem Cell Ther. 2014;7(4):127–35.

12. Whitsett JA, Wert SE, Weaver TE. Diseases of pulmonary surfactant homeostasis. Annu Rev Pathol. 2015;10:371–93.

13. Singh G, Katyal SL, Bedrossian CW, Rogers RM. Pulmonary alveolar proteinosis: staining for surfactant apoprotein in alveolar proteinosis and in conditions simulating it. Chest. 1983;83(1):82–6.

14. Delaval P, Brinchault G, Corre R, Jouneau S, Meunier C, Briens E. Lipoproteinose alveolaire pulmonaire [Pulmonary alveolar phospholipoproteinosis]. French. Rev Pneumol Clin. 2005;61(3):186–92.

15. Gu P, Fang X, Luo B, Chen H, Zeng Y, Lv H, et al. A noninvasive examination for the diagnosis of pulmonary alveolar proteinosis: induced sputum in conjunction with transmission electron microscopy. Int J Clin Exp Pathol. 2014;7(3):1200–5. Published 2014 Feb 15.

16. Smith BB, Torres NE, Hyder JA, Barbara DW, Gillespie SM, Wylam M, et al. Whole-lung lavage and pulmonary alveolar proteinosis: review of clinical and patient-centered outcomes. J Cardiothorac Vasc Anesth. 2019;33(9):2453–61.

17. Abdelmalak BB, Khanna AK, Culver DA, Popovich MJ. Therapeutic whole-lung lavage for pulmonary alveolar proteinosis: a procedural update. J Bronchology Interv Pulmonol. 2015;22(3):251–8.

18. Wylam ME, Ten R, Prakash UB, Nadrous HF, Clawson ML, Anderson PM. Aerosol granulocyte-macrophage colony-stimulating factor for pulmonary alveolar proteinosis. Eur Respir J. 2006;27(3):585–93.

19. Sheng G, Chen P, Wei Y, Chu J, Cao X, Zhang HL. Better approach for autoimmune pulmonary alveolar proteinosis treatment: inhaled or subcutaneous granulocyte-macrophage colony-stimulating factor: a meta-analyses. Respir Res. 2018;19(1):163. Published 2018 Aug 31.

A 55-Year-Old Woman With Dyspnea, Cough, and Acute Kidney Failure

15

Gwen E. Thompson, MD, and Ulrich Specks, MD

Case Presentation

A 55-year-old female smoker with no other past medical history had progressive fatigue, nonproductive cough, and dyspnea on exertion that began 3 weeks earlier. At an urgent care facility, she was given antibiotics for presumed community-acquired pneumonia. Her condition worsened, and 3 days later she presented to the emergency department. On physical examination she had tachypnea (respiratory rate to 32 breaths/min)

with mild respiratory distress; on lung auscultation crackles were heard at the bases bilaterally. Examination findings were otherwise unremarkable. Chest radiography showed diffuse infiltrates bilaterally (Figure 15.1). Laboratory test results (and reference ranges) were as follows: hemoglobin 5.1 g/dL (12.0-15.5 g/dL); white blood cell (WBC) count 12.9×10^9/L ($3.5\text{-}10.5 \times 10^9$/L); sodium 129 mmol/L (135-145 mmol/L); potassium 6.0 mmol/L (3.6-5.2 mmol/L); bicarbonate 8.0 mmol/L (22-29 mmol/L); serum urea nitrogen

Figure 15.1   Chest Radiograph

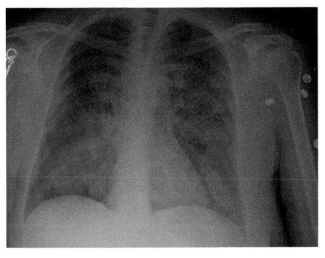

The radiograph shows diffuse pulmonary infiltrates bilaterally in a 55-year-old woman who had crackles at the bases bilaterally on auscultation.

154 mg/dL (6-21 mg/dL); creatinine 17 mg/dL (0.6-1.1 mg/dL); and lactate 0.7 mmol/L (0.6-2.3 mmol/L).

The patient underwent emergent hemodialysis. On bronchoscopy a progressively bloodier return was consistent with diffuse alveolar hemorrhage. Autoimmune serology screening was negative for antinuclear antibody and antineutrophil cytoplasmic antibody (ANCA) but positive for anti–glomerular basement membrane (GBM) antibody (8.0 U; reference range <1.0 U). A kidney biopsy showed cellular crescents with necrosis and linear immunoglobulin (Ig)G staining within the glomeruli consistent with anti-GBM disease. In addition to plasma exchange, therapy included methylprednisolone (1,000 mg intravenously daily) for 3 days and then prednisone (1 mg/kg orally daily) and cyclophosphamide (1.5 mg/kg orally daily). The patient underwent smoking cessation and her respiratory status improved, but she continued to need dialysis and her kidney function did not recover. During the next 1.5 months, she received the same daily doses of prednisone (1 mg/kg orally) and cyclophosphamide (1.5 mg/kg orally). Her anti-GBM antibody decreased to 1.1 U, and she had pancytopenia.

Questions

Multiple Choice (choose the best answer)

15.1. What management strategy should be used next?
   a. Increase the cyclophosphamide dosage
   b. Decrease the cyclophosphamide dosage
   c. Discontinue cyclophosphamide therapy
   d. Treat with plasma exchange again
   e. Start rituximab therapy

15.2. A 40-year-old male smoker presented with fatigue, nausea, and shortness of breath. He had acute kidney failure with bilateral patchy infiltrates on chest radiography. Findings on bronchoscopy confirmed diffuse alveolar hemorrhage. Laboratory test results indicated acute anemia and kidney failure; results were negative for perinuclear ANCA and cytoplasmic ANCA and positive for anti-GBM antibody. What diagnostic test would confirm the diagnosis and help with prognostication?
   a. No further testing is needed because the positive result for anti-GBM antibody confirms the diagnosis and is prognostic
   b. Kidney biopsy
   c. Transbronchial biopsy
   d. Urinalysis
   e. Video-assisted thorascopic lung biopsy

15.3. A 60-year-old female nonsmoker presented with acute kidney failure. Chest radiographs were unremarkable. Serologic tests were positive for anti-GBM antibody, and kidney biopsy results showed cellular crescents with necrosis and linear IgG staining within the glomeruli. These findings were confirmatory for anti-GBM disease. What is the first-line therapy for acute anti-GBM disease?
   a. Plasma exchange, glucocorticoids, and cyclophosphamide
   b. Plasma exchange, glucocorticoids, and rituximab
   c. Glucocorticoids and cyclophosphamide
   d. Glucocorticoids and rituximab
   e. Glucocorticoids alone

15.4. A 30-year-old male smoker presented with acute shortness of breath, hemoptysis, fatigue, and confusion. Test results showed that he had acute kidney failure and bilateral patchy infiltrates on chest radiography. Bronchoscopy confirmed diffuse alveolar hemorrhage. Anti-GBM antibody was 8.0 U (reference range <1.0 U). Kidney biopsy results, which showed linear IgG staining within the glomeruli, were confirmatory for anti-GBM disease. He began treatment with plasma exchange, cyclophosphamide, and a glucocorticoid taper. His clinical condition improved, and he regained kidney function. Nine months later he had been weaned from glucocorticoids, and his cyclophosphamide therapy was continued. Anti-GBM antibody is now undetectable. What maintenance agent should be used in anti-GBM disease?
   a. Azathioprine
   b. Methotrexate
   c. Rituximab
   d. Cyclophosphamide
   e. No maintenance agent is necessary

15.5. A 38-year-old male smoker presented with diffuse alveolar hemorrhage and acute kidney failure. Anti-GBM antibody was 6.0 U (reference range <1.0 U). Kidney biopsy results, which showed linear IgG staining within the glomeruli, were confirmatory for anti-GBM disease. Treatment was initiated with plasma exchange, cyclophosphamide, a glucocorticoid taper, and trimethoprim-sulfamethoxazole for *Pneumocystis jirovecii* prophylaxis. He improved clinically and regained kidney function. He underwent smoking cessation. One year later, the glucocorticoid therapy had been stopped, the disease had not relapsed, and anti-GBM antibody was undetectable. Therapy with cyclophosphamide and trimethoprim-sulfamethoxazole was therefore discontinued, but 1 month later the patient presented with shortness of breath and bilateral pulmonary infiltrates on chest radiography. What is the most likely cause of the pulmonary infiltrates?

a. Recurrent diffuse alveolar hemorrhage
b. Pneumocystis pneumonia
c. Fluid overload
d. Pulmonary alveolar proteinosis
e. Pulmonary fibrosis

Case Follow-up and Outcome

Cyclophosphamide therapy was stopped until the WBC count was greater than 4×10^9/L and was then resumed at two-thirds the original dose. Laboratory testing was conducted on a regular basis, and 1 month later the patient again had pancytopenia. Cyclophosphamide therapy was discontinued, and when her WBC count was greater than 4×10^9/L, therapy with rituximab was initiated. The disease was in remission 1 year after diagnosis, but the patient was dependent on dialysis and underwent kidney transplant.

Discussion

Pulmonary-renal syndromes present with acute kidney failure and diffuse alveolar hemorrhage. The most common diseases are ANCA-associated vasculitides and anti-GBM disease. Other diseases that rarely lead to kidney damage and pulmonary hemorrhage include systemic lupus erythematosus, IgA vasculitis (Henoch-Schönlein purpura), and infective endocarditis.

Anti-GBM disease is a rare disease caused by the pathogenic anti-GBM antibody against the noncollagenous 1 (NC1) domain of the alpha 3 chain of collagen type IV found in basement membranes. Normally these epitopes are not exposed. When they become exposed because of tissue injury or other mechanisms, pathogenic antibody formation is promoted, allowing local binding of the antibody to the exposed target epitopes. This elicits the inflammatory response that manifests as anti-GBM disease (1). Alpha 3 collagen expression is highest in the basement membranes of the glomeruli and alveoli. It is found in lower concentrations in the basement membranes of other tissues (such as the renal tubules, retina, and cochlea) and is absent in the majority of other organs (2). This differential composition of basement membranes in different organ tissues explains the selective disease manifestations of glomerulonephritis and pulmonary hemorrhage.

The diagnosis of anti-GBM disease includes a clinical presentation of acute kidney failure or pulmonary hemorrhage (or both) in the presence of anti-GBM antibodies. A confirmational biopsy is often completed because serologic testing of anti-GBM antibodies lacks sensitivity and specificity (3,4), and a kidney biopsy aids in prognostication. According to Levy et al (5), if a patient had a creatinine value of less than 5.7 mg/dL on presentation, patient and renal survival were high. If the creatinine value was greater than 5.7 mg/dL with no immediate need for dialysis, patient survival was 83% and renal survival was 82%. If the patient required immediate dialysis, the prognosis for survival worsened to 65% for patients and 8% for kidneys, and if those patients had 100% crescents on kidney biopsy, the kidney function did not recover (5).

The incidence of pulmonary hemorrhage in anti-GBM disease varies from 40% to 60% of patients across studies and is the sole clinical presentation in a small proportion of patients (6). The antigen must be exposed to the antibody for damage to occur, and with an intact basement membrane the antigen is hidden. Patients with pulmonary hemorrhage induced by anti-GBM disease frequently have an insulting factor such as tobacco smoking, pulmonary infection, drug use, or other chemical exposure (6).

Treatment of anti-GBM disease consists of plasma exchange and immunosuppression. In contrast to most other systemic autoimmune diseases, the pathogenic role of anti-GBM antibodies has been clearly proved for anti-GBM disease. This provides the rationale for the use of plasma exchange to remove these pathogenic autoantibodies (7), but the efficacy of plasma exchange in anti-GBM disease has been investigated in only 1 randomized controlled trial of 17 patients (8). Plasma exchange should be accompanied by concurrent immunosuppression with high doses of glucocorticoids and cyclophosphamide. Glucocorticoids are necessary to effectively suppress the acute inflammation and minimize kidney injury. After initial intravenous pulse bolus therapy (1,000 mg of methylprednisolone daily for 3-5 days), prednisone is given at 1 mg/kg (not to exceed 80 mg daily) and tapered after remission is achieved. The theoretical goal of cyclophosphamide or rituximab therapy is to prevent rebound antibody formation.

Patients receiving cyclophosphamide need to be monitored closely for adverse effects, such as cytopenias, and counseled to prevent hemorrhagic cystitis and infections. Prophylaxis for *P jiroveci* is imperative and should be continued for the duration of lymphopenia, which may outlast the duration of cyclophosphamide use (9). If cyclophosphamide is not tolerated, limited evidence suggests that rituximab may be an acceptable alternative agent (10).

The ideal duration of therapy is unknown. Unlike ANCA-associated vasculitis (11), anti-GBM disease rarely relapses (5). On average, the anti-GBM antibody resolves at 11 months without plasma exchange (12) and by 8 weeks with full treatment (13). Given this information, expert opinion is that duration of therapy should be 3 to 9 months, and anti-GBM antibody titers should be monitored for about 1 year.

Summary

Anti-GBM disease is a pulmonary-renal syndrome characterized by a pathogenic antibody directed against the basement membranes of the glomeruli and alveoli. The result is glomerulonephritis or pulmonary hemorrhage (or both). Diagnosis is based on clinical presentation, serologic markers, and pathologic confirmation. Prognosis is determined from renal factors. Treatment consists of plasma exchange and immunosuppression with glucocorticoids and cyclophosphamide as first-line agents.

Answers

15.1. Answer c.

The patient has pancytopenia due to use of cyclophosphamide. Cyclophosphamide is renally excreted, so dose adjustments should reflect kidney function, and the effect of cyclophosphamide should be monitored closely. Patients receiving cyclophosphamide should undergo monitoring that includes a complete blood cell count (CBC) with a differential WBC count weekly; aspartate aminotransferase (AST), alanine aminotransferase (ALT), and creatinine levels monthly; and urinalysis every 6 months. The goal is to keep the WBC count greater than 3.5×10^9/L for safety while ensuring lymphopenia for efficacy. This range is achieved by adjusting the cyclophosphamide dose. If cytopenia occurs, cyclophosphamide administration should be discontinued until the WBC count exceeds 4×10^9/L and then reinitiated at a lower dose. An initial dose reduction will not resolve the leukopenia; instead, cyclophosphamide therapy should be discontinued before the dose needs to be reduced. This approach is based on pharmacodynamic experience with the use of oral cyclophosphamide at the National Institutes of Health in the 1970s. Additional information is available in the medical literature (14).

15.2. Answer b.

The patient's clinical and serologic findings are highly suggestive of anti-GBM disease but not diagnostic. Anti-GBM antibody testing may have false-positive results and has variable sensitivity depending on the enzyme-linked immunosorbent assay used. Kidney biopsy should be pursued to establish a definite diagnosis and to assist in prognostication. However, given this patient's high probability of anti-GBM disease and severe presentation of the disease, therapy should be initiated while awaiting the biopsy results. Transbronchial biopsy is not helpful to establish the diagnosis. A urinalysis may show red blood cell casts, which would confirm the presence of active glomerulonephritis, but it would not provide information about the specific cause. Additional information is available in the medical literature (3-5).

15.3. Answer a.

The standard of care for patients with anti-GBM disease is the initiation of plasma exchange for antibody removal and concurrent immunosuppression with high doses of glucocorticoids and then a tapering of the glucocorticoids and administration of cyclophosphamide. Rituximab can be used when cyclophosphamide is contraindicated but is not considered first-line therapy. Additional information is available in the medical literature (10).

15.4. Answer e.

Patients rarely have a relapse of anti-GBM disease; hence, the risks of immunosuppressive agents outweigh the risk of relapse, and no maintenance therapy is needed. Azathioprine, methotrexate, and rituximab are agents used for maintenance in ANCA-positive vasculitis. Additional information is available in the medical literature (5,12,13).

15.5. Answer b.

The simultaneous discontinuation of cyclophosphamide and trimethoprim-sulfamethoxazole put this patient at risk for the development of pneumocystis pneumonia. Prophylaxis for *P jiroveci* should be continued for the duration of lymphopenia, which outlasts the duration of cyclophosphamide use. Recurrent diffuse alveolar hemorrhage would be unlikely with the low relapse rate of anti-GBM disease and with smoking cessation, which eliminates the insulting factor to the alveolar basement membrane. The patient has no known risk factors for fluid overload or pulmonary alveolar proteinosis. Pulmonary fibrosis can occur after prolonged or recurrent diffuse alveolar hemorrhage; however, with the acute nature of the infiltrate development in this patient, pulmonary fibrosis is unlikely. Additional information is available in the medical literature (9).

References

1. Pedchenko V, Bondar O, Fogo AB, Vanacore R, Voziyan P, Kitching AR, et al. Molecular architecture of the Goodpasture autoantigen in anti-GBM nephritis. N Engl J Med. 2010 Jul 22;363(4):343–54.

2. Derry CJ, Pusey CD. Tissue-specific distribution of the Goodpasture antigen demonstrated by 2-D electrophoresis and western blotting. Nephrol Dial Transplant. 1994;9(4):355–61.

3. Litwin CM, Mouritsen CL, Wilfahrt PA, Schroder MC, Hill HR. Anti-glomerular basement membrane disease: role of enzyme-linked immunosorbent assays in diagnosis. Biochem Mol Med. 1996 Oct;59(1):52–6.

4. Sinico RA, Radice A, Corace C, Sabadini E, Bollini B. Anti-glomerular basement membrane antibodies in the diagnosis of Goodpasture syndrome: a comparison of different assays. Nephrol Dial Transplant. 2006 Feb;21(2):397–401.

5. Levy JB, Turner AN, Rees AJ, Pusey CD. Long-term outcome of anti-glomerular basement membrane antibody disease treated with plasma exchange and immunosuppression. Ann Intern Med. 2001 Jun 5;134(11):1033–42.

6. Lazor R, Bigay-Game L, Cottin V, Cadranel J, Decaux O, Fellrath JM, et al; Groupe d'Etudes et de Recherche sur les Maladies Orphelines Pulmonaires (GERMOP); Swiss Group for Interstitial and Orphan Lung Diseases (SIOLD). Alveolar hemorrhage in anti-basement membrane antibody disease: a series of 28 cases. Medicine (Baltimore). 2007 May;86(3):181–93.

7. Lerner RA, Glassock RJ, Dixon FJ. The role of anti-glomerular basement membrane antibody in the pathogenesis of human glomerulonephritis. J Am Soc Nephrol. 1999 Jun;10(6):1389–404.

8. Johnson JP, Moore J Jr, Austin HA 3rd, Balow JE, Antonovych TT, Wilson CB. Therapy of anti-glomerular basement membrane antibody disease: analysis of prognostic significance of clinical, pathologic and treatment factors. Medicine (Baltimore). 1985 Jul;64(4):219–27.

9. Fauci AS, Dale DC, Wolff SM. Cyclophosphamide and lymphocyte subpopulations in Wegener's granulomatosis. Arthritis Rheum. 1974 Jul-Aug;17(4):355–61.

10. Syeda UA, Singer NG, Magrey M. Anti-glomerular basement membrane antibody disease treated with rituximab: a case-based review. Semin Arthritis Rheum. 2013 Jun;42(6):567–72.

11. Specks U, Merkel PA, Seo P, Spiera R, Langford CA, Hoffman GS, et al; RAVE-ITN Research Group. Efficacy of remission-induction regimens for ANCA-associated vasculitis. N Engl J Med. 2013 Aug 1;369(5):417–27.

12. Flores JC, Taube D, Savage CO, Cameron JS, Lockwood CM, Williams DG, et al. Clinical and immunological evolution of oligoanuric anti-GBM nephritis treated by haemodialysis. Lancet. 1986 Jan 4;1(8471):5–8.

13. Savage CO, Pusey CD, Bowman C, Rees AJ, Lockwood CM. Antiglomerular basement membrane antibody mediated disease in the British Isles 1980-4. Br Med J (Clin Res Ed). 1986 Feb 1;292(6516):301–4.

14. Dale DC, Fauci AS, Wolff SM. The effect of cyclophosphamide on leukocyte kinetics and susceptibility to infection in patients with Wegener's granulomatosis. Arthritis Rheum. 1973 Sep-Oct;16(5):657–64.

A 51-Year-Old Man With Fatigue, Dyspnea, and Lung Nodules[a]

Matthew Koslow, MD, Misbah Baqir, MBBS, and Jay H. Ryu, MD

Case Presentation

A 51-year-old man was evaluated for multiple pulmonary nodules that were discovered during evaluation of fatigue and dyspnea. The patient, a farmer in rural Minnesota, had a history of rheumatoid arthritis for the past 7 years treated with leflunomide, prednisone (10 mg daily), and hydroxychloroquine. He was a former smoker with 30-pack-year exposure. His father died of lung cancer at age 76 years.

On physical examination the patient was slender and not in respiratory distress (resting oxygen saturation, 98%; heart rate, 78 beats/min; and respiratory rate, 16 breaths/min). Pedal edema was absent, and lung sounds were clear on auscultation. His metacarpophalangeal and proximal interphalangeal joints were mildly tender on palpation; he had ulnar deviation but no joint effusion or swelling. A subcutaneous nodule was present on the extensor surface of the right elbow.

Pulmonary function test results (and percentage of predicted value) were as follows: forced expiratory volume in the first second of expiration (FEV_1), 2.9 L (72%); forced vital capacity (FVC), 4.11 L (81%); total lung capacity, 6.98 L (99.5%); and mean diffusing capacity of lung for carbon monoxide, 25.3 (82%), which was corrected for hemoglobin concentration. FEV_1/FVC was 70.5, and oxygen saturation as measured by pulse oximetry at rest was 95% and unchanged with exercise.

Multiple bilateral pulmonary opacities were present on posteroanterior and lateral chest radiographs (Figure 16.1). Computed tomography (CT) of the chest showed 13 pulmonary nodules with smooth borders, mostly located in the periphery with occasional satellite nodules and cavitation; the largest nodule measured 14 mm (Figure 16.2). On laboratory testing, rheumatoid factor was elevated (1,420 IU/mL), but results were within reference ranges for inflammatory markers, a complete blood cell count, and a comprehensive metabolic panel.

[a] Portions previously published in Koslow M, Young JR, Yi ES, Baqir M, Decker AP, Johnson GB, et al. Rheumatoid pulmonary nodules: clinical and imaging features compared with malignancy. Eur Radiol. 2019;29(4):1684-92; used with permission.

Figure 16.1   Multiple Bilateral Pulmonary Opacities on Chest Radiographs

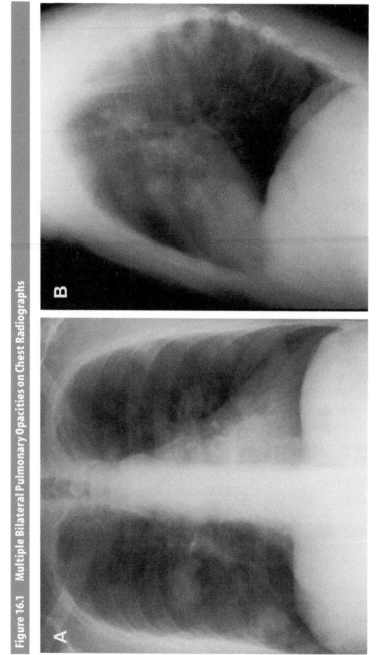

A, Posteroanterior view. B, Lateral view.

Figure 16.2   Rheumatoid Lung Nodules on CT of the Chest

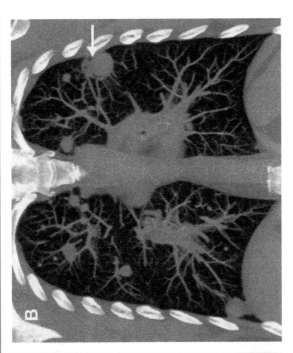

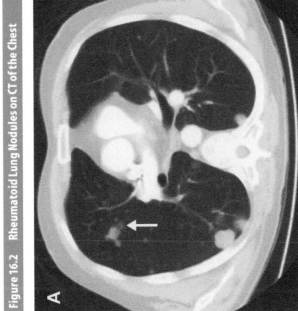

A, Axial view. B, Coronal maximum intensity projection. These images show several circumscribed solid nodules, satellite nodules (A, arrow), and developing cavitation (B, arrow).

(From Koslow M, Young JR, Yi ES, Baqir M, Decker AP, Johnson GB, et al. Rheumatoid pulmonary nodules: clinical and imaging features compared with malignancy. Eur Radiol. 2019;29[4]:1684-92; used with permission.)

Multiple Choice (choose the best answer)

16.1. Which of the following laboratory tests would provide the most useful information for evaluation of the lung nodules?
a. Hypersensitivity panel
b. Serologic testing for endemic fungi
c. Anti–cyclic citrullinated peptide antibody
d. Positron emission tomography (PET)-CT
e. Magnetic resonance imaging (MRI) of the thorax

16.2. What is the estimated probability that 1 of the lung nodules will be diagnosed as cancer in the next 2 to 4 years?
a. 65%
b. 35%
c. 15%
d. 10%
e. <5%

16.3. Which of the following imaging features is *not* a characteristic of rheumatoid lung nodules?
a. Cavitary nodule
b. Satellite nodules
c. Subsolid nodule
d. Subpleural location
e. Smooth borders

16.4. Which of the following does *not* characterize the 2017 Fleischner Society guidelines for the management of pulmonary nodules?
a. They do not apply to patients younger than 35 years or to patients who are immunocompromised or are known to have cancer
b. They encourage fewer follow-up examinations for stable nodules
c. For subsolid nodules, the duration of follow-up has been extended to 5 years
d. The minimum threshold size for recommending follow-up is based on an estimated cancer risk of at least 5%
e. CT scans of the thorax should be reconstructed and archived with contiguous thin sections (≤.5 mm; typically, 1.0 mm)

16.5. For a solitary noncalcified nodule larger than 8 mm, which of the following recommendations is appropriate?
a. Short 3-month follow-up with CT
b. PET-CT
c. Tissue sampling
d. CT, PET-CT, or tissue sampling at 3 months
e. CT at 3 to 6 months

Case Follow-up and Outcome

CT-guided biopsy was performed on the right lung nodule adjacent to the chest wall. On histopathology the nodule was necrotic, hyalinized, and fibrotic. Stains and cultures were negative for infectious organisms. The patient was subsequently followed with serial CT of the chest, which showed the slow progression over several years of a left peripheral nodule from solid to cavitary (Figure 16.3).

Discussion

Pulmonary nodules present a diagnostic challenge because they commonly occur and they raise concern for lung cancer (1). Prediction models have been developed for estimating the probability that a lung nodule will be diagnosed as cancer (2,3). Nodule features associated with lung cancer include increasing nodule size, upper lobe location, and spiculated border. Decreased risk for cancer is associated with a perifissural

Figure 16.3   Cavitation of Rheumatoid Lung Nodule on Axial CT Images of the Thorax

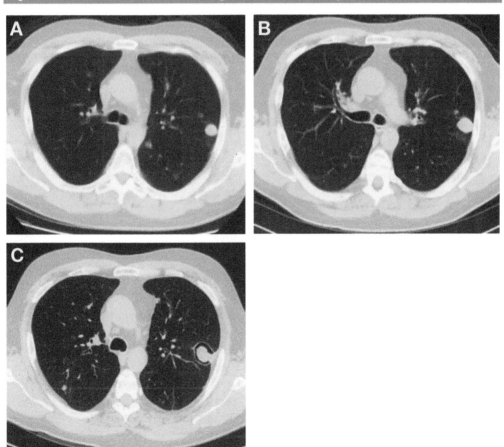

A, Peripheral solid nodule is apparent in the left thorax. B, Two years later, the nodule is larger. C, Five years later, the same nodule indicates cavitary disease.

(From Koslow M, Young JR, Yi ES, Baqir M, Decker AP, Johnson GB, et al. Rheumatoid pulmonary nodules: clinical and imaging features compared with malignancy. Eur Radiol. 2019;29[4]:1684-92; used with permission.)

location and an increasing number of nodules (≥5 nodules) (4). The 2017 Fleischner Society guidelines for the management of incidental pulmonary nodules detected on CT are based on nodule characteristics and the patient's underlying risk for malignancy. These guidelines are not intended for patients who have a known primary cancer at risk for metastases nor for immunocompromised patients who have an increased risk for infection (5), and they are not intended for children or patients younger than 35 years because lung cancer is rare in those patient populations.

The differential diagnosis for multiple pulmonary nodules includes vasculitis (eg, granulomatosis with polyangiitis and microscopic polyangiitis), infection (eg, endemic fungal infection such as pulmonary histoplasmosis, blastomycosis, and coccidiomycosis), and other benign lesions (eg, amyloidosis). Laboratory testing may be helpful in the initial evaluation. Antineutrophil cytoplasmic antibody tests should be performed for any patient who has signs or symptoms suggestive of vasculitis in addition to an examination for extrapulmonary sites of disease involvement (6). Serologic testing for pulmonary fungal infections is useful for patients who have epidemiologic risk factors for endemic fungal infection and a compatible clinical presentation (7).

Patients with rheumatoid arthritis require additional diagnostic consideration because rheumatoid lung nodules can mimic cancer (8). In a blinded review of CT and PET-CT of histologically proven pulmonary nodules in rheumatoid patients, the clinical and imaging features of rheumatoid lung nodules were distinct compared to those of lung malignancy (9). Rheumatoid lung nodules were solid and typically round with smooth borders. They were located peripherally, and satellite nodules were often nearby (Figure 16.2); they cavitated over time but rarely became calcified (Figure 16.3). On CT, rheumatoid nodules in a subpleural location coalesced and formed a confluent rind of soft tissue (Figure 16.4). Rheumatoid lung nodules, compared to malignant disease, showed low to moderate fluorodeoxyglucose F 18 (FDG) avidity and were rarely associated with large, draining lymph nodes that had FDG avidity (Figure 16.5). Patients with rheumatoid lung nodules were younger and more likely to have subcutaneous nodules and seropositivity compared to patients with lung malignancy.

The authors of that study proposed a *rheumatoid lung nodule score* for imaging. For a rheumatoid lung nodule, the presence of at least 3 of 6 features (≥4 nodules, peripheral location, cavitation, satellite nodules, smooth border, and subpleural rind of soft tissue) provided maximal sensitivity (77%) and specificity (92%) (area under the curve [AUC]=0.85; 95% CI, 0.75-0.94) (9). Results improved when those 6 features were used in combination with 2 other key findings (subcutaneous rheumatoid lung nodule and seropositivity) and at least 4 of the 8 clinical and imaging features were present (sensitivity, 95%; specificity, 85%; AUC = 0.90 [95% CI, 0.83-0.98]). However, data related to subcutaneous rheumatoid nodules or serology (or both) were incomplete for 15 of 50 patients with malignancy but were present for all but 1 patient with rheumatoid lung nodule.

For the patient described above in the case presentation, CT of the chest showed 13 nodules that were solid with smooth borders, were peripherally located, and had occasional satellite nodules and cavitation. On the basis of these imaging features, the rheumatoid lung nodule score would predict rheumatoid lung nodule with at least 92% specificity. Conversely, this patient is a 51-year-old man with risk factors for malignancy (age, smoking history, and family history). The estimated probability for lung cancer is 2.4% (3). Although this estimated risk is low, the minimum threshold for recommending follow-up is based on an estimated cancer risk of 1%, according to the 2017 Fleischner Society guidelines. PET-CT is not recommended for the evaluation of multiple pulmonary nodules but rather for a single nodule (≥8 mm) (5).

Figure 16.4   Necrobiotic Cavitary Nodules on Axial CT Images of the Thorax

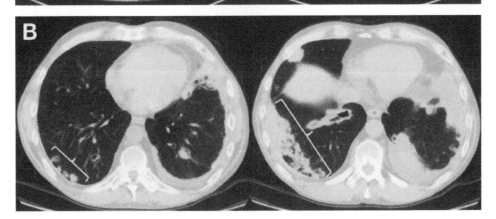

A, Arrows indicate 2 necrobiotic cavitary lesions that have thick internal debris. B, White brackets indicate a thick subpleural rind of soft tissue formed from the coalescence of subpleural nodules.

(From Koslow M, Young JR, Yi ES, Baqir M, Decker AP, Johnson GB, et al. Rheumatoid pulmonary nodules: clinical and imaging features compared with malignancy. Eur Radiol. 2019;29[4]:1684-92; used with permission.)

Summary

The evaluation of pulmonary nodules requires consideration of several factors, including the patient's underlying risk for malignancy, nodule characteristics, and systemic conditions associated with pulmonary manifestations. Society guidelines and prediction equations may support management decisions, which should ultimately be made on a case-by-case basis (5).

Figure 16.5   Benign and Malignant Lung Nodules on PET-CT

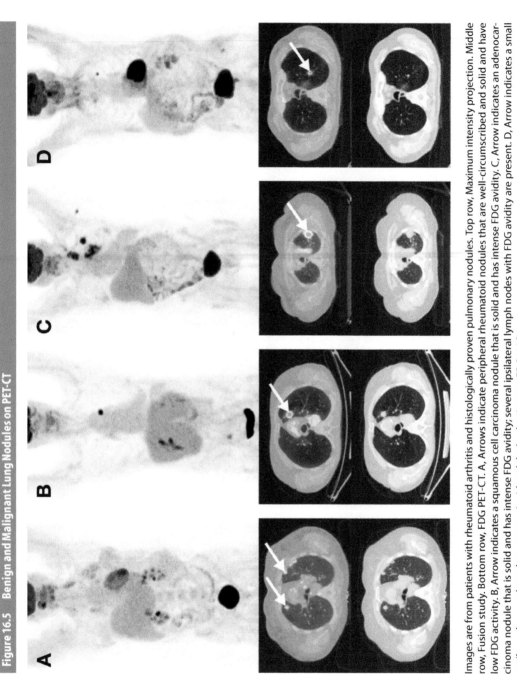

Images are from patients with rheumatoid arthritis and histologically proven pulmonary nodules. Top row, Maximum intensity projection. Middle row, Fusion study. Bottom row, FDG PET-CT. A, Arrows indicate peripheral rheumatoid nodules that are well-circumscribed and solid and have low FDG activity. B, Arrow indicates a squamous cell carcinoma nodule that is solid and has intense FDG avidity. C, Arrow indicates an adenocarcinoma nodule that is solid and has intense FDG avidity; several ipsilateral lymph nodes with FDG avidity are present. D, Arrow indicates a small peribronchovascular pulmonary carcinoid nodule that has intense FDG avidity.

(From Koslow M, Young JR, Yi ES, Baqir M, Decker AP, Johnson GB, et al. Rheumatoid pulmonary nodules: clinical and imaging features compared with malignancy. Eur Radiol. 2019;29[4]:1684-92; used with permission.)

Answers

16.1. Answer b.

Serologic testing for common endemic fungal diseases, such as pulmonary histoplasmosis, would be useful if a patient has a compatible clinical presentation and epidemiologic risk factors. Positive immunodiffusion results are reported as M or H precipitants or bands. The M band is more common, whereas the H band is often seen with disseminated infection. Where the disease is endemic, seropositivity by immunodiffusion is low (<1%), so that background seropositivity is not a major limitation, although false-negative results may occur when patients are immunosuppressed.

The radiologic pattern is not characteristic of hypersensitivity pneumonitis. Anti–cyclic citrullinated peptide antibody is a nonspecific biomarker associated with rheumatoid arthritis, and positive results may occur in other autoimmune diseases, tuberculosis, and other chronic infections. PET-CT is useful for differentiating between benign and malignant solitary noncalcified nodules (≥8 mm) and for detecting occult metastases in patients with potentially resectable lung nodules or masses, but PET-CT is not recommended for evaluating multiple pulmonary nodules. The value of MRI is limited in the evaluation of parenchymal lung lesions, but it can be useful for lesions in the chest wall, diaphragm, or pleurae. Additional information is available in the medical literature (7).

16.2. Answer e.

Lung cancer is the leading cause of cancer death, and screening for early detection and treatment of lung cancer may decrease the number of deaths. However, screening studies of smokers at high risk for malignancy suggest that the majority of nodules detected on CT are benign. Risk of cancer is higher among patients who have any of the following characteristics: older age, female, emphysema, family history of cancer, and nodules that are relatively few in number, large in size, spiculated, partly solid, or located in the upper lobe. On CT of the chest, the patient described above had 13 nodules, a striking number. The Brock University cancer prediction equation, which accounts for the number of nodules, would estimate a low probability (<5%) that a lung nodule would be diagnosed as cancer within 2 to 4 years. The patient described above, who had rheumatoid arthritis, had other features that are characteristic of rheumatoid lung nodules and further decrease the likelihood of malignancy, although such findings have not been validated in prospective studies. Additional information is available in the medical literature (3,9).

16.3. Answer c.

Benign nodules typically have well-defined, smooth borders, whereas spiculated or lobulated borders increase the concern for malignancy. Patients with underlying rheumatoid arthritis, rather than malignancy, are more likely to have smooth nodules, cavitary nodules, subpleural nodules, and satellite nodules. Subsolid nodules, defined as having attenuation that is less than that of soft tissue, are not characteristic of rheumatoid lung nodules but are characteristic of early adenocarcinoma. Additional information is available in the medical literature (9,10).

16.4. Answer d.

The purpose of the 2017 Fleischner Society guidelines was to decrease unnecessary follow-up examinations and to allow radiologists, clinicians, and patients to have more discretion in making decisions. The recommendations refer specifically to adult patients who are at least 35 years old and who have incidental lung nodules on CT. The guidelines are not intended for patients who are known to have primary cancers, who are at risk for metastases, who are immunocompromised and are at risk for infection, or who are younger than 35 years. For patients who have persistent part-solid nodules with a solid component smaller than 6 mm in diameter, the recommendation is to extend follow-up to 5 years because such nodules may progress to adenocarcinoma over many years. On imaging, thin sections (≤1.5 cm) enable accurate characterization of small pulmonary nodules, whereas thick sections increase volume averaging, preclude accurate characterization, and can affect management.

The Fleischner recommendations are based on estimations of risk of malignancy for nodules and for individuals. For example, solid lung nodules that have a cancer risk of less than 1% are excluded from routine CT follow-up. In addition to accounting for nodule size and morphology, the recommendations for nodule management also consider estimations of individual risk for malignancy. Risk is assigned according to categories proposed by the American College of Chest Physicians, which consider exposure to smoke and other carcinogens; the presence of emphysema, fibrosis, or an upper lobe location; and a patient's sex, age, and family history of lung cancer. Additional information is available in the medical literature (5,11).

16.5. Answer d.

For a solitary, solid noncalcified nodule larger than 8 mm in diameter, the Fleischner Society recommendations include 3-month follow-up and evaluation with CT, PET-CT, tissue sampling, or a combination of these options since any of them may be appropriate depending on size, morphology, comorbidity, and other factors. For example, a patient who has an 8-mm solitary nodule has an average estimated risk of cancer of about 3%, but certain patients may have a much higher risk because of the nodule's morphology and location. CT at 3 to 6 months is not recommended because the estimated risk for such nodules exceeds the guideline cutoff that excludes nodules from routine CT follow-up if they carry a risk of cancer that is less than 1%. Additional information is available in the medical literature (12).

References

1. Golden SE, Wiener RS, Sullivan D, Ganzini L, Slatore CG. Primary care providers and a system problem: a qualitative study of clinicians caring for patients with incidental pulmonary nodules. Chest. 2015;148(6):1422–9.

2. Swensen SJ, Silverstein MD, Ilstrup DM, Schleck CD, Edell ES. The probability of malignancy in solitary pulmonary nodules: application to small radiologically indeterminate nodules. Arch Intern Med. 1997;157(8):849–55.

3. McWilliams A, Tammemagi MC, Mayo JR, Roberts H, Liu G, Soghrati K, et al. Probability of cancer in pulmonary nodules detected on first screening CT. N Engl J Med. 2013;369(10):910–9.

4. Heuvelmans MA, Walter JE, Peters RB, de Bock GH, Yousaf-Khan U, van der Aalst CM, et al. Relationship between nodule count and lung cancer probability in baseline CT lung cancer screening: the NELSON study. Lung Cancer. 2017;113:45–50.

5. MacMahon H, Naidich DP, Goo JM, Soo Lee K, Leung ANC, Mayo JR, et al. Guidelines for management of incidental pulmonary nodules detected on CT images: from the Fleischner Society 2017. Radiology. 2017;284(1):228–43.

6. Finkielman JD, Lee AS, Hummel AM, Viss MA, Jacob GL, Homburger HA, et al; WGET Research Group. ANCA are detectable in nearly all patients with active severe Wegener's granulomatosis. Am J Med. 2007;120(7):643.e9–643.e6.43E14.

7. Wheat J, French ML, Kohler RB, Zimmerman SE, Smith WR, Smith WR, et al. The diagnostic laboratory tests for histoplasmosis: analysis of experience in a large urban outbreak. Ann Intern Med. 1982;97(5):680–5.

8. Jolles H, Moseley PL, Peterson MW. Nodular pulmonary opacities in patients with rheumatoid arthritis: a diagnostic dilemma. Chest. 1989;96(5):1022–5.

9. Koslow M, Young JR, Yi ES, Baqir M, Decker AP, Johnson GB, et al. Rheumatoid pulmonary nodules: clinical and imaging features compared with malignancy. Eur Radiol. 2019;29(4):1684–92.

10. Naidich DP, Bankier AA, MacMahon H, Schaefer-Prokop CM, Pistolesi M, Goo JM, et al. Recommendations for the management of subsolid pulmonary nodules detected at CT: a statement from the Fleischner Society. Radiology. 2013 Jan;266(1):304–17. Epub 2012 Oct 15.

11. Gould MK, Donington J, Lynch WR, Mazzone PJ, Midthun DE, Naidich DP, et al. Evaluation of individuals with pulmonary nodules: when is it lung cancer? Diagnosis and management of lung cancer, 3rd ed: American College of Chest Physicians evidence-based clinical practice guidelines. Chest. 2013 May;143(5 Suppl):e93S–e120S.

12. Gould MK, Fletcher J, Iannettoni MD, Lynch WR, Midthun DE, Naidich DP, et al; American College of Chest Physicians. Evaluation of patients with pulmonary nodules: when is it lung cancer?: ACCP evidence-based clinical practice guidelines (2nd edition). Chest. 2007 Sep;132(3 Suppl):108S–30S.

A 48-Year-Old Woman With Shortness of Breath and Cough

Hasan A. Albitar, MD, and Alice Gallo de Moraes, MD

Case Presentation

A 48-year-old woman, who had never smoked, presented to the emergency department with shortness of breath associated with intermittent dry cough. She had a previous medical history of hypothyroidism, medically complicated obesity (body mass index, 53; calculated as weight in kilograms divided by height in meters squared), obstructive sleep apnea, bilateral deep vein thrombosis complicated by bilateral subsegmental pulmonary emboli, and glioblastoma multiforme (GBM), for which she underwent surgical resection and subsequent administration of pembrolizumab and temozolomide.

The patient said that she had not had any chest pain, fever, or chills. Her medications included enoxaparin, levothyroxine, ondasetron, pembrolizumab, temozolomide, and citalopram. She was normotensive and afebrile, she had a normal heart rate and respiratory rate, but she was hypoxemic and required oxygen at a flow rate of 6 L/min through a nasal cannula to maintain an oxygen saturation of 94%. On pulmonary examination she had crackles bilaterally, and she had decreased breath sounds at the lung bases bilaterally. Abdominal, cardiac, musculoskeletal, and neurologic examination findings were unremarkable.

Computed tomography (CT) of the chest showed new diffuse, mixed interstitial, and ground-glass infiltrates throughout both lungs and small pleural effusions bilaterally. CT was negative for acute pulmonary embolism and showed no enlargement of the previous emboli.

A complete blood cell count showed anemia, mild leukocytosis with neutrophilic predominance, and a normal platelet count. The brain-type naturietic peptide (BNP) level was less than 20 pg/mL (reference range <20 pg/mL), the creatinine concentration was 0.6 mg/dL (reference range, 0.6-1.1 mg/dL), and electrolyte values were within the reference ranges. The patient began therapy with vancomycin, cefepime, and levofloxacin for presumed pneumonia and was admitted to the hospital for further evaluation.

All the following tests had negative results: sputum Gram staining; fungal staining; bacterial and fungal cultures; fungal serologies for *Blastomyces*, *Aspergillus*, *Coccidioides*, and *Histoplasma*; hypersensitivity pneumonitis panel; and *Legionella pneumophila* urinary antigen and *Streptococcus pneumoniae* urinary antigen. A trial of diuretics with intravenous furosemide was initiated, but the patient's symptoms and oxygen saturations did not improve. The patient continued to have dyspnea, and she continued to require oxygen at a flow rate of 6 L/min through a nasal cannula despite the trial of diuretics and administration of antibiotics for 5 days.

Multiple Choice (choose the best answer)

17.1. Which of the following is the most appropriate next step?
   a. Continue the patient's current antibiotic regimen
   b. Start corticosteroid therapy
   c. Discontinue enoxaparin and switch to a direct oral anticoagulant (DOAC)
   d. Perform bronchoscopy with bronchoalveolar lavage (BAL)
   e. Perform surgical lung biopsy

17.2. What would be the most likely diagnosis if results of flexible bronchoscopy included normal endobronchial findings, nonbloody BAL fluid return (total nucleated cell count, 9.9×10^9/L; predominance of lymphocytes and macrophages), and negative results for additional testing for bacterial and fungal organisms?
   a. Idiopathic pulmonary fibrosis (IPF)
   b. Lymphangioleiomyomatosis (LAM)
   c. Desquamative interstitial pneumonia (DIP)
   d. Malignant lung infiltration
   e. Pembrolizumab-induced pneumonitis

17.3. What is the most appropriate initial therapy for this condition?
   a. Discontinue pembrolizumab only
   b. Initiate corticosteroids and discontinue pembrolizumab indefinitely
   c. No further treatment is warranted at this time

   d. Continue pembrolizumab and initiate corticosteroids
   e. Discontinue pembrolizumab indefinitely and initiate infliximab

17.4. Which of the following correctly describes pulmonary immune-related adverse events (irAEs)?
   a. The risk of pneumonitis is the same with immune checkpoint inhibitor (ICI) monotherapy and ICI combination therapy
   b. Patients most commonly present with fevers
   c. Surgical lung biopsy is required for the diagnosis of pneumonitis
   d. Pneumonitis is a diagnosis of exclusion
   e. The mortality rate for patients with pneumonitis is less than 1%

17.5. Which of the following is correct about ICI-induced pneumonitis?
   a. There is no correlation between the presence of ICI-induced pneumonitis and tumor response to therapy
   b. The nonspecific interstitial pneumonia (NSIP) pattern is not seen in patients with ICI-induced pneumonitis
   c. Response rate and progression-free survival are better among patients who have non–small cell lung cancer treated with nivolumab and who have irAEs
   d. Patients who have received thoracic radiotherapy do not have an increased risk of ICI-induced pneumonitis
   e. Chest CT findings are often diagnostic among patients who have ICI-associated pneumonitis

Case Follow-up and Outcome

The patient underwent flexible bronchoscopy. Endobronchial examination findings were normal, and the BAL fluid return was nonbloody. Results of BAL fluid testing showed a total nucleated cell count of 9.9×10^9/L with a predominance of lymphocytes and macrophages. The results of additional testing of BAL fluid were negative for Gram staining and bacterial cultures, mycobacterial culture and acid-fast staining, viral cultures, fungal staining and cultures, *Legionella* culture, and *Nocardia* staining and cytology. The patient continued to be symptomatic and continued to require oxygen at a flow rate of 5 to 6 L/min through a nasal cannula. After the exclusion of infectious and malignant processes, the most likely diagnosis was pembrolizumab-induced pneumonitis. The patient began therapy with methylprednisolone 1 mg/kg intravenously with a subsequent prolonged taper over 6 weeks with prednisone. Her symptoms improved considerably with corticosteroid therapy, and her oxygen requirements also improved. She was discharged home with oxygen at a flow rate of 2 L/min through a nasal cannula.

Discussion

ICIs are used for treatment of several malignancies, including non–small cell lung cancer, melanoma, and lymphoma. The use of an ICI, such as pembrolizumab, can cause unique adverse reactions referred to as irAEs. These include gastrointestinal, dermatologic, endocrine, and pulmonary irAEs. Pneumonitis is an uncommon but potentially fatal complication encountered with ICIs (1).

The use of ICIs is expected to expand in the future, so clinicians should be familiar with the diagnosis and treatment of pneumonitis in patients treated with ICIs. The incidence of ICI-induced pneumonitis has varied among studies, but a recent meta-analysis showed an overall incidence of 2.7% (2). The median time to onset of ICI-induced pneumonitis has also varied among studies, ranging from 3 to 19 months (3).

Most commonly, patients with ICI-induced pneumonitis present with cough, dyspnea, and tachypnea with or without hypoxia (4). The diagnosis of pneumonitis can be challenging because of the similarities in presentation with other disorders, such as pneumonia, radiation-induced pneumonitis, and lung involvement with malignancy. There are no laboratory tests specific for ICI-induced pneumonitis. While chest CT findings are not specific for ICI-induced pneumonitis, commonly encountered CT patterns include bilateral consolidation in addition to ground-glass opacities in a peripheral distribution as is found with cryptogenic organizing pneumonia. Other chest CT findings can resemble the pattern found with NSIP (5). The imaging findings in pneumonitis may take up to 2 months to resolve (5). In suspected cases of ICI-induced pneumonitis, BAL is helpful to rule out infections. BAL findings are nonspecific, so a definitive diagnosis cannot be reached on the basis of the results. Therefore, the diagnosis is a diagnosis of exclusion.

Pneumonitis is graded (grades 1-5) according to the National Cancer Institute Common Terminology Criteria for Adverse Events (CTCAE) grading system (6), and the American Society of Clinical Oncology (ASCO) guidelines describe treatment (7). For grade 1 pneumonitis, an ICI should be held until chest CT is repeated in 3 to 4 weeks. Grade 2 pneumonitis is treated by holding immunotherapy until the symptoms resolve and adding prednisone 1 to 2 mg/kg with a prolonged taper over 4 to 6 weeks. For grade 3 or 4 pneumonitis, immunotherapy should be permanently discontinued in addition to beginning treatment with methylprednisolone 1 to 2 mg/kg intravenously with a subsequent prolonged corticosteroid taper over 4 to 6 weeks. ICI-induced pneumonitis carries a risk of mortality that is as high as 36% in some studies (8).

Summary

With its high risk of morbidity and mortality, ICI-induced pneumonitis must be considered in all patients receiving an ICI and presenting with respiratory distress and hypoxemic respiratory failure.

Answers

17.1. Answer d.

Bronchoscopy with BAL can provide valuable information and is less invasive than surgical lung biopsy. For this patient, bronchoscopy with BAL would be the most appropriate next step to further rule out infections and alveolar hemorrhage. Continuing the patient's current antimicrobial regimen would be inappropriate because she did not improve after 5 days of treatment and because an infection has not been definitively established. There is no clear indication to start corticosteroid therapy, and further testing is warranted to establish the diagnosis. Switching enoxaparin to a DOAC would also be inappropriate because CT of the chest showed that the size of the known pulmonary emboli was stable, and CT was negative for acute pulmonary embolism. Moreover, low-molecular-weight heparin has traditionally been the preferred agent for long-term anticoagulation in patients with cancer. Although surgical lung biopsy might be helpful, it is invasive and would not be an appropriate next step. Additional information is available in the medical literature (9).

17.2. Answer e.

The patient described above, who recently began therapy with pembrolizumab, presented with respiratory symptoms in addition to new chest CT findings of ground-glass opacities. After infectious and malignant processes were excluded, the most likely diagnosis would be pembrolizumab-induced pneumonitis. IPF typically affects older patients in their sixth and seventh decades. Typical high-resolution CT (HRCT) findings include reticular opacities with traction bronchiectasis in a subpleural distribution with honeycombing. Therefore, IPF is unlikely in this patient. LAM manifests as a diffuse cystic lung disease due to infiltration of smooth muscle cells into the pulmonary parenchyma. It can occur sporadically in young women or in association with tuberous sclerosis. Other findings in LAM include spontaneous pneumothorax and angiomyolipomas. This patient lacks all these features, so LAM is unlikely. DIP is uncommon and typically affects smokers. The fact that the patient has never smoked would be an argument against DIP as an explanation for her presentation. Extracranial metastasis of GBM is rare, so a metastatic process is less likely. Additional information is available in the medical literature (1,10-12).

17.3. Answer b.

The patient described above had pneumonitis that would be classified grade 3 according to the National Cancer Institute CTCAE version 4.0. The ASCO recommendations state that patients with grade 3 or 4 pneumonitis should be treated with high doses of corticosteroids with a prolonged taper of 4 to 6 weeks in addition to permanent discontinuation of therapy with ICIs, such as pembrolizumab. Since the patient had grade 3 pneumonitis, discontinuing use of pembrolizumab without giving corticosteroids would be inappropriate, and proceeding without treatment would also be inappropriate. According to ASCO, infliximab can be used in refractory pneumonitis that is unresponsive to high doses of corticosteroids. Additional information is available in the medical literature (6,7).

17.4. Answer d.

The diagnosis of pneumonitis requires ruling out infections, radiation pneumonitis, and malignant lung infiltration. The overall incidence of pneumonitis is higher when combination therapy with more than 1 ICI is used. In a meta-analysis, the use of combination ICI therapy nearly doubled the risk of pneumonitis. Patients with pneumonitis present more commonly with shortness of breath and cough than with fevers. Surgical lung biopsy is invasive and is not required to establish the diagnosis of ICI-induced pneumonitis. The reported mortality rate for patients with pneumonitis varies among studies, but it is generally 9% to 36%. Additional information is available in the medical literature (2,8,13).

17.5. Answer c.

New evidence indicates that the presence of irAEs is associated with better tumor response to therapy and better progression-free survival. This was demonstrated in studies of patients who had non–small cell lung cancer treated with nivolumab. As discussed above, NSIP is a pattern that may be seen when patients have ICI-induced pneumonitis and nonspecific CT findings, which can be encountered with various disorders. The incidence of ICI-induced pneumonitis is higher among patients who have a history of chest radiotherapy and among those who have a smoking history and COPD. Additional information is available in the medical literature (14-16).

References

1. Abdel-Rahman O, Fouad M. Risk of pneumonitis in cancer patients treated with immune checkpoint inhibitors: a meta-analysis. Ther Adv Respir Dis. 2016;10(3):183–93.
2. Nishino M, Giobbie-Hurder A, Hatabu H, Ramaiya NH, Hodi FS. Incidence of programmed cell death 1 inhibitor-related pneumonitis in patients with advanced cancer: a systematic review and meta-analysis. JAMA Oncol. 2016;2(12):1607–16.
3. Naidoo J, Wang X, Woo KM, Iyriboz T, Halpenny D, Cunningham J, et al. Pneumonitis in patients treated with anti-programmed death-1/programmed death ligand 1 therapy [published correction appears in J Clin Oncol. 2017 Aug 1;35(22):2590]. J Clin Oncol. 2017;35(7):709–17.
4. Nishino M, Ramaiya NH, Awad MM, Sholl AL, Maattala JA, Taibi M, et al. PD-1 Inhibitor-related pneumonitis in advanced cancer patients: radiographic patterns and clinical course. Clin Cancer Res. 2016;22(24):6051–60.
5. Tirumani SH, Ramaiya NH, Keraliya A, Bailey ND, Ott PA, Hodi FS, et al. Radiographic profiling of immune-related adverse events in advanced melanoma patients: treated with Ipilimumab. Cancer Immunol Res. 2015;3(10):1185–92.
6. National Cancer Institute. Common terminology criteria for adverse events (CTCAE). [cited 2020 Sep 16]. Updated 2020 Mar 27. Available from: https://ctep.cancer.gov/protocolDevelopment/electronic_applications/ctc.htm#ctc_40.
7. Brahmer JR, Lacchetti C, Schneider BJ, Atkins MB, Brassil KJ, Caterino JM, et al; National Comprehensive Cancer Network. Management of immune-related adverse events in patients treated with immune checkpoint inhibitor therapy: American Society of Clinical Oncology Clinical Practice Guideline. J Clin Oncol. 2018;36(17):1714–68.
8. Fujimoto D, Kato R, Morimoto T, Shimizu R, Sato Y, Kogo M, et al. Characteristics and prognostic impact of pneumonitis during systemic anti-cancer therapy in patients with advanced non-small-cell lung cancer. PLoS One. 2016;11(12):e0168465. Published 2016 Dec 22.
9. Kearon C, Akl EA, Ornelas J, Blaivas A, Jimenez D, Bounameaux H, et al. Antithrombotic therapy for VTE disease: CHEST Guideline and Expert Panel Report [published correction appears in Chest. 2016 Oct;150(4):988]. Chest. 2016;149(2):315–52.
10. Ryu JH, Moua T, Daniels CE, Hartman TE, Yi ES, Utz JP, et al. Idiopathic pulmonary fibrosis: evolving concepts. Mayo Clin Proc. 2014;89(8):1130–42.
11. Kalassian KG, Doyle R, Kao P, Ruoss S, Raffin TA. Lymphangioleiomyomatosis: new insights [published correction appears in Am J Respir Crit Care Med 1997 Aug;156(2 Pt 1):670]. Am J Respir Crit Care Med. 1997;155(4):1183–6.
12. Hoffman HA, Li CH, Everson RG, Strunck JL, Yong WH, Lu DC. Primary lung metastasis of glioblastoma multiforme with epidural spinal metastasis: Case report. J Clin Neurosci. 2017;41:97–9.
13. Delaunay M, Cadranel J, Lusque A, Meyer N, Gounant V, Moro-Sibilot D, et al. Immune-checkpoint inhibitors associated with interstitial lung disease in cancer patients [published correction appears in Eur Respir J. 2017 Nov 9;50(5):1750050]. Eur Respir J. 2017;50(2):1700050. Published 2017 Aug 10.
14. Toi Y, Sugawara S, Kawashima Y, Aiba T, Kawana S, Saito R, et al. Association of immune-related adverse events with clinical benefit in patients with advanced non-small-cell lung cancer treated with nivolumab. Oncologist. 2018 Nov;23(11):1358–65. Epub 2018 Jun 22.
15. Haratani K, Hayashi H, Chiba Y, Kudo K, Yonesaka K, Kato R, et al. Association of immune-related adverse events with nivolumab efficacy in non-small-cell lung cancer. JAMA Oncol. 2018 Mar 1;4(3):374–8.
16. Johkoh T, Lee KS, Nishino M, Travis WD, Ryu JH, Lee HY, et al. Chest CT diagnosis and clinical management of drug-related pneumonitis in patients receiving molecular targeting agents and immune checkpoint inhibitors: a position paper from the Fleischner Society. Chest. 2021 Mar;159(3):1107–25. Epub 2021 Jan 12.

A 59-Year-Old Woman With Progressive Dyspnea Undergoing Evaluation for Lung Transplant

18

Zhenmei Zhang, MD, and Steve G. Peters, MD

A 59-year-old woman with progressive symptoms of lung disease was referred for consideration of lung transplant. Lung disease was diagnosed when she was 10 years old, but in the past decade, she has had slowly progressive hypoxemia and has required supplemental oxygen. She described worsening shortness of breath, and pulse oximetry showed desaturation with any activity.

She never smoked cigarettes and did not have a family history of pulmonary disease. She described no occupational or environmental exposures. Her medical history included scoliosis, obesity for which she underwent sleeve gastrectomy 5 years earlier, and gastroesophageal reflux disease. On examination, the patient was not in acute distress but appeared chronically ill. Oxygen saturation as measured by pulse oximetry was 96% with 3 L/min supplemental oxygen. On cardiac examination, she had a regular rhythm without murmurs, and on lung examination, she had shallow inspiration and decreased basilar breath sounds without adventitial sounds.

Radiography of the chest showed diffuse calcific densities bilaterally throughout the lungs and mild interlobular septal thickening (Figure 18.1). Computed tomography (CT) showed extensive thickening and calcification of the interlobular and intralobular septa throughout both lungs with ground-glass attenuation and consolidation in both lower lobes (Figure 18.2). Pulmonary function testing results (and percentage of the predicted value) showed severe restriction with total lung capacity, 2.17 L (44%); forced expiratory volume in the first second of expiration, 1.03 L (40%); and forced vital capacity, 1.14 L (35%). Low lung volumes prevented measurement of the diffusing capacity of lung for carbon monoxide.

Figure 18.1   Chest Radiograph

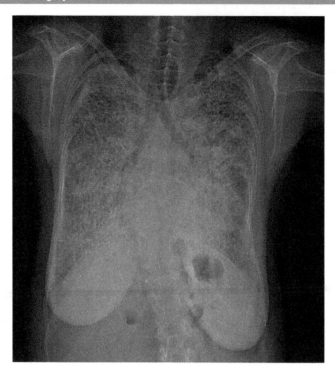

Anteroposterior view shows diffuse calcific densities bilaterally throughout the lungs and mild interlobular septal thickening.

Figure 18.2   CT of the Chest

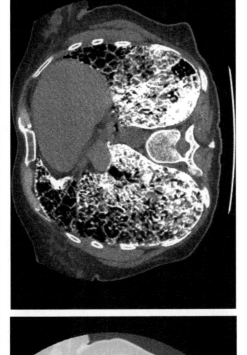

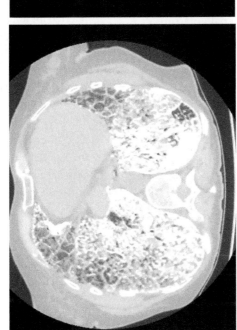

Axial sections show extensive thickening and calcification of the interlobular and intralobular septa throughout the lungs. Left, Lung window view. Right, Mediastinal window view.

Multiple Choice (choose the best answer)

18.1. On the basis of this patient's history and imaging findings, what is the most likely diagnosis?
   a. Pulmonary alveolar proteinosis
   b. Pulmonary alveolar microlithiasis (PAM)
   c. Broncholithiasis
   d. Idiopathic pulmonary fibrosis
   e. Pulmonary edema

18.2. Given this patient's pulmonary history and consideration for lung transplant, which of the following should be the next procedure?
   a. Coronary angiography
   b. Positron emission tomography (PET)-CT
   c. Ventilation-perfusion scan
   d. Transthoracic echocardiography
   e. Right-sided heart catheterization

18.3. Right-sided heart catheterization showed systolic pulmonary arterial pressure, 89 mm Hg; mean pulmonary arterial pressure (mPAP), 52 mm Hg; pulmonary arterial wedge pressure (PAWP), 8 mm Hg; and pulmonary vascular resistance (PVR), 12.87 Wood units. With these results, how should the patient's pulmonary hypertension be categorized?
   a. No evidence of pulmonary hypertension
   b. Precapillary pulmonary hypertension
   c. Postcapillary pulmonary hypertension

   d. Combined precapillary and postcapillary pulmonary hypertension
   e. Indeterminate from the provided information

18.4. Which of the following is *not* a contraindication for lung transplant?
   a. Active nicotine dependence
   b. Body mass index (BMI; calculated as weight in kilograms divided by height in meters squared) greater than 35
   c. Lung disease due to smoking-related emphysema
   d. Malignancy within the past 2 years
   e. Severe, untreatable disease in organ systems other than the lung

18.5. Which of the following is true about lung transplant evaluation?
   a. Lung transplant referral should be delayed until patients show clear progression of disease despite optimal medical therapy
   b. Patients 65 years or older should not be referred for lung transplant evaluation
   c. Systemic glucocorticoids should not be used in patients listed for lung transplant
   d. Posttransplant survival is similar for recipients of bilateral lung transplant and recipients of single-lung transplant
   e. The lung allocation score (LAS) can be used to compare medical urgency and the expected posttransplant survival rate between a lung transplant candidate and other patients on the waiting list

Case Follow-up and Outcome

The disease that was diagnosed when the patient was 10 years old was PAM. During the patient's transplant evaluation, transthoracic echocardiography showed mild right ventricular enlargement with mildly reduced systolic function. Estimated right ventricular systolic pressure was 64 mm Hg, the septum was *D* shaped, the left ventricular chamber size was normal, the calculated ejection fraction was 56%, and the tricuspid valve had mild to moderate regurgitation. During the 6-minute walk test, she walked 344 m. Subsequent right-sided heart catheterization showed normal mean right atrial pressure (4 mm Hg), extremely high right ventricular systolic pressure (87 mm Hg), high end-diastolic pressure (10 mm Hg), and extremely high pulmonary artery systolic pressure (83 mm Hg) and mPAP (52 mm Hg). Cardiac output was borderline low (4.04 L/min). With nitric oxide, the pulmonary artery systolic pressure decreased to 49 mm Hg, and mPAP decreased to 28 mm Hg. She began treatment with sildenafil and macitentan for pulmonary arterial hypertension. On follow-up right-sided heart catheterization, pulmonary artery pressure was 62/20 mm Hg, mPAP was 37 mm Hg, and cardiac output had improved to 6.2 L/min. A suitable donor was later identified, and the patient underwent bilateral lung transplant about 18 months after her initial evaluation in the transplant clinic.

Discussion

PAM is a rare autosomal recessive disorder that is characterized by intra-alveolar accumulation of calcium phosphate microliths. The disease is thought to be due to *SLC34A2* sequence variations, which lead to the inability of alveolar epithelial type II cells to clear phosphate ions, with subsequent deposition of calcium phosphate in the alveolar space (1). PAM affects people of all ages, the disease course varies among patients,

and the presentation is markedly heterogeneous. Most patients are asymptomatic in the initial stages of the disease, and the severity of symptoms such as dyspnea and cough is often less pronounced than the chest radiographs would suggest (2). Abnormalities on chest radiographs are often the first sign of underlying PAM. The typical radiographic finding is a "sandstorm" appearance of scattered calcified micronodules that are more prominent in the lung bases. As more micronodules form, the increased density of the lung parenchyma may obscure the heart borders and produce the radiographic manifestation described as the vanishing heart phenomenon (2).

High-resolution CT shows micronodular calcifications in bronchovascular bundles and in subpleural and perilobular regions (3). Ground-glass opacities can also be present, and with the resultant interlobular septal thickening from extensive calcifications, the opacities may resemble the "crazy-paving" pattern seen in pulmonary alveolar proteinosis, but discrete calcifications visualized on the mediastinal window can help distinguish the 2 diagnoses (4,5). The findings from tissue biopsy, if performed, typically show numerous microliths in the alveolar spaces and a thickened, concentric lamellar interstitium (4). The radiologic findings can often be diagnostic for PAM, but definitive diagnosis requires at least 1 additional clinical feature such as the finding of microliths on sputum or bronchoalveolar lavage, histopathologic findings, a positive family history, or genetic testing that shows a sequence variation in *SLC34A2* (2). Pulmonary function tests often show a restrictive pattern with decreased diffusing capacity, but the findings can be normal in the early stages of the disease.

Disease progression is not reversed by any current medical or genetic therapy. Lung transplant is the only available treatment for end-stage disease; the first successful bilateral lung transplant for PAM, described in 1992, was performed in a patient in France (6). Whether PAM can recur after lung transplant is unknown, but to date, no cases of recurrence in transplanted lungs have been reported (5).

According to the most recent guidelines from the International Society for Heart and Lung Transplantation (ISHLT), patients with chronic end-stage lung disease should be considered for lung transplant if their risk of death from lung disease within 2 years exceeds 50% if transplant is not pursued, if their likelihood of surviving at least 90 days after transplant exceeds 80%, and if their likelihood of surviving 5 years after transplant and having adequate graft function exceeds 80% (7). Since lung transplant is a risky and complex procedure, before a patient is listed for lung transplant, a comprehensive multidisciplinary evaluation must be performed and should include a consideration of contraindications and disease-specific factors. Currently, the most common indications for lung transplant are chronic obstructive pulmonary disease with or without α_1-antitrypsin deficiency, interstitial lung disease, and cystic fibrosis (8).

Since May 2005, the LAS has been used to address the order of patients on the waiting list. Both the waiting list urgency and the likelihood of posttransplant survival are considered in the calculation of the score, with a higher number (on a continuous scale of 0-100) indicating a greater urgency and a bigger potential benefit from lung transplant. Parameters in the LAS calculation include measurements such as forced vital capacity, patient age, serum creatinine level, New York Heart Association functional classification, pulmonary diagnosis, 6-minute walk distance, measurements of the severity of pulmonary hypertension, and the supplemental oxygen requirement (9). Evaluation to determine the presence and category of pulmonary hypertension is important for potential transplant recipients because the presence of pulmonary hypertension has been associated with worse survival while the patient is on the waiting list and after transplant, and patients may need to be considered for heart-lung transplant if considerable cardiac dysfunction is evident (10,11). The median survival is 6 years, and patients who are alive 1 year after transplant have a conditional median survival of 8.1 years. Recipients of bilateral lung transplant have had better survival than recipients of unilateral transplant at 1 year after transplant, and the survival advantage increases further in subsequent years (8).

Summary

PAM is a rare autosomal recessive disorder that is characterized by intra-alveolar accumulation of microliths and a sandstorm appearance on chest radiography. The only currently available and effective therapy for PAM is lung transplant. Appropriate patients with progressive, chronic lung disease should be referred to transplant centers in a timely manner to complete the comprehensive multidisciplinary evaluation.

Answers

18.1. Answer b.

The imaging findings are key to the diagnosis of PAM. Chest radiographs typically show a sandstorm appearance with scattered calcific micronodules that are more prominent in the lung bases. High-resolution CT shows micronodular calcifications that are more pronounced in bronchovascular bundles and in subpleural and perilobular regions. This imaging pattern on radiography and CT of the chest is commonly diagnostic for PAM. None of the other answer choices are consistent with the imaging findings. Additional information is available in the medical literature (3).

18.2. Answer d.

Given the patient's long-standing history of pulmonary disease and the extent of hypoxia, evaluation for pulmonary hypertension would be important because the presence of pulmonary hypertension has been associated with decreased survival. Before right-sided heart catherization, transthoracic echocardiography can be a reasonable, initial, noninvasive screening tool for confirmation and categorization of pulmonary hypertension. Coronary angiography, PET-CT, and ventilation-perfusion scans may be performed before lung transplant depending on the specific patient indicators. Additional information is available in the medical literature (12).

18.3. Answer b.

Pulmonary hypertension is defined as mPAP greater than 20 mm Hg. PAWP and PVR during right-sided heart catherization can be used to further categorize pulmonary hypertension. Precapillary pulmonary hypertension is defined as PAWP of 15 mm Hg or less in combination with PVR of at least 3 Wood units, and these values are consistent with the findings for this patient. Isolated postcapillary pulmonary hypertension is defined as mPAP that exceeds 20 mm Hg, PAWP that exceeds 15 mm Hg, and PVR less than 3 Wood units. When patients have PAWP that exceeds 15 mm Hg and PVR of at least 3 Wood units, the pulmonary hypertension is categorized as combined precapillary and postcapillary. Additional information is available in the medical literature (13).

18.4. Answer c.

Lung transplant should be considered for patients with end-stage pulmonary disease who have a high risk of death from pulmonary disease if lung transplant is not performed within 2 years and who are expected to survive after lung transplant. Smoking-related emphysema leading to chronic end-stage lung disease is an indication for consideration for lung transplant. The ISHLT has provided a list of absolute contraindications for lung transplant (Box 18.A4). Additional information is available in the medical literature (7).

18.5. Answer e.

The LAS is a numerical value that can affect waiting list and posttransplant survival. This score accounts for several parameters, such as age, lung disease diagnosis, functional status, oxygen requirement, forced vital capacity, and 6-minute walk test distance, and a higher score indicates more urgency for transplant and greater potential benefit. Since the evaluation process for lung transplant takes coordination and time, the process should be initiated before the patient becomes critically ill. For example, the process can begin as soon as the patient receives the initial diagnosis of interstitial lung disease. Age older than 65 years is a relative contraindication and is considered with other comorbidities when

Box 18.A4

ISHLT Absolute Contraindications for Lung Transplant

Active or recent history of malignancy within the past 2 years

Severe, untreatable dysfunction of another major organ system unless combined transplant can be performed

Uncorrected atherosclerotic disease with end-organ ischemia or dysfunction and/or coronary artery disease not amenable to revascularization

Acute medical instability

Uncorrectable bleeding diathesis

Poorly controlled chronic infection with highly virulent and/or resistant microbes

Active *Mycobacterium tuberculosis* infection

Chest wall or spinal deformity that could cause severe restriction after transplant

BMI ≥ 35

Current or history of nonadherence to medical therapy that is perceived to increase the risk of nonadherence after transplant

Psychiatric or psychologic conditions associated with an inability to cooperate with the health care team or to adhere to complex medical therapy

Absence of a reliable social support system

Severely limited functional status with poor rehabilitation potential

Substance abuse or dependence that involves alcohol, tobacco, marijuana, or other illicit substances

Modified from Weill et al (7); used with permission.

transplant eligibility is considered. Low-dose prednisone (≤20 mg daily) has been used safely in patients waiting for lung transplant and is not a contraindication to transplant. The median survival for primary lung transplant is 6.0 years, and survival is better for bilateral transplant recipients than single-lung recipients starting at 1 year posttransplant. Additional information is available in the medical literature (7-9,14).

References

1. Huqun, Izumi S, Miyazawa H, Ishii K, Uchiyama B, Ishida T, et al. Mutations in the SLC34A2 gene are associated with pulmonary alveolar microlithiasis. Am J Respir Crit Care Med. 2007;175(3):263–8.
2. Kosciuk P, Meyer C, Wikenheiser-Brokamp KA, McCormack FX. Pulmonary alveolar microlithiasis. Eur Respir Rev. 2020;29(158):2000–24.
3. Saito A, McCormack FX. Pulmonary Alveolar Microlithiasis. Clin Chest Med. 2016;37(3):441–8.
4. Siddiqui NA, Fuhrman CR. Best cases from the AFIP: Pulmonary alveolar microlithiasis. Radiographics. 2011;31(2):585–90.
5. Castellana G, Castellana G, Gentile M, Castellana R, Resta O. Pulmonary alveolar microlithiasis: review of the 1022 cases reported worldwide. Eur Respir Rev. 2015;24(138):607–20.
6. Bonnette P, Bisson A, el Kadi NB, Colchen A, Leroy M, Fischler M, et al. Bilateral single lung transplantation. Complications and results in 14 patients. Eur J Cardiothorac Surg. 1992;6(10):550–4.
7. Weill D, Benden C, Corris PA, Dark JH, Davis RD, Keshavjee S, et al. A consensus document for the selection of lung transplant candidates: 2014-- an update from the Pulmonary Transplantation Council of the International Society for Heart and Lung Transplantation. J Heart Lung Transplant. 2015;34(1):1–15.
8. Chambers DC, Yusen RD, Cherikh WS, Goldfarb SB, Kucheryavaya AY, Khusch K, et al. The Registry of the International Society for Heart and Lung Transplantation: Thirty-fourth Adult Lung And Heart-Lung Transplantation Report-2017; Focus Theme: Allograft ischemic time. J Heart Lung Transplant. 2017;36(10):1047–59.
9. Gottlieb J. Lung allocation. J Thorac Dis. 2017;9(8): 2670–4.
10. Hayes D, Jr., Black SM, Tobias JD, Kirkby S, Mansour HM, Whitson BA. Influence of Pulmonary Hypertension on Patients With Idiopathic Pulmonary Fibrosis Awaiting Lung Transplantation. Ann Thorac Surg. 2016;101(1):246–52.
11. Kim CY, Park JE, Leem AY, Song JH, Kim SY, Chung KS, et al. Prognostic value of pre-transplant mean pulmonary arterial pressure in lung transplant recipients: a single-institution experience. J Thorac Dis. 2018;10(3):1578–87.
12. Hayes D, Jr., Black SM, Tobias JD, Mansour HM, Whitson BA. Influence of pulmonary hypertension on survival in advanced lung disease. Lung. 2015;193(2):213–21.
13. Simonneau G, Montani D, Celermajer DS, Denton CP, Gatzoulis MA, Krowka M, et al. Haemodynamic definitions and updated clinical classification of pulmonary hypertension. Eur Respir J. 2019;53(1):1801–913.
14. McAnally KJ, Valentine VG, LaPlace SG, McFadden PM, Seoane L, Taylor DE. Effect of pre-transplantation prednisone on survival after lung transplantation. J Heart Lung Transplant. 2006;25(1):67–74.

A 52-Year-Old Woman With Arthralgias, Hair Loss, and Skin Ulcers

Cyril Varghese, MD, MS, and Jay H. Ryu, MD

Case Presentation

A 52-year-old woman, who had a history of Hashimoto disease and relapsing-remitting multiple sclerosis treated with glatiramer acetate, had a 6-month history of arthralgias and unexplained hair loss. A rash developed and progressed into ulcerations in the digits, elbows, inner thighs, and buttocks (Figure 19.1). The patient's antihistone antibody titer was weakly positive, so glatiramer-induced lupus was considered, and treatment was begun with prednisone at 60 mg daily and a subsequent dose taper.

Punch biopsy at the margin of an ulcerative lesion showed vacuolar interface dermatitis consistent with a connective tissue disease such as dermatomyositis. Creatine kinase and aldolase values were within the reference ranges. The myositis marker panel showed a high titer of anti–melanoma differentiation-associated gene 5 (MDA5) antibody.

The patient was admitted to the hospital because of the ulcers. Therapy was begun with intravenous (IV) methylprednisolone, IV immunoglobulin, and IV cyclophosphamide. When shortness of breath developed, she was transferred to the intensive care unit, where she was intubated because of increasing oxygen requirements. Ten days after admission, high-resolution computed tomography (HRCT) of the chest showed lower lobe–predominant consolidation and ground-glass opacities (Figure 19.2). Sputum and blood cultures were negative for an infectious cause. Because her clinical condition was not improving, plasma exchange (PLEX) therapy was initiated. Within 48 hours after the first PLEX cycle, her condition improved, and extubation was successful.

Figure 19.1   Typical Deep Cutaneous Ulcers in a Patient With Anti-MDA5 ADM

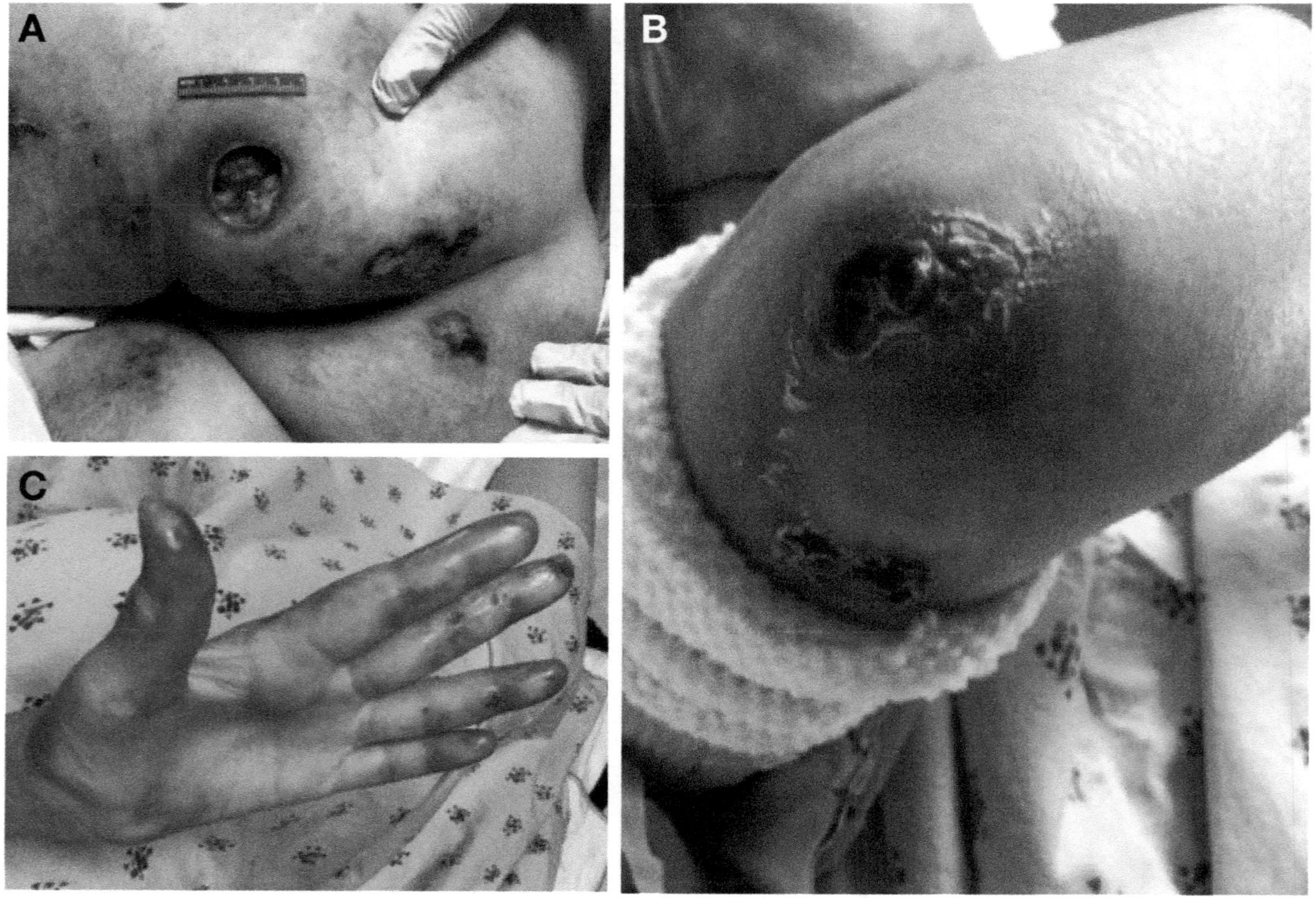

A, Buttocks. B, Right elbow. C, Left hand.

Figure 19.2   Lower Lobe Consolidation and Ground-glass Opacities on HRCT Axial View

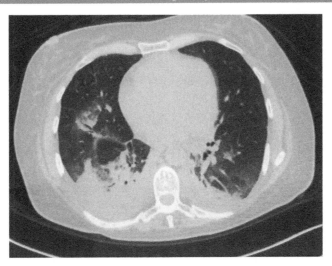

These opacities are hallmarks of ILD Related to Anti-MDA5.

Questions

Multiple Choice (choose the best answer)

19.1. Inflammatory myositis is associated with malignancy. Compared to the frequency of myositis without malignancy, how common is interstitial lung disease (ILD) in malignancy-associated myositis?
a. More common
b. Less common
c. About the same
d. No association
e. Inflammatory myositis is always associated with an occult malignancy

19.2. What is a hallmark of anti-MDA5 amyopathic dermatomyositis (ADM)?
a. Profound weakness
b. High serum aldolase levels
c. Cutaneous ulcers
d. Responsiveness to high doses of IV corticosteroids
e. Mechanic's hands

19.3. In which population is anti-MDA5 most prevalent?
a. White
b. Black
c. Hispanic
d. Asian
e. Southeast Asian

19.4. Which is an HRCT feature of anti-MDA5–positive ILD?
a. Peripheral reticulation
b. Interlobular septal thickening
c. Traction bronchiectasis
d. Lower lobe–predominant consolidation
e. "Crazy-paving" pattern

19.5. Which of the following is used to identify the severity and measure the response to treatment of anti-MDA5 ADM and its related systemic manifestations?
a. Antinuclear antibody titer
b. Anti-Jo-1 antibody titer
c. Ferritin level
d. Anti-MDA5 level
e. Both ferritin and anti-MDA5 levels

Case Follow-up and Outcome

After 7 cycles of PLEX (conducted on alternate days), the patient no longer needed supplemental oxygen, the cutaneous lesions and other systemic signs began to improve, and the anti-MDA5 antibody titer decreased. The patient made a full recovery. At 1-year follow-up, she was well with no recurrence of skin lesions or ILD.

Discussion

Patients with ADM, a subset of dermatomyositis, have cutaneous features without signs of overt myopathy as assessed with serum muscle enzymes, electromyography, or muscle biopsy (1). Patients with a subset of ADM, initially identified in Chinese and Japanese populations, have anti-MDA5 autoantibody (2-4). Clinical features that should increase awareness for this subtype of ADM include cutaneous ulcers that have a deep punched-out appearance with a predilection for the digital pulp, nail folds, and overlying Gottron papules; in addition, a rapidly progressive ILD is present in 50% to 100% of patients who have positive anti-MDA5 results (5). Therefore, essential screening for ILD should include pulmonary function testing or HRCT (or both). HRCT features include lower lobe–predominant consolidation, ground-glass opacities, and an absence of reticular fibrosis (6).

Optimal treatment of this disease has not been determined. Patients with mild cutaneous lesions may respond to treatment with mycophenolate mofetil, which may also anecdotally attenuate progression to ILD (7). In patients with refractory cutaneous lesions, IV immunoglobulin has been used in addition to mycophenolate mofetil (8). Rapidly progressive ILD is by far the most feared complication of anti-MDA5 ADM, and numerous strategies, including use of cyclophosphamide, rituximab, and polymyxin B hemoperfusion, have been tried with various results (4,9). The use of PLEX to remove the anti-MDA5 antibody may be an effective salvage strategy as shown with the patient described above. Serum anti-MDA5 titers and ferritin levels decrease in response to successful treatment (10).

Summary

Anti-MDA5 antibody–positive ADM is a unique subset of dermatomyositis characterized by deep ulcerative cutaneous lesions, rapidly progressive ILD, and high mortality. A high degree of awareness is required for quick identification and management, which includes immunosuppression and removal of anti-MDA5 antibodies from the plasma in patients with refractory disease.

Answers

19.1. Answer b.

Although inflammatory myositis has long been associated with malignancies, ILD itself is less common in patients with inflammatory myositis associated with malignancy. Anti-TIF1γ is associated with several malignancies, including lymphoma and breast, ovarian, and gastrointestinal tract cancers. Additional information is available in the medical literature (11-14).

19.2. Answer c.

ADM associated with anti-MDA5 has a characteristic cutaneous phenotype with deep skin and oral ulcerations and non-scarring alopecia. Patients generally do not have muscle involvement, so they tend to not have weakness or high serum aldolase levels. ADM associated with anti-MDA5 is usually not responsive to many first-line immunosuppressive agents, including systemic corticosteroids, as reported for the patient described above. A patient with mechanic's hands is more likely to have antisynthetase syndrome than anti-MDA5 ADM. Additional information is available in the medical literature (5,9).

19.3. Answer d.

ADM associated with anti-MDA5 is a rare disease, so the exact prevalence in different racial and geographic groups is unknown.

However, many of the initial reports described the disease in people of Asian descent, specifically in Chinese and Japanese populations. Although the disease has now been identified in people of other races, it is not more common in those races. Additional information is available in the medical literature (4,6,7,9,10).

19.4. Answer d.

Predominant HRCT features in ADM associated with anti-MDA5 have been described. In a study of 25 patients with dermatomyositis and ILD, HRCT findings from 12 patients with anti-MDA5 patients were compared to findings from 13 without the antibody. Lower lobe consolidation or ground-glass attenuation was seen in 50% of the patients with anti-MDA5, and lower lobe–predominant reticulation was more common in patients without anti-MDA5. Additional information is available in the medical literature (6).

19.5. Answer e.

Although decreased anti-MDA5 levels have been associated with improving clinical course, anti-MDA5 testing may not be readily available. However, ferritin, a nonspecific marker of inflammation, has been correlated to disease activity in ADM associated with anti-MDA5, so the correct and complete answer is that both ferritin and anti-MDA5 levels are used. Additional information is available in the medical literature (10).

References

1. Moghadam-Kia S, Oddis CV, Sato S, Kuwana M, Aggarwal R. Antimelanoma differentiation-associated gene 5 antibody: expanding the clinical spectrum in North American patients with dermatomyositis. J Rheumatol. 2017;44(3):319–25.
2. Sato S, Hirakata M, Kuwana M, Suwa A, Inada S, Mimori T, et al. Autoantibodies to a 140-kd polypeptide, CADM-140, in Japanese patients with clinically amyopathic dermatomyositis. Arthritis Rheum. 2005;52(5):1571–6.
3. Chen Z, Cao M, Plana MN, Liang J, Cai H, Kuwana M, et al. Utility of anti-melanoma differentiation-associated gene 5 antibody measurement in identifying patients with dermatomyositis and a high risk for developing rapidly progressive interstitial lung disease: a review of the literature and a meta-analysis. Arthritis Care Res (Hoboken). 2013;65(8):1316–24.
4. Hamaguchi Y, Kuwana M, Hoshino K, Hasegawa M, Kaji K, Matsushita T, et al. Clinical correlations with dermatomyositis-specific autoantibodies in adult Japanese patients with dermatomyositis: a multicenter cross-sectional study. Arch Dermatol. 2011;147(4):391–8.
5. Kurtzman DJB, Vleugels RA. Anti-melanoma differentiation-associated gene 5 (MDA5) dermatomyositis: a concise review with an emphasis on distinctive clinical features. J Am Acad Dermatol. 2018;78(4):776–85.
6. Tanizawa K, Handa T, Nakashima R, Kubo T, Hosono Y, Watanabe K, et al. HRCT features of interstitial lung disease in dermatomyositis with anti-CADM-140 antibody. Respir Med. 2011;105(9):1380–7.
7. Hayashi M, Kikuchi T, Takada T. Mycophenolate mofetil for the patients with interstitial lung diseases in amyopathic dermatomyositis with anti-MDA-5 antibodies. Clin Rheumatol. 2017;36(1):239–40.
8. Femia AN, Eastham AB, Lam C, Merola JF, Qureshi AA, Vleugels RA. Intravenous immunoglobulin for refractory cutaneous dermatomyositis: a retrospective analysis from an academic medical center. J Am Acad Dermatol. 2013;69(4):654–7.
9. Teruya A, Kawamura K, Ichikado K, Sato S, Yasuda Y, Yoshioka M. Successful polymyxin B hemoperfusion treatment associated with serial reduction of serum anti-CADM-140/MDA5 antibody levels in rapidly progressive interstitial lung disease with amyopathic dermatomyositis. Chest. 2013;144(6):1934–6.
10. Gono T, Kawaguchi Y, Ozeki E, Ota Y, Satoh T, Kuwana M, et al. Serum ferritin correlates with activity of anti-MDA5 antibody-associated acute interstitial lung disease as a complication of dermatomyositis. Mod Rheumatol. 2011;21(2):223–7.
11. Ungprasert P, Bethina NK, Jones CH. Malignancy and idiopathic inflammatory myopathies. N Am J Med Sci. 2013 Oct;5(10):569–72.
12. Ikeda S, Arita M, Misaki K, Mishima S, Takaiwa T, Nishiyama A, et al. Incidence and impact of interstitial lung disease and malignancy in patients with polymyositis, dermatomyositis, and clinically amyopathic dermatomyositis: a retrospective cohort study. Springerplus. 2015 May 28;4:240.
13. Douglas WW, Tazelaar HD, Hartman TE, Hartman RP, Decker PA, Schroeder DR, et al. Polymyositis-dermatomyositis-associated interstitial lung disease. Am J Respir Crit Care Med. 2001 Oct 1;164(7):1182–5.
14. Oldroyd A, Sergeant JC, New P, McHugh NJ, Betteridge Z, Lamb JA, et al; UKMyoNet. The temporal relationship between cancer and adult onset anti-transcriptional intermediary factor 1 antibody-positive dermatomyositis. Rheumatology (Oxford). 2019 Apr 1;58(4):650–5.

A 61-Year-Old Man With Dyspnea on Minimal Exertion

Rachana Krishna, MBBS, and Jay H. Ryu, MD

Case Presentation

A 61-year-old man presented with shortness of breath on exertion that began 2 months earlier with a gradual onset. Symptoms progressed until he became dyspneic with minimal exertion and could not work. He said that he did not have cough, wheezing, chest pain, fevers, or chills. His past medical history was notable for hypertension, hyperlipidemia, obesity (body mass index 33), epilepsy, ischemic heart disease that required coronary stents, and chronic low back pain. He estimated that he has been smoking cigarettes (1 pack daily) for the past 34 years. He worked at a milk powder processing plant, he did not have any pets at home, and he did not have any recent travel or unusual exposures. His medications included aspirin, atorvastatin, levetiracetam, lisinopril, metoprolol, and fish oil supplements. His family history was notable for emphysema in his mother.

On physical examination, the patient's oxygen saturation was low (93%), and he required supplemental oxygen (2 L/min). On auscultation of his lungs, the patient had fine bibasilar crackles without wheezing. Other examination findings were unremarkable.

Results of lung function testing indicated mild restriction with severely reduced diffusion capacity (Table 20.1).

On computed tomography (CT) of the chest, the patient had diffuse ground-glass opacities bilaterally, predominantly in the upper lobes, with areas of small cystic changes and centrilobular emphysema (Figure 20.1). Areas of interstitial opacities and mild traction bronchiectasis were also present.

Results of surgical lung biopsy from the right upper lobe showed alveolated parenchyma with an irregular nodular area consisting of fibrosis with mixed inflammation, an increased concentration of eosinophils, and a background of diffuse intra-alveolar pigmented histiocytes. Many cells had positive staining with CD1a and Langerin immunostains.

Table 20.1 Results of Lung Function Testing		
Component	Value	Percentage of predicted value
FVC, L	2.40	76
FEV$_1$, L	2.08	82
FEV$_1$/FVC, %	87	NA
TLC, L	3.55	61
DLco, mL/min/mm Hg	7.93	32

Abbreviations: DLco, diffusing capacity of lung for carbon monoxide; FEV$_1$, forced expiratory volume in first second of expiration; FVC, forced vital capacity; NA, not applicable; TLC, total lung capacity.

Figure 20.1   CT of the Chest, Axial View

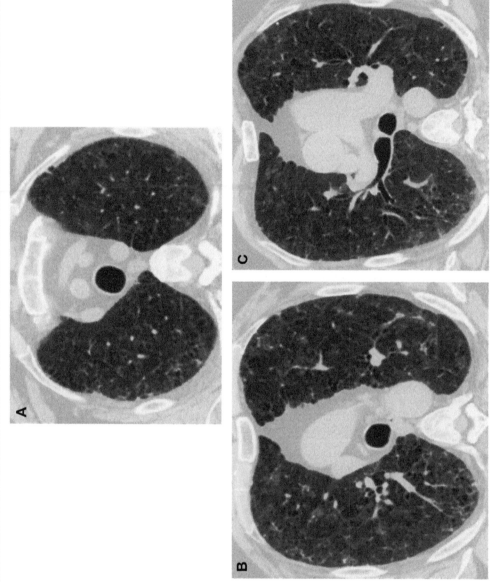

A-C, Bilateral, diffuse ground-glass opacities are seen predominantly in the upper lobes in addition to small cystic changes and centrilobular emphysema.

Questions

Multiple Choice (choose the best answer)

20.1. Which of the following statements is true about this patient's condition?

a. Extrapulmonary organ involvement occurs in more than 50% of patients with this condition

b. Smoking cessation can result in regression of the disease

c. Hemoptysis is the most common presentation

d. Bronchoscopy with bronchoalveolar lavage usually provides a definitive diagnosis

e. Lower lobes of the lungs are more commonly involved in this condition

20.2. Which of the following is *not* a known complication of this patient's condition?

a. Spontaneous pneumothorax

b. Pulmonary hypertension

c. Diabetes insipidus

d. Kidney cancer

e. Lung cancer

20.3. Which of the following organs has been reported to be involved in this patient's condition?

a. Kidney

b. Parotid gland

c. Muscle

d. Bone

e. Thyroid

20.4. Which of the following treatments is *not* used in this patient's condition?

a. Corticosteroids

b. Smoking cessation

c. Sirolimus

d. Cladribine

e. Oxygen supplementation

20.5. Which of the following has *not* been associated with decreased survival of patients with this condition?

a. Low DLCO (<72% of the predicted value)

b. Male sex

c. Low FEV_1 (<60% of the predicted value)

d. Increased residual volume (>120%)

e. Older age

Case Follow-up and Outcome

A diagnosis of pulmonary Langerhans cell histiocytosis (PLCH) was made on the basis of the clinical context and findings from surgical lung biopsy. The patient was thought to have smoking-related lung disease because pathology findings included areas of respiratory bronchiolitis, and emphysema was apparent on imaging.

After the diagnosis, the patient quit smoking, and he was given supplemental oxygen therapy. He did not have any extrapulmonary manifestations of Langerhans cell histiocytosis. Because his DLCO was severely low, the patient was followed clinically after smoking cessation. If his condition did not improve, corticosteroid therapy would be a consideration.

Discussion

The differential diagnosis for a patient with diffuse cystic lung disease includes PLCH, lymphangioleiomyomatosis, lymphocytic interstitial pneumonia, Birt-Hogg-Dube syndrome, and pulmonary amyloidosis. Patients with smoking-related interstitial lung disease can present with cysts in the lungs in PLCH, but they can also have nodules and ground-glass infiltrates on imaging from respiratory bronchiolitis and desquamative interstitial pneumonia (DIP). Respiratory bronchiolitis, DIP, and PLCH may all be present along with emphysema in patients who smoke (1,2).

PLCH is a rare disease in which tissues are infiltrated by a cluster of Langerhans cells that are organized in loose granulomas (3). Langerhans cells are bone marrow–derived dendritic cells that usually process and present skin-derived antigens. They are also in airway epithelium, where they process inhaled antigens. Aberrant accumulation of Langerhans cells can result in granuloma formation with eosinophilic infiltration. These cells, which stain positive with CD1a

and Langerin immunostains, are useful markers to aid in the diagnosis of this condition on lung biopsy (1).

PLCH in adults is related to smoking and is usually limited to the lungs. Extrapulmonary disease occurs in about 10% to 15% of patients (1). The most common extrapulmonary manifestations are involvement of bone with lytic lesions in the skull or axial skeleton, pituitary involvement with diabetes insipidus, and less commonly skin, liver, and lymph node involvement (4). Childhood-onset Langerhans cell histiocytosis usually has multiorgan involvement and, unlike adult-onset disease, is not strongly associated with smoking.

PLCH usually occurs in young adults (peak age, 20-40 years). Adults with PLCH usually present with dyspnea or cough, but the disease may also be recognized incidentally on imaging performed for other reasons (4). Some patients with PLCH (15%-20%) present with chest pain from spontaneous pneumothorax, and hemoptysis is a rare presentation. Constitutional symptoms of fevers and weight loss may also occur, but if these features are present, the possibility of malignancy must be investigated and excluded (1,3,4).

CT of the lungs of patients with PLCH shows nodules, including cavitating nodules, and thin-walled cysts in the parenchyma. These cysts may have various sizes and irregular shapes. Findings are predominantly in the upper and middle lung lobes with relative sparing of the lung bases. If patients have coexisting respiratory bronchiolitis or DIP from smoking, ground-glass opacities may also be seen (2).

Lung function testing usually shows decreased DLCO in 80% to 90% of patients. Spirometry may indicate obstruction or restriction (or both). Diagnostic characteristics associated with shorter survival include lower values for DLCO, FEV_1, and FEV_1/FVC and a higher residual volume (4). Bronchoscopy with bronchoalveolar lavage may be helpful if the concentration of CD1a-positive cells is at least 5%, but that finding is seen in no more than about a third of patients. Transbronchial lung biopsy may increase the yield to 50%; the gold standard is surgical lung biopsy (5).

Management of PLCH, like other smoking-related interstitial lung diseases, mainly involves smoking cessation. In a majority of patients, smoking cessation may result in stabilization of the disease or even improvement in lung function and imaging findings (4). If a patient's condition continues to progressively worsen despite smoking cessation, treatment with corticosteroids may be considered. Pulmonary hypertension is a well-known complication of PLCH, and vasodilator therapy has been used for pulmonary arterial hypertension in patients with PLCH (6).

Vinblastine and cladribine have been used when the disease progresses despite smoking cessation, especially if a patient has multisystem involvement (3,7,8). If the disease continues to progress, some patients may require lung transplant. Secondary hematologic malignancies and lung cancer also occur at a higher rate in adults with PLCH (4). *BRAF* V600E mutation has been described in about a third of patients with PLCH, and targeted therapies for this mutation are available if malignancy is present (9).

Summary

PLCH is a diffuse cystic lung disease related to smoking in adults. The disease may coexist with other smoking-related conditions, including respiratory bronchiolitis, DIP, and emphysema. Decreased DLCO is the most common finding on pulmonary function testing. Extrapulmonary involvement, mainly with bone and pituitary involvement, occurs in 10% to 15% of adults with smoking-related PLCH. Treatment of PLCH is mainly smoking cessation; rarely, corticosteroids and cladribine are used if the disease continues to progress despite smoking cessation. Complications of PLCH include spontaneous pneumothorax, pulmonary hypertension, and increased risk of malignancies.

Answers

20.1. Answer b.

After patients with PLCH stop smoking, some have progressive disease, but in others the nodular opacities seen on imaging regress and resolve. In a series with 21 patients, nodular opacities regressed in about half the patients, but in some patients the opacities evolved to cystic changes. Extrapulmonary symptoms occur in less than 20% of patients with PLCH. Bronchoscopy is helpful for diagnosis of PLCH in only about a third of patients; for diagnosis, bronchoalveolar lavage fluid should show at least 5% CD1a-positive cells. PLCH is characterized by involvement of upper and mid lung lobes with nodules and cysts, but the lower lobes are relatively spared. Additional information is available in the medical literature (1,5,10).

20.2. Answer d.

Spontaneous pneumothorax, pulmonary hypertension, diabetes insipidus, and lung and hematologic malignancies are all known complications of PLCH. Renal cell carcinoma is associated with Birt-Hogg-Dube syndrome, which is another cystic lung disease. Renal angiomyolipoma is associated with lymphangioleiomyomatosis. Additional information is available in the medical literature (1).

20.3. Answer d.

Extrapulmonary manifestations, which occur in less than 20% of adults with PLCH, include bone cysts, diabetes insipidus, and, less commonly, skin rash. Parotid gland involvement with sicca symptoms can occur in Sjögren syndrome, which can cause lymphocytic interstitial pneumonia, but not in PLCH. Renal angiomyolipomas are associated with lymphangiomyomatosis. Thyroid and muscle involvement is not seen in PLCH. Additional information is available in the medical literature (1).

20.4. Answer c.

Smoking cessation is the mainstay of treatment in PLCH. In patients with progressive disease despite smoking cessation, oral corticosteroids have been used, and some patients have had good response to cladribine. Oxygen therapy is used in patients with advanced disease and hypoxemia. Sirolimus is used in the treatment of lymphangioleiomyomatosis but not in the treatment of PLCH. Additional information is available in the medical literature (3,7).

20.5. Answer b.

Low DLCO, reduced FEV_1, increased residual volume, and older age are all associated with worse outcomes in PLCH. However, male sex has not been associated with worse outcomes than female sex. Additional information is available in the medical literature (4).

References

1. Vassallo R, Ryu JH, Colby TV, Hartman T, Limper AH. Pulmonary Langerhans'-cell histiocytosis. N Engl J Med. 2000;342(26):1969–78.
2. Vassallo R, Jensen EA, Colby TV, Ryu JH, Douglas WW, Hartman TE, et al. The overlap between respiratory bronchiolitis and desquamative interstitial pneumonia in pulmonary Langerhans cell histiocytosis: high-resolution CT, histologic, and functional correlations. Chest. 2003;124(4):1199–205.
3. Vassallo R, Harari S, Tazi A. Current understanding and management of pulmonary Langerhans cell histiocytosis. Thorax. 2017;72(10):937–45.
4. Vassallo R, Ryu JH, Schroeder DR, Decker PA, Limper AH. Clinical outcomes of pulmonary Langerhans'-cell histiocytosis in adults. N Engl J Med. 2002;346(7):484–90.
5. Baqir M, Vassallo R, Maldonado F, Yi ES, Ryu JH. Utility of bronchoscopy in pulmonary Langerhans cell histiocytosis. J Bronchology Interv Pulmonol. 2013;20(4):309–12.
6. Le Pavec J, Lorillon G, Jais X, Tcherakian C, Feuillet S, Dorfmuller P, et al. Pulmonary Langerhans cell histiocytosis-associated pulmonary hypertension: clinical characteristics and impact of pulmonary arterial hypertension therapies. Chest. 2012;142(5):1150–7.
7. Grobost V, Khouatra C, Lazor R, Cordier JF, Cottin V. Effectiveness of cladribine therapy in patients with pulmonary Langerhans cell histiocytosis. Orphanet J Rare Dis. 2014;9:191. Published 2014 Nov 30.
8. Aerni MR, Aubry MC, Myers JL, Vassallo R. Complete remission of nodular pulmonary Langerhans cell histiocytosis lesions induced by 2-chlorodeoxyadenosine in a non-smoker. Respir Med. 2008;102(2):316–9.
9. Roden AC, Hu X, Kip S, Castellar ERP, Rumilla KM, Vrana J, et al. BRAF V600E expression in Langerhans cell histiocytosis: clinical and immunohistochemical study on 25 pulmonary and 54 extrapulmonary cases. Am J Surg Pathol. 2014;38(4):548–51.
10. Brauner MW, Grenier P, Tijani K, Battesti JP, Valeyre D. Pulmonary Langerhans cell histiocytosis: evolution of lesions on CT scans. Radiology. 1997 Aug;204(2):497–502.

A 67-Year-Old Woman With Progressive Dyspnea and Atypical Infiltrates

Aahd F. Kubbara, MBBS, and Teng Moua, MD

Case Presentation

A 67-year-old woman presented with a 9-month history of progressive dyspnea without other associated signs or symptoms. Dyspnea started after she traveled to an elevation of 6,600 feet (2,012 m) but did not improve upon returning to her home elevation of 1,000 feet (305 m). Her past medical history was notable for chronic lymphocytic leukemia (CLL), which was diagnosed 2 years earlier and was being observed without treatment. She also had mild immunoglobulin deficiency treated with occasional replacement therapy. She was a lifetime nonsmoker. On physical examination she had a heart rate of 114 beats/min, a grade 1/6 systolic murmur, and clear lung sounds bilaterally.

When the dyspnea became progressively worse, she was referred for cardiac and pulmonary evaluation. During cardiac stress testing, oxygen saturation decreased to 80%. Computed tomography (CT) of the chest showed patchy peripheral ground-glass opacities with mild interlobular septal thickening and focal areas of ground-glass nodularity (Figure 21.1). Two months later, subsequent CT of the chest did not show any notable changes. With these findings, the broad differential diagnosis included alveolar hemorrhage, hypersensitivity pneumonitis, and chronic microaspiration, which was considered because the patient had an esophageal hiatal hernia. Pulmonary lymphoproliferative disease was also considered given her history of CLL. Hypersensitivity pneumonitis serology panels were negative for mold and avian antigens.

The patient's pulmonary function test (PFT) results included the following: forced expiratory volume in the first second of expiration (FEV_1) was 67% of the predicted value; forced vital capacity (FVC), 63%; diffusing capacity of lung for carbon monoxide (DLCO), 31%; and total lung capacity (TLC), 78% (Table 21.1). The FEV_1/FVC ratio was normal, and the patient did not have an acute bronchodilator response. Transthoracic echocardiography showed normal left ventricular function, an ejection fraction of 67%, an estimated right ventricular systolic pressure of 32 mm Hg, and no valvular abnormalities.

The CT findings supported the possibility of hypersensitivity pneumonitis, so a trial of corticosteroid therapy was started with prednisone (30 mg daily for 30 days and then 20 mg daily for 30 days), but the patient remained symptomatic. After 2 months of treatment, CT of the chest showed a new left lower lobe nodular opacity with cystic lucencies (Figure 21.2). Percutaneous CT-guided biopsy of this lesion showed abundant necrotic change within alveolated parenchyma but no malignancy. Her white blood cell count was 10.4×10^9/L.

Figure 21.1   CT of the Chest Showing Diffuse Ground-Glass Opacities

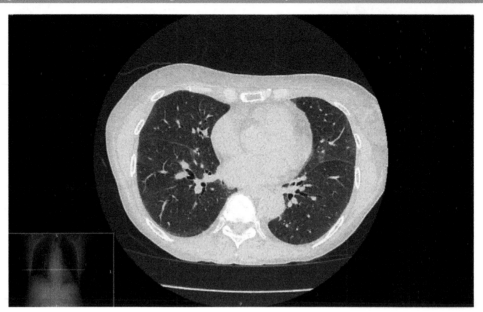

Table 21.1   PFT Results

Component	Value	Reference value	Percentage of predicted value
TLC, L	3.52	4.53	78
VC, L	1.73	2.67	65
FRC pleth, L	2.06	2.57	80
RV, L	1.80	1.90	95
RV, % of TLC	51	42	121
FVC, L	1.67	2.67	63
FEV_1, L	1.39	2.09	67
FEV_1/FVC, %	83.3	78.7	106
$FEF_{25\%-75\%}$, L/min	1.92	1.85	104
PEF, L/min	6.2	5.2	119
FET, s	7.71	NA	NA
MVV, L/min	53	88	60
Dlco, mL/min/mm Hg	6.2	19.8	31
Dlco cSB, mL/min/mm Hg	5.9	19.8	30
Hb, g/dL	15.0	11.6–15.0	NA
VA_{SB}, L	2.71	4.54	60

Abbreviations: cSB, single breath corrected for hemoglobin; $FEF_{25\%-75\%}$, forced expiratory flow, midexpiratory phase; FET, forced expiratory time; FEV_1, forced expiratory volume in first second of expiration; FRC pleth, functional residual capacity measured by plethysmography; FVC, forced vital capacity; Hb, hemoglobin; max, maximum; MVV, maximum voluntary ventilation; NA, not applicable; PEF, peak expiratory flow; RV, residual volume; TLC, total lung capacity; VA_{SB}, single-breath alveolar volume; VC, vital capacity.

Figure 21.2   CT of the Chest Showing Left Basal Nodular Lesion

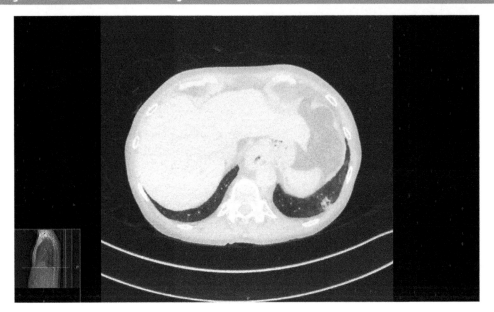

Questions

Multiple Choice (choose the best answer)

21.1. On the basis of this patient's CT images and PFT results, what would be the best next step?
  a. Initiation of chemotherapy for underlying CLL
  b. Follow-up CT of the chest and PFTs in 3 months
  c. Bronchoscopy with bronchoalveolar lavage to rule out infection
  d. Serologic testing for autoimmune disease
  e. Open lung biopsy for diagnosis of underlying interstitial lung disease

21.2. Of the following types of pulmonary amyloidosis, which is the most common pattern of disease involvement?
  a. Tracheobronchial amyloidosis
  b. Diffuse alveolar septal amyloidosis
  c. Pulmonary vascular amyloidosis
  d. Pleural amyloidosis
  e. Nodular pulmonary amyloidosis

21.3. Which statement related to the final diagnosis is correct?
  a. Most patients with pulmonary amyloidosis are symptomatic
  b. Diffuse alveolar septal amyloidosis usually involves AA amyloid

  c. Pulmonary hypertension is the most common cause of death among patients with pulmonary amyloidosis
  d. Amyloidosis-related pleural effusion is usually transudative
  e. A diagnosis of pulmonary amyloidosis can be made from clinical and radiologic findings alone

21.4. Which of the following correctly describes the prognosis for patients with pulmonary amyloidosis?
  a. The prognosis for patients with nodular amyloidosis is generally good
  b. For patients with localized amyloidosis, conservative excision is usually noncurative
  c. Tracheobronchial amyloidosis is mostly a benign process
  d. In patients with pulmonary amyloidosis related to hematologic malignancy, chemotherapy improves local amyloid deposits
  e. Diffuse alveolar septal amyloidosis carries a favorable prognosis

21.5. When amyloidosis is confirmed after biopsy, what is the best next test for delineating an underlying cause of pulmonary involvement?
  a. Bone marrow biopsy
  b. Serum and urine protein electrophoresis
  c. Amyloid subtyping, preferably with mass spectrometry–based proteomic analysis
  d. Cardiac magnetic resonance imaging
  e. Total body positron emission tomography–CT

Case Follow-up and Outcome

Wedge biopsy of the nodular area in the right upper, middle, and lower lobes showed diffuse alveolar septal amyloidosis with Congo red (Figure 21.3). There were no immunophenotypic features of involvement from CLL. On liquid chromatography tandem mass spectrometry, the peptide profile was consistent with AL (κ)-type amyloid deposition, and the concentration of serum κ free light chains was high (62 mg/dL; upper limit of reference range, 1.94 mg/dL). Bone marrow biopsy showed 20% plasma cell involvement. The patient was referred to the hematology department for directed management with induction therapy, including cyclophosphamide, bortezomib, and dexamethasone, with consideration for autologous stem cell transplant.

Discussion

Amyloidosis is rare, with an incidence rate of 6 to 10 cases per 1 million people in the US (1). It is characterized by deposition of misfolded protein fibrils in the extracellular space. Although amyloidosis can affect any organ system, 50% of patients have pulmonary involvement (2). Radiologic findings can be protean and nonspecific, so a high degree of awareness is required, and a final diagnosis relies on biopsy confirmation.

The decision to pursue surgical biopsy in patients with diffuse parenchymal lung disease is challenging when patients present with atypical or nonspecific clinical and radiologic findings. Clinicians often need to ensure relative procedural safety and acceptability, balancing the risk of potential complications with potential

Figure 21.3   Congo Red Staining of Lung Biopsy Specimen

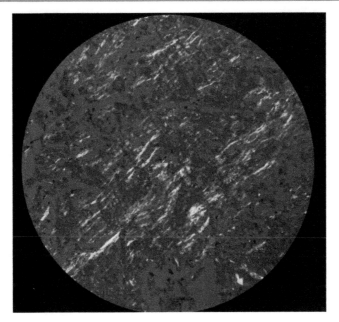

changes to treatment if biopsy is required for an initial diagnosis or a more specific diagnosis. Despite the common use of corticosteroids empirically, many parenchymal lung diseases that can be defined only with histopathology are not responsive to corticosteroids; these include amyloidosis, desquamative interstitial pneumonia, and aspiration-related interstitial disease. In contrast, diseases such as idiopathic nonspecific interstitial pneumonia, chronic hypersensitivity pneumonitis, and immunoglobulin G4–related disease may be responsive to immunosuppression but are often confidently diagnosed only with histopathology (3).

The 3 predominant parenchymal or airway patterns of pulmonary amyloidosis are diffuse alveolar septal, nodular, and tracheobronchial (4). Additionally, amyloidosis may be associated with pleural effusions that are related to coexisting cardiac amyloidosis or adjacent pulmonary disease. In two-thirds of amyloid effusions, the pleural fluid findings are transudative (4).

Pulmonary amyloidosis is often asymptomatic and found incidentally on imaging, although progression of the disease may eventually lead to pulmonary symptoms. The tracheobronchial pattern may be more frequently symptomatic because associated airway stenosis may cause cough, wheeze, hemoptysis, or dyspnea. Many patients initially receive a misdiagnosis of asthma (3).

Nodular pulmonary amyloidosis is often considered localized because systemic involvement is frequently absent. The amyloid deposits are usually subpleural and bilateral and of various sizes. Associated causes usually include lymphoproliferative disorders, specifically mucosa-associated lymphoid tissue lymphoma (MALToma) and similar conditions (5). If an underlying process is not identified and no systemic amyloidosis is apparent, even with negative immunohistochemical staining, a specific peptide profile may be evident with mass spectrometry analysis of the amyloid deposits (5). In contrast to systemic amyloidosis, nodular pulmonary amyloidosis often involves predominantly κ light chains rather than λ (5). Several types of amyloid protein cause the nodular pattern of involvement; the most common types are localized AL and AL/AH (5). Overall, the prognosis is favorable for patients with nodular amyloidosis.

Unlike nodular pulmonary amyloidosis, diffuse alveolar septal amyloidosis is typically associated with systemic disease. Various radiologic patterns that have been described include reticular opacities, interlobular septal thickening, micronodules, and, rarely, ground-glass opacities (6). Treatment is directed toward an underlying cause and usually involves cytotoxic chemotherapy.

Tracheobronchial amyloidosis tends to be an organ-limited disease that often causes symptoms of airway stenosis. AL-type deposits are typically identified. Symptomatic proximal airway disease is controlled with the use of laser, forceps débridement, or external beam radiotherapy (7).

Summary

Diagnosis of pulmonary amyloidosis tends to be delayed because the condition is rare and few symptoms develop, although incidental radiologic findings may be extensive. The 3 types of pulmonary amyloidosis have distinctive radiologic and clinical presentations, underlying causes, and prognoses. Nodular amyloidosis tends to be associated with a local lymphoproliferative disorder and usually carries a favorable prognosis. Diffuse alveolar septal amyloidosis is typically associated with underlying systemic disease and, with its histologic pattern of alveolar damage, tends to impair gas exchange and lead more commonly to dyspnea and hypoxemia. Tracheobronchial amyloidosis may result in airway compromise and hemoptysis. Of these, diffuse alveolar septal forms carry the worst prognosis.

Answers

21.1. Answer e.

Fine-needle aspiration biopsy did not help to establish the diagnosis for this patient who has clinical and radiologic features of pulmonary amyloidosis. Although she has impaired pulmonary function, she can likely tolerate open lung biopsy. Chemotherapy is not indicated for amyloidosis since identification of the nodular subtype (if known) would suggest resection. Watchful follow-up is not favored because of the symptoms and impaired pulmonary function. Infection and autoimmune disease were not supported by the clinical presentation and results of fine-needle aspiration biopsy. Additional information is available in the medical literature (4).

21.2. Answer e.

In a case series of 48 patients with pulmonary amyloidosis, over 55% had the nodular pulmonary type. All the remaining patterns of involvement have been reported less commonly. Additional information is available in the medical literature (8).

21.3. Answer d.

Up to two-thirds of pleural effusions related to amyloidosis have been reported to be transudative. Most patients are asymptomatic, and amyloid lung findings would be incidental on imaging. AL amyloid is the pattern commonly found in the diffuse alveolar septal type. Among patients with pulmonary amyloidosis, the cause of death is usually extrapulmonary. As an example, among patients with diffuse alveolar septal types, the most common cause of death is cardiac amyloidosis. Finally, the diagnosis of pulmonary amyloidosis requires a biopsy. Additional information is available in the medical literature (4).

21.4. Answer a.

In a study that involved 207 lung specimens, disease-specific 10-year survival among patients with nodular amyloidosis was 96.0% but only 51.9% among patients with systemic AL amyloidosis. Surgical resection of nodular amyloidosis tends to be curative. Tracheobronchial amyloidosis can lead to subglottic stenosis with life-threatening complications. If amyloid deposits related to malignancy have already appeared, treating the underlying malignancy will not reverse them. Diffuse alveolar septal amyloidosis is associated with poorer outcomes and increased mortality. Additional information is available in the medical literature (9).

21.5. Answer c.

Mass spectrometry has demonstrated high sensitivity and specificity and is considered superior to other methods for amyloid subtyping. All the remaining answer choices have lower sensitivity and specificity for determining the amyloid subtype and mechanism of amyloid production. Additional information is available in the medical literature (10).

References

1. Kyle RA, Linos A, Beard CM, Linke RP, Gertz MA, O'Fallon WM, et al. Incidence and natural history of primary systemic amyloidosis in Olmsted County, Minnesota, 1950 through 1989. Blood. 1992;79(7): 1817–22.

2. Gandham AK, Gayathri AR, Sundararajan L. Pulmonary amyloidosis: a case series. Lung India. 2019; 36(3):229–32.

3. Mikolasch TA, Garthwaite HS, Porter JC. Update in diagnosis and management of interstitial lung disease. Clin Med (Lond). 2017;17(2):146–53.

4. Milani P, Basset M, Russo F, Foli A, Palladini G, Merlini G. The lung in amyloidosis. Eur Respir Rev. 2017;26(145):170046.

5. Grogg KL, Aubry MC, Vrana JA, Theis JD, Dogan A. Nodular pulmonary amyloidosis is characterized by localized immunoglobulin deposition and is frequently associated with an indolent B-cell lymphoproliferative disorder. Am J Surg Pathol. 2013;37(3):406–12.

6. Pickford HA, Swensen SJ, Utz JP. Thoracic cross-sectional imaging of amyloidosis. AJR Am J Roentgenol. 1997;168(2):351–5.

7. O'Regan A, Fenlon HM, Beamis JF Jr, Steele MP, Skinner M, Berk JL. Tracheobronchial amyloidosis: the Boston University experience from 1984 to 1999. Medicine (Baltimore). 2000;79(2):69–79.

8. Hui AN, Koss MN, Hochholzer L, Wehunt WD. Amyloidosis presenting in the lower respiratory tract: clinicopathologic, radiologic, immunohistochemical, and histochemical studies on 48 cases. Arch Pathol Lab Med. 1986 Mar;110(3):212–8.

9. Baumgart JV, Stuhlmann-Laeisz C, Hegenbart U, Nattenmuller J, Schonland S, Kruger S, et al. Local vs. systemic pulmonary amyloidosis: impact on diagnostics and clinical management. Virchows Arch. 2018 Nov;473(5):627–37. Epub 2018 Aug 22.

10. Khoor A, Colby TV. Amyloidosis of the lung. Arch Pathol Lab Med. 2017 Feb;141(2):247–54.

Sleep Medicine, Neuromuscular and Skeletal

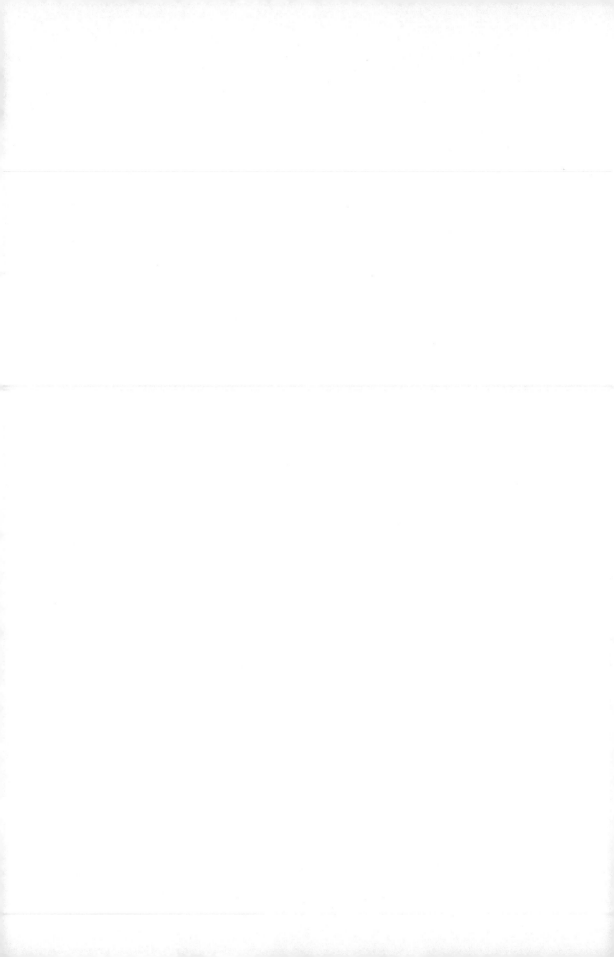

A 60-Year-Old Man With Persistent Coma

Yosuf W. Subat, MD, MPH, and Hilary M. DuBrock, MD

Case Presentation

A 60-year-old man with altered mental status was admitted to the hospital. Five weeks before admission, he had undergone left total knee arthroplasty at another hospital. The patient's medical history was notable for psoriatic arthritis (for which he was taking adalimumab), osteoarthritis, and chronic pain (treated with opioids). After the arthroplasty was completed without complications, the patient was discharged to his home, where his dog reportedly licked the surgical wounds frequently. Two weeks postoperatively, the patient presented to the emergency department at that same hospital with erythema, pain, and swelling of the left knee. Arthrocentesis yielded purulent fluid, and cultures grew *Pasteurella multocida*. The patient underwent incision and drainage with prosthetic exchange. After he began treatment with ceftriaxone, the left knee improved.

The patient recovered relatively well at home over the next 3 weeks, but then he had progressive visual impairment, slurred speech, and imbalance, which prompted a return to the same emergency department. Shortly after he was readmitted to that hospital, the patient had progressive confusion and somnolence, which required intubation for airway protection. Findings were unremarkable from computed tomography (CT) of the head and electroencephalography (EEG). Extensive laboratory evaluation performed at that hospital included a basic metabolic panel, a liver function panel, a

ammonia level, thyrotropin level, morning cortisol level, blood and urine cultures, and urine toxicology screening, but the results were not abnormal. The patient was intubated and sedated with propofol and fentanyl. Examination results were not documented. The next day, the sedative medications were stopped, but the patient appeared to be persistently comatose for the next 5 days. Magnetic resonance imaging (MRI) of the brain and subsequent EEG findings were unremarkable. According to the report from that hospital, the patient had an absence of oculocephalic and pupillary reflexes.

The patient was transferred to a tertiary care center for further evaluation and management. Upon arrival at the medical intensive care unit, the patient was already intubated but was not receiving any sedative medications. The neurology consultation service evaluated the patient and documented the following physical examination findings: temperature 38.4 °C, heart rate 145 beats/min, and blood pressure 162/102 mm Hg. Oxygen saturation was 96% with supplemental oxygen (30% fraction of inspired oxygen). The patient could open his eyes and cough on command but otherwise could not follow simple commands. He had anisocoria. Oculocephalic reflexes were absent, corneal reflexes were intact, and pupillary reflexes were sluggish. He could not move his extremities spontaneously and did not withdraw from painful stimuli. Reflexes were absent in all extremities. The left knee had no evidence of swelling, warmth, or erythema, and the surgical incisions had healed well. Findings were unremarkable from the remainder of the physical examination and bedside point-of-care ultrasonography.

Results were normal for complete blood cell count (CBC), kidney and liver function tests, electrolyte levels, and arterial blood gas tests. The C-reactive protein level was increased (20.4 mg/L). Blood, urine, and tracheal culture results were negative. Findings were unremarkable from radiography of the chest, electrocardiography, and follow-up CT of the head. Although there was no evidence of active infection at the left knee, arthrocentesis was performed because of the possibility that the patient, who was receiving immunosuppressive therapy with adalimumab, could have had persistent septic arthritis with an attenuated inflammatory response. On arthrocentesis, the patient had a total nucleated cell count of 79,000/μL with 87% neutrophils, but the Gram stain and culture results were negative. Therapy with ceftriaxone was continued.

Lumbar puncture results were as follows: clear cerebrospinal fluid (CSF); total nucleated cell count, 1/μL; total protein 62 mg/dL (reference range, 0-35 mg/dL); glucose 80 mg/dL (serum glucose 84 mg/dL); and negative findings with Gram stain. Opening pressure was normal. The increased CSF protein level in combination with a normal CSF white blood cell (WBC) count is known as *albuminocytologic dissociation*, which is the characteristic CSF profile in acute inflammatory demyelinating polyneuropathy (AIDP), also known as Guillain-Barré syndrome (GBS) (1). The impression was probable AIDP, Miller Fisher syndrome (MFS), or Bickerstaff brainstem encephalitis (BBE).

Electromyographic (EMG) findings were consistent with an acute, mixed axonal and demyelinating polyradiculoneuropathy. Follow-up MRI of the brain showed focal enhancement of cranial nerves III and V bilaterally with subcortical and periventricular hyperintensities (Figure 22.1). Serum anti-GQ1b antibody results, which were highly positive (1:12,800), provided confirmation of a diagnosis of MFS, a variant of GBS (2).

Figure 22.1   MRI of the Brain With Contrast Enhancement

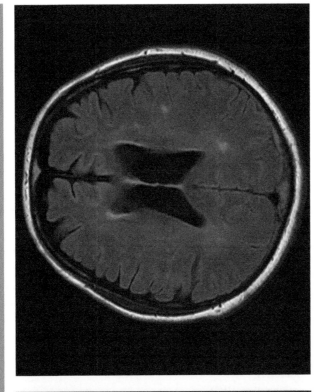

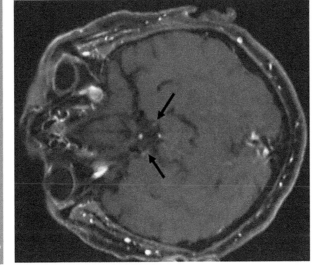

Axial views show bilateral enhancement of cranial nerve III (left; arrows) and multiple new subcortical and periventricular white matter hyperintensities (right).

Questions

Multiple Choice (choose the best answer)

22.1. A patient has subacute, progressive symmetric weakness beginning in both lower extremities. Lumbar puncture provides the following CSF profile: total nucleated cell count, 2/μL; protein, 107 mg/dL (reference range, 0-35 mg/dL); glucose, 70 mg/dL (serum glucose, 74 mg/dL); Gram stain, negative; and opening pressure, 7 cm H_2O. Which of the following diagnoses is most likely?
   a. AIDP
   b. Herpes simplex virus (HSV) encephalitis
   c. HIV-1 meningitis
   d. Anti–N-methyl-D-aspartate (NMDA) receptor encephalitis
   e. Cryptococcal meningitis

22.2. Which of the following is appropriate initial treatment of AIDP?
   a. High doses of glucocorticoids
   b. Broad-spectrum antibiotics
   c. Intravenous immunoglobulin (IVIG)
   d. IVIG and plasma exchange (PLEX)
   e. Levetiracetam

22.3. Results from which of the following tests could support a diagnosis of MFS?
   a. CSF protein 14-3-3
   b. Neuron-specific enolase (NSE)
   c. CSF β_2-transferrin
   d. Serum anti-GQ1b antibody titer
   e. CSF lactate

22.4. Which of the following diagnostic tests is *not* indicated in the initial evaluation of a patient who is comatose?
   a. CT of the head without intravenous (IV) contrast agent
   b. EEG
   c. Intracranial pressure (ICP) monitoring
   d. Lumbar puncture
   e. Arterial blood gas tests

22.5. Which of the following initial interventions is indicated for all patients who present to the emergency department with coma from an unknown cause?
   a. Broad-spectrum antibiotics
   b. Naloxone
   c. Flumazenil
   d. Activated charcoal
   e. Glucose and thiamine

Case Follow-up and Outcome

The patient received 5 days of treatment with IVIG (0.4 g/kg daily). The hypertension, tachycardia, and hyperthermia were thought to be related to dysautonomia due to MFS because it commonly occurs with AIDP. The dysautonomia resolved with the initiation of gabapentin therapy. Ceftriaxone was continued for 6 weeks for septic arthritis. The patient underwent tracheostomy and percutaneous endoscopic gastrostomy (PEG) tube placement during treatment with IVIG (9 days after intubation). He was liberated from the ventilator the day after IVIG therapy was completed. Over the next 3 weeks, he had an excellent recovery with improvement in his strength and vision. The tracheostomy and PEG tubes were decannulated, and the patient was discharged to inpatient rehabilitation. He made a full recovery without long-term deficits.

Discussion

MFS is a variant of AIDP, and patients typically present with ataxia, ophthalmoplegia, and areflexia (2). It was first described in 1956 by a Canadian neurologist, Charles Miller Fisher (3). Similar to AIDP, the condition typically develops after an antecedent illness. MFS is thought to result from a postinfectious autoimmune process and lead to molecular mimicry and subsequent cross-reactivity to peripheral nerves (2).

Positive titers for antibodies against GQ1b, the ganglioside component of nerves, are present in 85% to 90% of patients who have MFS and are strongly associated with oculomotor nerve involvement (4,5). Gangliosides are important components of peripheral nerves and are positioned on the outer surface of the neuronal plasma membrane. Cranial nerves have differential expression of GQ1b, with increased expression on cranial nerves III, IV, and VI, which is consistent with the common finding

of ophthalmoplegia (6). In addition, anti-GQ1b antibodies have pathogenic effects at the peripheral nerves and neuromuscular junction (7).

Anti-GQ1b antibody positivity is present in an array of AIDP variants, including MFS, BBE, and acute ophthalmoparesis (8). BBE can resemble MFS, but BBE often occurs with central nervous system (CNS) involvement, including hyperreflexia and encephalopathy. Patients with MFS can also present with similarities to typical AIDP (also called GBS), with quadriparesis and diaphragmatic weakness. The patient described above in the Case Presentation had the classic triad of MFS (ataxia, ophthalmoplegia, and areflexia) and symptoms of GBS, which probably indicated an overlap of MFS and GBS (9). The overlap of these syndromes has been well characterized, highlighting a common immunologic pathophysiology over a continuous range (10).

Like GBS, MFS typically occurs after an antecedent illness. Infection with *Campylobacter jejuni* has been shown to be the antecedent illness in 31% of cases of GBS and 18% of MFS cases (11). The hypothesis of molecular mimicry in MFS is supported by evidence showing that anti-GQ1b antibodies cross-react with surface epitopes on the lipopolysaccharide of *C jejuni* (12). Like *C jejuni*, *P multocida* is a gram-negative bacterium surrounded by a lipopolysaccharide, but cross-reactivity with anti-GQ1b antibodies has not been demonstrated.

One previous case of MFS after an antecedent illness with *P multocida* has been reported (13). That patient was a 70-year-old woman who had a *P multocida* infection in a prosthetic joint after a cat bite. She presented with ataxia, ophthalmoplegia, and areflexia but with preserved strength and sensation. She received IVIG for 5 days, and her neurologic status gradually improved over several weeks, with full recovery after 5 months.

Although MFS is typically self-limited, IVIG and PLEX are the 2 primary treatments that have been reported to improve recovery. No studies have compared IVIG therapy and PLEX therapy in MFS; therefore, therapy for AIDP variants often resembles that for GBS. Several clinical trials have shown similar effectiveness between IVIG therapy and PLEX therapy for GBS and no additional benefit with combination therapy (14,15).

Although MFS is a rare diagnosis, the case described above highlights the importance of considering a broad differential diagnosis when patients present with coma. A long list of diagnoses can cause or mimic coma, so an extensive evaluation should be performed. Initial evaluation should involve a laboratory evaluation that includes a CBC with a differential count, a basic metabolic panel, coagulation factor tests, liver function tests, arterial blood gas tests, and drug screening. Additional testing can include thyroid function testing, cortisol level, blood cultures, peripheral smear, carboxyhemoglobin level, and screening for medications (eg, acetaminophen and salicylates), toxins, and substance use, depending on the clinical context. Neuroimaging with CT of the head initially, potentially with subsequent MRI of the brain, can be used to evaluate for devastating neurologic causes of coma, such as intracranial hemorrhage, large ischemic stroke, and tumors. The use of EEG is important to rule out nonconvulsive status epilepticus as a cause of coma. Lumbar puncture is also important to evaluate for conditions that can mimic coma, including CNS infections, autoimmune encephalitis, nonconvulsive status epilepticus, subarachnoid hemorrhage, and inflammatory and demyelinating conditions such as AIDP or MFS.

Summary

The classic presentation of patients who have MFS, a variant of AIDP, is the triad of ataxia, ophthalmoplegia, and areflexia. MFS most often occurs after an antecedent illness that is most likely caused by an autoimmune process involving molecular mimicry. The diagnosis of AIDP is supported by a CSF profile that shows an albuminocytologic dissociation (ie, an increased CSF protein level with a normal CSF WBC count) and EMG findings that show demyelination. Serum anti-GQ1b antibody levels are increased in nearly 90% of patients with MFS. AIDP is often self-limited, but treatment with IVIG or PLEX can shorten the recovery time.

Answers

22.1. Answer a.

This CSF profile shows a high protein level with a normal WBC count (ie, *albuminocytologic dissociation*), which commonly occurs with AIDP (also called GBS). Albuminocytologic dissociation is present in the majority of patients who have AIDP (50%-75%), and the prevalence increases 2 to 3 weeks after symptom onset. This finding may be due to increased permeability of the blood-nerve barrier caused by inflammation in AIDP. However, AIDP should not be ruled out in the absence of albuminocytologic dissociation, which is not present in nearly half the patients with AIDP, especially in the first week after symptom onset.

The CSF profile in HSV encephalitis would most likely show lymphocytic pleocytosis and high levels of protein and red blood cells. HIV-1 meningitis would also probably cause lymphocytic pleocytosis and high protein levels. Anti-NMDA receptor encephalitis would most commonly show CSF lymphocytic pleocytosis or oligoclonal bands. Typical findings with cryptococcal meningitis include a WBC count less than 50/μL with a mononuclear predominance, low or normal glucose level, and a high opening pressure (>20 cm H_2O).

Additional information is available in the medical literature (1,16).

22.2. Answer c.

AIDP is often self-limited, but the only treatments that have been shown to shorten recovery time are IVIG and PLEX. In several studies IVIG and PLEX have had similar efficacy, but combination therapy has not shown a clear benefit. Glucocorticosteroid therapy is not effective in treating AIDP or the MFS subtype. Antibiotic therapy is not indicated for AIDP, which is typically caused

by a postinfectious autoimmune process rather than an active infection; however, antibiotics should be used if concomitant infection is present. Antiepileptic medications have no specific use in AIDP. Additional information is available in the medical literature (14,15,17).

22.3. Answer d.

Titers for serum anti-GQ1b (ganglioside antibody) are commonly positive with variants of AIDP, such as MFS or BBE. Anti-GQ1b antibody levels would strongly support a diagnosis of MFS, which can present with ataxia, ophthalmoplegia, and areflexia. Positive titers for antibodies against GQ1b, the ganglioside component of nerve, are present in 85% to 90% of patients who have MFS and are strongly associated with oculomotor nerve involvement.

The presence of protein 14-3-3 in the CSF would support a diagnosis of Creutzfeldt-Jakob disease (CJD), a prion disease. NSE is a nonspecific marker of neuronal destruction that can be increased in several conditions, including CJD, rapidly progressive dementias, and large strokes. Testing for β_2-transferrin can be performed on fluid that is suspected of originating from the CSF, such as in suspected CSF leaks (eg, basilar skull fracture), or on pleural fluid if a dural-pleural fistula is suspected. Detection of β_2-transferrin in known CSF is unhelpful because it would certainly be present. CSF lactate has shown diagnostic accuracy in the differentiation of bacterial meningitis from aseptic meningitis.

Additional information is available in the medical literature (4,6).

22.4. Answer c.

Monitoring of ICP is not recommended as part of the initial evaluation of a patient who is comatose. ICP monitoring is often used when patients have had traumatic brain injury, but it is not the most appropriate method of evaluation for causes of increased ICP, which can cause coma. Initial neuroimaging with CT of the head and possibly subsequent MRI of the brain would be a better approach to screen for conditions that can cause increased ICP and coma, such as intracranial hemorrhage, large ischemic stroke, and tumors.

The differential diagnosis is broad for conditions that can cause or mimic coma. Initial evaluation should involve an extensive laboratory evaluation that includes a CBC with a differential count, a basic metabolic panel, coagulation factor tests, liver function tests, arterial blood gas tests, and drug screening. Additional blood tests such as thyroid testing, cortisol level, blood cultures, blood smear, carboxyhemoglobin level, and screening for medications (eg, acetaminophen and salicylates) should also be considered depending on the clinical context. EEG is important to rule out nonconvulsive status epilepticus, and lumbar puncture is important in the evaluation for conditions that can mimic coma, including CNS infections, subarachnoid hemorrhage, and inflammatory and demyelinating conditions.

Additional information is available in the medical literature (18).

22.5. Answer e.

Glucose and thiamine are indicated for all patients who present to the emergency department with coma or stupor from an unknown cause because hypoglycemia is a common and reversible cause. Thiamine is given in conjunction with glucose to prevent or treat acute Wernicke encephalopathy. Broad-spectrum antibiotic therapy should be initiated for patients if an infection is likely. If a drug overdose is likely, appropriate therapy would be naloxone for opioid intoxication and flumazenil for benzodiazepine intoxication. Although many physicians often use glucose and thiamine in combination with naloxone and flumazenil, a systematic review showed that naloxone and flumazenil should not be used reflexively in all patients because of possible adverse effects and cost-ineffectiveness. However, that study did support the empirical use of glucose and thiamine in all patients. Activated charcoal and gastric lavage could be considered for patients with acute drug overdose or poisoning but should not be used in all patients. Additional information is available in the medical literature (18).

References

1. Yuki N, Hartung HP. Guillain-Barre syndrome. N Engl J Med. 2012;366(24):2294–304.
2. Lo YL. Clinical and immunological spectrum of the Miller Fisher syndrome. Muscle Nerve. 2007;36(5):615–27.
3. Fisher M. An unusual variant of acute idiopathic polyneuritis (syndrome of ophthalmoplegia, ataxia and areflexia). N Engl J Med. 1956;255(2):57–65.
4. Chiba A, Kusunoki S, Obata H, Machinami R, Kanazawa I. Serum anti-GQ1b IgG antibody is associated with ophthalmoplegia in Miller Fisher syndrome and Guillain-Barre syndrome: clinical and immunohistochemical studies. Neurology. 1993;43(10):1911–7.
5. Willison HJ, Veitch J, Paterson G, Kennedy PG. Miller Fisher syndrome is associated with serum antibodies to GQ1b ganglioside. J Neurol Neurosurg Psychiatry. 1993;56(2):204–6.
6. Chiba A, Kusunoki S, Obata H, Machinami R, Kanazawa I. Ganglioside composition of the human cranial nerves, with special reference to pathophysiology of Miller Fisher syndrome. Brain Res. 1997;745(1-2):32–6.
7. Willison HJ, O'Hanlon G, Paterson G, O'Leary CP, Veitch J, Wilson G, et al. Mechanisms of action of anti-GM1 and anti-GQ1b ganglioside antibodies in Guillain-Barre syndrome. J Infect Dis. 1997;176 Suppl 2:S144–9.
8. Shahrizaila N, Yuki N. Bickerstaff brainstem encephalitis and Fisher syndrome: anti-GQ1b antibody syndrome. J Neurol Neurosurg Psychiatry. 2013;84(5):576–83.
9. van Doorn PA. Diagnosis, treatment and prognosis of Guillain-Barre syndrome (GBS). Presse Med. 2013;42(6 Pt 2):e193–201.
10. Verboon C, van Berghem H, van Doorn PA, Ruts L, Jacobs BC. Prediction of disease progression in Miller Fisher and overlap syndromes. J Peripher Nerv Syst. 2017;22(4):446–50.
11. Yuki N, Takahashi M, Tagawa Y, Kashiwase K, Tadokoro K, Saito K. Association of Campylobacter jejuni serotype with antiganglioside antibody in Guillain-Barre syndrome and Fisher's syndrome. Ann Neurol. 1997;42(1):28–33.
12. Jacobs BC, Endtz H, van der Meche FG, Hazenberg MP, Achtereekte HA, van Doorn PA. Serum anti-GQ1b IgG antibodies recognize surface epitopes on Campylobacter jejuni from patients with Miller Fisher syndrome. Ann Neurol. 1995;37(2):260–4.
13. Bennetto LP, Lyons P. Miller Fisher syndrome associated with Pasteurella multocida infection. J Neurol Neurosurg Psychiatry. 2004;75(12):1786–7.
14. Hughes RA, Wijdicks EF, Barohn R, Benson E, Cornblath DR, Hahn AF, et al. Practice parameter: immunotherapy for Guillain-Barre syndrome: report of the Quality Standards Subcommittee of the American Academy of Neurology. Neurology. 2003;61(6):736–40.
15. Patwa HS, Chaudhry V, Katzberg H, Rae-Grant AD, So YT. Evidence-based guideline: intravenous immunoglobulin in the treatment of neuromuscular disorders: report of the Therapeutics and Technology Assessment Subcommittee of the American Academy of Neurology. Neurology. 2012;78(13):1009–15.
16. Fokke C, van den Berg B, Drenthen J, Walgaard C, van Doorn PA, Jacobs BC. Diagnosis of Guillain-Barre syndrome and validation of Brighton criteria. Brain. 2014;137(Pt 1):33–43.
17. Hughes RA, Brassington R, Gunn AA, van Doorn PA. Corticosteroids for Guillain-Barre syndrome. Cochrane Database Syst Rev. 2016;10:CD001446.
18. Hoffman RS, Goldfrank LR. The poisoned patient with altered consciousness: controversies in the use of a 'coma cocktail.' JAMA. 1995;274(7):562–9.

An 83-Year-Old Woman With Obstructive Sleep Apnea at High Altitude

23

Kara L. Dupuy-McCauley, MD, and Bernardo J. Selim, MD

Case Presentation

An 83-year-old woman from the Midwest with a previous diagnosis of obstructive sleep apnea (OSA) presented to the sleep clinic for evaluation of resistant hypertension. She and her husband enjoyed spending time in Colorado and visited the state annually. Their dwelling in Colorado was at an elevation of about 2,550 m (8,500 ft), and she noticed that whenever she was at high altitude she would have poorly controlled hypertension and require the use of multiple medications to decrease her blood pressure to acceptable ranges. At presentation, the hypertension had persisted despite the patient's return to baseline elevation. She had been referred for consultation because poorly controlled sleep apnea was the suspected contributing factor for resistant hypertension.

When she first received a diagnosis of sleep apnea, polysomnography had shown moderate OSA (apnea-hypopnea index of 24 respiratory events per hour) associated with oscillatory oxygen desaturation. The sleep-disordered breathing responded to therapy with continuous positive airway pressure (CPAP) at 7 cm H_2O, so CPAP was prescribed. At her return visit a month later, her level of daytime alertness (according to the Epworth Sleepiness Scale) and sleep quality had improved. Over time, however, although she received adequate OSA treatment as assessed from the CPAP download report while at home in the Midwest, the patient had persistent hypertension and daytime sleepiness while in Colorado. Additionally, her husband related that he had seen episodes of apnea and periodic breathing, which seemed to occur predominately in Colorado. Because of the geographic association of her symptoms, an overnight oximetry test was performed with use of CPAP while the patient breathed room air (fraction of inspired oxygen, 0.21) during her stay in Colorado. Oximetry results showed a low overall baseline oxygen saturation (88%; range, 81%-95%) with nearly continual oscillatory waveform variability suggestive of central sleep apnea (CSA) (Figure 23.1).

The patient's sleep history was updated. She had never smoked, and her weight had been stable. She stated that she did not have nasal congestion and, although she had a large diaphragmatic hernia, that she did not have symptoms of gastroesophageal reflux when she used a wedge pillow while sleeping. She was disturbed by her nocturia, which occurred 1 to 5 times per night, but she did not have prolonged wakefulness. She said that she did not have symptoms of restless legs syndrome or pain that disturbed her sleep. She woke up around 8 to 9 AM with a dry mouth but no headache. Her blood pressure remained poorly controlled despite the use of 3 antihypertensive medications. She was receiving maximum doses

Figure 23.1   Overnight Oximetry Results

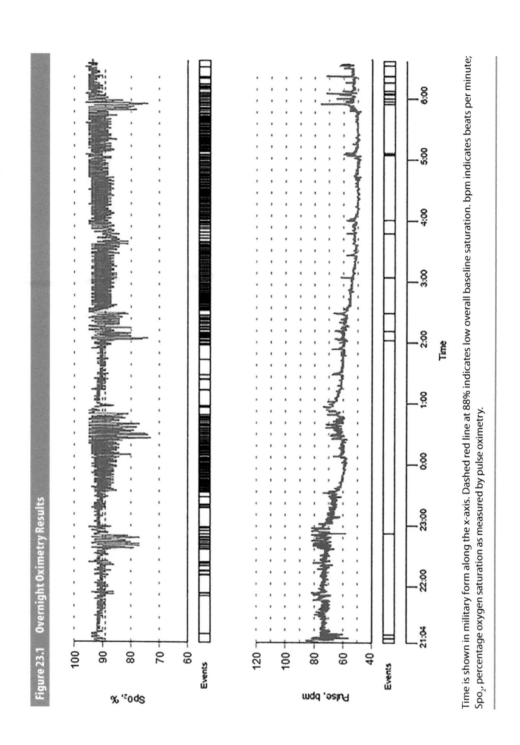

Time is shown in military form along the x-axis. Dashed red line at 88% indicates low overall baseline saturation. bpm indicates beats per minute; Spo₂, percentage oxygen saturation as measured by pulse oximetry.

of hydrochlorothiazide, amlodipine, and lisinopril with only intermittent control of her blood pressure. She did not have any cardiac symptoms, and results from a recent electrocardiogram and echocardiogram were within normal limits.

On physical examination, her nares were patent, and the oropharynx was crowded by a low-hanging soft palate (Mallampati class IV). Findings were normal from examination of her nervous system, heart, and lungs.

Questions

Multiple Choice (choose the best answer)

23.1. Which of the following mechanisms is involved with central apnea and periodic breathing at high altitude?
   a. Increased chemosensitivity to decreasing levels of carbon dioxide
   b. Decrease in arterial oxygen tension (hypobaric hypoxemia)
   c. Increased severity of upper airway obstruction precipitating centrally mediated disordered breathing events
   d. Decreased chemosensitivity to increasing levels of carbon dioxide
   e. Decrease in partial pressure of atmospheric oxygen leading to increased sympathetic tone

23.2. Which of the following statements correctly describes the behavior of OSA at high altitude?
   a. At high altitude, the frequency of obstructive events increases concomitantly with the appearance of central events
   b. At high altitude, obstructive events are nearly always replaced entirely by central events
   c. Both the complete replacement of obstructive events with central events and the appearance of central events in addition to obstructive events have been shown in studies, but changes in the nature and severity may depend on the altitude or the severity of sleep-disordered breathing at the patient's baseline elevation

   d. High altitude tends to bring about severe central events in patients who have severe OSA at the baseline elevation; this is in contrast to mild OSA, in which the patient typically begins to have mild centrally mediated disordered breathing events
   e. Obstructive apnea is known to markedly worsen at high altitude

23.3. Which of the following is a literature-supported therapy for CSA due to other causes but not for high-altitude periodic breathing?
   a. Gradual ascent to high altitude
   b. Acetazolamide
   c. Oxygen supplementation
   d. Benzodiazepines
   e. Adaptive servo-ventilation (ASV)

23.4. What changes occur in sleep architecture at high altitude?
   a. Increased arousals, decrease in stage N1 sleep (light sleep), decrease in rapid eye movement (REM) sleep, and increase in stage N3 sleep
   b. Increased arousals, increase in stage N1 sleep (light sleep), variable effects on REM sleep, and decrease in stage N3 sleep
   c. Decreased arousals, increase in stage N1 sleep (light sleep), increase in REM sleep, and increase in stage N3 sleep
   d. Increased arousals, decrease in stage N1 sleep (light sleep), variable effects on REM sleep, and decrease in stage N3 sleep
   e. Decreased arousals, increase in stage N1 sleep (light sleep), increase in REM sleep, and decrease in stage N3 sleep

23.5. Acute mountain sickness (AMS), another clinical syndrome associated with ascent to high altitude, can include headache, loss of appetite, nausea, vomiting, decreased mental acuity, and insomnia. Which medication can be used to prevent AMS and to treat high-altitude periodic breathing, and how should it be administered?

a. Acetazolamide administered on the day before ascent and 2 days after ascent to high altitude (or longer if ascent is still in progress)

b. Dexamethasone administered twice daily during ascent and until the person is acclimated

c. Temazepam administered nightly while the person is at high altitude

d. Sildenafil administered twice daily during ascent

e. Ibuprofen administered every 8 hours on the day before ascent and 2 days after ascent to high altitude (or longer if ascent is still in progress)

Case Follow-up and Outcome

After the patient completed an overnight oximetry test at high altitude while she was receiving CPAP therapy with no supplemental oxygen, a diagnosis of high-altitude periodic breathing was confirmed. Oxygen supplementation at 2 L was added to her previously prescribed CPAP therapy while she was in Colorado. This intervention targeted hypobaric hypoxemia, an inciting factor for periodic breathing due to high altitude, and proved effective. Shortly thereafter, the patient was able to return to her initial doses of antihypertensive medications for the first time in 10 years with good control of her blood pressure.

Discussion

Unlike the more familiar subtype of CSA, Cheyne-Stokes respiration associated with congestive heart failure, periodic breathing at high altitude occurs in breath clusters with large tidal volumes after each apneic episode. Although a few healthy persons may have periodic breathing at altitudes as low as 1,500 m (5,000 ft), a larger percentage (25%) have periodic breathing at 2,500 m (8,333 ft), and it occurs in virtually everyone at 4,000 m (13,333 ft) (1). High-altitude periodic breathing may occur when a person is asleep or awake even in the absence of a previous diagnosis of sleep-disordered breathing (2). Periodic breathing at high altitude puts the person at risk for daytime symptoms. Cyclical oxygen desaturation leads to frequent nighttime arousals, and sleep quality is degraded as sleep architecture is distorted. The person has decreased sleep efficiency, less stage N3 and REM sleep, and typically a decrease in total sleep time (2).

At high altitude, periodic breathing occurs commonly even in healthy persons (2-4), and for patients who already have a diagnosis of OSA, obstructive events can be replaced by episodes of central apnea or occur in addition to them

(2,5,6). At high altitude, the atmospheric partial pressure of oxygen is lower (hypobaric hypoxia), and hypocapnic chemosensitivity to $Paco_2$ is increased below the apneic threshold (2,4). The net result of these changes is that a smaller variation in gas tension elicits larger changes in ventilation. The first ventilatory change that occurs is an increase in respiratory rate and tidal volume as a result of hypoxia (2,4). As opposed to the periodic breathing in congestive heart failure, which waxes and wanes gradually, periodic breathing at high altitude occurs in smaller clusters with a rapid increase in tidal volume (4). A ventilatory overshoot decreases the $Paco_2$ and induces apnea upon restoration of normoxia (2). During each episode of apnea, $Paco_2$ increases while Pao_2 decreases, once again stimulating respiration (4).

The use of supplemental oxygen can attenuate the hypoxia that incites this chain of events and therefore lessen the propensity for periodic breathing (2). When the oxygen saturation level is restored to normal, periodic breathing continues with apneic periods until the $Paco_2$ returns to normal (4). This periodic pattern of breathing causes repeated arousals that, along with the change in sleep architecture, worsen daytime symptoms. In addition to worsening daytime sleepiness, OSA can increase blood pressure possibly because of sustained hypoxia and repetitive sympathetic activation with each arousal from sleep (6).

At high altitude, sleep apnea is rarely controlled with a patient's home CPAP settings, and some patients require supplemental oxygen and an increase in pressure to decrease the severity of OSA (ie, a decrease in the residual apnea-hypopnea index) (7). Few evidence-based treatment options exist. If descent from high altitude is not an option, adjunctive treatment with acetazolamide or oxygen (or both) has been shown to be effective; however, availability, adverse effects, and practical limitations of the intervention should be considered. Both oxygen and acetazolamide have been shown to improve nocturnal oxygen saturation and decrease central disordered breathing events (6,8). Patients with OSA may still need CPAP to treat obstructive breathing events at high altitude, and in this case, supplemental oxygen or acetazolamide could be used in combination with CPAP therapy (9).

Summary

Sleep-disordered breathing, a prevalent diagnosis, can worsen at high altitude because of increased frequency of centrally mediated disordered breathing events and subsequent increased arousal from sleep with changes in sleep architecture. Consequences may include worse blood pressure control, decreased daytime alertness, and sleep fragmentation (insomnia). Before travel to high altitude, patients should be counseled about the potential for worsening of OSA and the emergence of high-altitude periodic breathing from CSA. If descent from high altitude is not feasible, a change in CPAP or APAP pressure settings with or without either supplemental oxygen or acetazolamide should be considered.

Answers

23.1. Answer b.

High-altitude periodic breathing is driven by hypobaric hypoxemia, which stimulates the peripheral chemoreceptors and results in increased ventilation in patients who have an enhanced ventilatory response to both hypercapnia (not hypocapnia) and hypoxia. Patients with CSA can have pharyngeal narrowing and occlusion during centrally mediated disordered breathing events, but that is not the cause of periodic breathing at high altitude. Patients who have periodic breathing at high altitude typically have increased (not decreased) chemosensitivity to carbon dioxide. While CSA can increase sympathetic output, it is not the cause of high-altitude periodic breathing. Additional information is available in the medical literature (2,10,11).

23.2. Answer c.

The behavior of OSA at high altitude has not been clearly delineated. Studies have suggested that the severity of OSA tends not to increase at high altitude and may even decrease in some cases. In mild OSA, central events can replace obstructive events, but in moderate to severe OSA, central events may occur with obstructive events. Additional information is available in the medical literature (2).

23.3. Answer e.

Therapy with low doses of temazepam has variable effects on high-altitude periodic breathing, but it does improve sleep quality by shortening sleep latency, decreasing arousals, increasing sleep efficiency, and increasing REM sleep. Temazepam has been shown to objectively improve sleep quality for climbers sleeping above 4,000 m (13,333 ft). Although gradual ascent allows for natural acclimatization to high altitude over a few days, with a subsequent decrease in periodic breathing events, it is not always a practical way to manage altitude-induced breathing disturbances and would not be a pertinent recommendation for patients with CSA who are not at high altitude. Acetazolamide improves high-altitude periodic breathing by increasing arterial oxygenation during sleep and decreasing the duration of periodic breathing through renal excretion of bicarbonate, which leads to metabolic acidosis and stimulation of the respiratory center, increasing the P_{CO_2} reserve. In persons with high-altitude periodic breathing, oxygen supplementation increases the arterial oxygen tension, which leads to a more stable breathing pattern by eliminating the overshoot and undershoot caused by hyperventilation in response to hypoxia. Oxygen supplementation has been shown to be effective therapy for high-altitude periodic breathing. Although ASV is an accepted therapy for other kinds of CSA, treatment of high-altitude periodic breathing with ASV has not been shown to be clearly efficacious for decreasing symptoms or decreasing disordered breathing events. Additional information is available in the medical literature (2,8,12-14).

23.4. Answer b.

Many small studies of sleep architecture at high altitude have been published. They generally show an increase in lighter sleep (stage N1), a decrease in slow-wave sleep (stage N3), variable effects on REM sleep, and increased arousals from sleep due to central events associated with high-altitude periodic breathing but also postarousal centrally mediated breathing pauses. Additional information is available in the medical literature (2).

23.5. Answer a.

AMS and high-altitude pulmonary edema (HAPE) often occur with acute exposure to high altitude. Acetazolamide can be used to treat high-altitude periodic breathing and prevent AMS. Dexamethasone is effective in treating AMS but has no known effect on high-altitude periodic breathing. Although temazepam improves sleep quality and lessens the severity of high-altitude periodic breathing, it has no known effect on AMS. Sildenafil can prevent HAPE but does not treat AMS or periodic breathing. Ibuprofen can be used for headache associated with ascent to high altitude but is not effective for prophylaxis or treatment of AMS or high-altitude periodic breathing. Additional information is available in the medical literature (15).

References

1. Burgess KR, Ainslie PN. Central sleep apnea at high altitude. Adv Exp Med Biol. 2016;903:275–83.
2. Principles and practice of sleep medicine. Kryger M, Roth T, Dement WC, editors. 6th ed. Philadelphia (PA): Elsevier; c2017. 1730 pp.
3. Rey de Castro J, Liendo A, Ortiz O, Rosales-Mayor E, Liendo C. Ventilatory cycle measurements and loop gain in central apnea in mining drivers exposed to intermittent altitude. J Clin Sleep Med. 2017;13(1):27–32.
4. Javaheri S, Dempsey JA. Central sleep apnea. Compr Physiol. 2013;3(1):141–63.
5. Burgess KR, Cooper J, Rice A, Wong K, Kinsman T, Hahn A. Effect of simulated altitude during sleep on moderate-severity OSA [published correction appears in Respirology. 2006 Mar;11(2):228]. Respirology. 2006;11(1):62–9.
6. Nussbaumer-Ochsner Y, Schuepfer N, Ulrich S, Bloch KE. Exacerbation of sleep apnoea by frequent central events in patients with the obstructive sleep apnoea syndrome at altitude: a randomised trial. Thorax. 2010;65(5):429–35.
7. Nishida K, Lanspa MJ, Cloward TV, Weaver LK, Brown SM, Bell JE, et al. Effects of positive airway pressure on patients with obstructive sleep apnea during acute ascent to altitude. Ann Am Thorac Soc. 2015;12(7):1072–8.
8. Orr JE, Heinrich EC, Djokic M, Gilbertson D, Deyoung PN, Anza-Ramirez C, et al. Adaptive servoventilation as treatment for central sleep apnea due to high-altitude periodic breathing in nonacclimatized healthy individuals. High Alt Med Biol. 2018 Jun;19(2):178–84. Epub 2018 Mar 13.
9. Latshang TD, Nussbaumer-Ochsner Y, Henn RM, Ulrich S, Lo Cascio CM, Ledergerber B, et al. Effect of acetazolamide and autoCPAP therapy on breathing disturbances among patients with obstructive sleep apnea syndrome who travel to altitude: a randomized controlled trial. JAMA. 2012;308(22):2390–8.
10. Badr MS, Toiber F, Skatrud JB, Dempsey J. Pharyngeal narrowing/occlusion during central sleep apnea. J Appl Physiol (1985). 1995 May;78(5):1806–15.
11. Bradley TD, Floras JS. Sleep apnea and heart failure: Part II: central sleep apnea. Circulation. 2003 Apr 8;107(13):1822–6.
12. Dubowitz G. Effect of temazepam on oxygen saturation and sleep quality at high altitude: randomised placebo controlled crossover trial. BMJ. 1998 Feb 21;316(7131):587–9.
13. Swenson ER, Leatham KL, Roach RC, Schoene RB, Mills WJ Jr, Hackett PH. Renal carbonic anhydrase inhibition reduces high altitude sleep periodic breathing. Respir Physiol. 1991 Dec;86(3):333–43.
14. Lahiri S, Maret K, Sherpa MG. Dependence of high altitude sleep apnea on ventilatory sensitivity to hypoxia. Respir Physiol. 1983 Jun;52(3):281–301.
15. Luks AM, McIntosh SE, Grissom CK, Auerbach PS, Rodway GW, Schoene RB, et al; Wilderness Medical Society. Wilderness Medical Society consensus guidelines for the prevention and treatment of acute altitude illness. Wilderness Environ Med. 2010 Jun;21(2):146–55. Epub 2010 Mar 10. Erratum in: Wilderness Environ Med. 2010 Dec;21(4):386.

An 82-Year-Old Woman With Acute Hypoxic Respiratory Failure

Michelle B. Herberts, MD, Jessica Lau, MD, and William F. Dunn, MD

Case Presentation

An 82-year-old woman with a past medical history that included tobacco use, hypertension, hyperlipidemia, and pulmonary embolism (diagnosed 2 months previously) was admitted to the pulmonology service with acute hypoxic respiratory failure. Over the past 4 months, she had progressively worsening shortness of breath, orthopnea, lower extremity edema, fatigue, and unintentional weight loss. At the onset of her symptoms, she underwent evaluation with a ventilation-perfusion scan, which indicated a low probability for a pulmonary embolism. She was prescribed oral diuretics for her leg edema and orthopnea. When she was evaluated for dyspnea again 2 months after symptom onset, computed tomographic (CT) angiography of the chest showed an embolism of the right pulmonary artery. She was treated with anticoagulation, but her symptoms of weakness, orthopnea, and dyspnea persisted. During outpatient pulmonary consultation, she was hypoxic (oxygen saturation as measured by pulse oximetry [Spo_2], 72% while breathing room air) and was sent to the hospital for direct admission to the pulmonology service.

Upon arrival at the hospital, the patient was hemodynamically stable and Spo_2 was 98% while she was breathing 2 L/min with a nasal cannula. On physical examination she had inspiratory crackles in the lung bases and bilateral lower extremity edema. Initial radiography of the chest showed bilateral pulmonary effusions, and she was given diuretics intravenously. She reported that the dyspnea improved, but she continued to have persistent orthopnea. Subsequently she underwent ultrasonography of the lower extremities, which was negative for acute venous thromboembolism. Echocardiography showed an ejection fraction of 70% to 75%, no regional wall abnormalities, and right ventricular systolic pressure of 48 mm Hg. On further examination, she had muscle fasciculations in her left jaw and chest. Electromyography showed evidence of a diffuse process affecting anterior horn cells and active and chronic denervation in the cervical, thoracic, and lumbosacral segments. After consultation with the neurology service, the conclusion was that the clinical presentation in combination with the electrophysiologic findings were suggestive of amyotrophic lateral sclerosis (ALS).

Questions

Multiple Choice (choose the best answer)

24.1. What is the typical finding when patients present with ALS?
   a. Limb weakness
   b. Dysarthria and dysphagia
   c. Cognitive disturbances
   d. Respiratory failure
   e. Upper extremity tremor

24.2. When motor neuron disease is being considered, which of the following laboratory evaluations is *not* needed?
   a. Complete blood cell count
   b. Kidney function panel
   c. Thyrotropin test
   d. HIV test
   e. Cadmium levels

24.3. What is the most common patient population for sporadic ALS?
   a. White patients
   b. Patients from East Asia
   c. Hispanic patients
   d. Black patients
   e. ALS does not affect 1 population more commonly than others

24.4. Exposure to which of the following has been identified as a potential risk factor for development of sporadic ALS?
   a. Asbestos
   b. Lead
   c. Carbon monoxide
   d. Arsenic
   e. Cadmium

24.5. What pulmonary measure has been found to be most helpful prognostically for patients with ALS?
   a. Forced vital capacity (FVC)
   b. Maximum expiratory pressure (MEP)
   c. Forced expiratory volume in the first second of expiration (FEV_1)
   d. Sniff nasal inspiratory pressure (SNIP)
   e. Total lung capacity

Case Follow-up and Outcome

The patient became somnolent a few days after admission and was found to be hypercapnic (Pco_2, 92 mm Hg). Earlier that day a bedside FVC maneuver showed FVC of 0.85 L (44% of the predicted value). She was then transferred to the intensive care unit for initiation of bilevel positive airway pressure (BiPAP) therapy. CT of the head and spine did not show any acute abnormalities. After she was evaluated by the sleep medicine service, she began nocturnal BiPAP therapy at home. Her condition remained stable, and she was discharged home with resources for ALS specialists and resources in her community.

Discussion

ALS is a progressively worsening neuromuscular disease that usually leads to death 2 to 5 years after diagnosis (1). Although it has no established diagnostic criteria, ALS is characterized by progressively worsening motor weakness without sensory symptoms. Patients usually present with symptoms of limb weakness but may have a chief complaint of dysphagia, dysarthria, behavioral disturbance, or early respiratory failure (2). Signs of upper and lower motor neuron dysfunction are usually present on examination with hyperreflexia, fasciculations, and muscle weakness and atrophy (2).

ALS can be familial or sporadic. Sporadic ALS is more common and accounts for approximately 90% of cases (2,3), and it is more common among White men older than 60 years (2). The other approximately 10% of cases are the familial type, and affected patients usually present at a younger age, they may have only lower motor neuron signs, and they may have more signs of dementia (1,2). Genetic causes for familial ALS are being studied, and the superoxide dismutase 1 gene (SOD1) is the first gene identified (2).

Patients with ALS have progressive respiratory muscular weakness that can lead to hypercapnic respiratory failure, ineffective cough, and recurrent respiratory infections. Death usually occurs approximately 2 to 5 years after the diagnosis and is usually due to respiratory failure (2). Current treatment options include supportive therapy with respiratory support, an exercise regimen, and secretion management. As more genetic targets of ALS become known, novel treatments are being discovered (2). At present only 2 medications, riluzole and edaravone, have been approved by the US Food and Drug Administration for ALS treatment (1).

Respiratory failure and sleep-disordered breathing are relatively common as ALS progresses, and early identification of these disorders is beneficial (4). Noninvasive ventilation has been shown to improve quality of life and morbidity among patients with ALS (3,4). SNIP measurement has been deemed most helpful in prognostication, but often FVC is useful for monitoring patients' lung function. Indications for when to initiate noninvasive ventilation include the following: respiratory symptoms, FVC less than 50% of the predicted value, minimal inspiratory pressure less than 60 cm H_2O or SNIP less than 40 cm H_2O, $Paco_2$ greater than 45 mm Hg, and nocturnal oximetry desaturation less than 88% for 5 minutes or more (5). Once these criteria have been met, initiation of noninvasive ventilation has been shown to increase tracheostomy-free survival and slow the rate of respiratory decline (6).

Summary

When a patient presents with orthopnea, hypoxia, and muscle weakness, ALS should be considered in the differential diagnosis. Patients usually present with lower extremity weakness but can present with bulbar symptoms or respiratory failure. Complications associated with ALS include acute hypoxic and hypercapnic respiratory failure that often requires positive pressure ventilation. Noninvasive ventilator support can improve the quality of life and mortality rates of patients with ALS. Sleep-disordered breathing is also common among patients with ALS, and early identification of this disorder is beneficial.

Answers

24.1. Answer a.

In approximately two-thirds of patients, the earliest sign of ALS is limb weakness. Bulbar weakness and dysphagia are presenting symptoms in one-third of patients. A minority of patients may present with behavioral disturbances and respiratory failure. Additional information is available in the medical literature (2).

24.2. Answer e.

Anemia, kidney dysfunction, thyroid dysfunction, and HIV infection can all cause weakness that must be ruled out during assessment for ALS. Cadmium levels, however, are not related to weakness and do not need to be included in the patient evaluation. Additional information is available in the medical literature (7).

24.3. Answer a.

The prevalence of ALS has been shown to be highest in the White population (5.4 per 100,000) and is more than twice the prevalence in the Black population (2.4 per 100,000). Additional information is available in the medical literature (1).

24.4. Answer b.

High levels of lead in blood and bone have been found among patients who have a diagnosis of ALS. For each doubling of the lead concentration in the blood, the risk of ALS increases 2.6-fold. No correlations have been identified for the other answer choices listed. Additional information is available in the medical literature (8).

24.5. Answer d.

Among the answer choices, SNIP has been shown to decrease the most before initiation of noninvasive ventilation and to provide the most accurate prognostic information. Additional information is available in the medical literature (9).

References

1. Mehta P, Kaye W, Raymond J, Wu R, Larson T, Punjani R, et al. Prevalence of amyotrophic lateral sclerosis: United States, 2014. MMWR Morb Mortal Wkly Rep. 2018 Feb 23;67(7):216–8.
2. Ajroud-Driss S, Siddique T. Sporadic and hereditary amyotrophic lateral sclerosis (ALS). Biochim Biophys Acta. 2015;1852(4):679–84.
3. Sancho J, Servera E, Banuls P, Marin J. Predictors of need for noninvasive ventilation during respiratory tract infections in medically stable, non-ventilated subjects with amyotrophic lateral sclerosis. Respir Care. 2015 Apr;60(4):492–7.
4. Selim BJ, Wolfe L, Coleman JM 3rd, Dewan NA. Initiation of noninvasive ventilation for sleep related hypoventilation disorders: advanced modes and devices. Chest. 2018 Jan;153(1):251–65.
5. Nichols NL, Van Dyke J, Nashold L, Satriotomo I, Suzuki M, Mitchell GS. Ventilatory control in ALS. Respir Physiol Neurobiol. 2013 Nov 1;189(2):429–37.
6. Berlowitz DJ, Howard ME, Fiore JF Jr, Vander Hoorn S, O'Donoghue FJ, Westlake J, et al. Identifying who will benefit from non-invasive ventilation in amyotrophic lateral sclerosis/motor neurone disease in a clinical cohort. J Neurol Neurosurg Psychiatry. 2016 Mar;87(3):280–6.
7. Foster LA, Salajegheh MK. Motor neuron disease: pathophysiology, diagnosis, and management. Am J Med. 2019 Jan;132(1):32–37. Epub 2018 Aug 1.
8. Fang F, Peters TL, Beard JD, Umbach DM, Keller J, Mariosa D, et al. Blood lead, bone turnover, and survival in amyotrophic lateral sclerosis. Am J Epidemiol. 2017;186(9):1057–64.
9. Tilanus TBM, Groothuis JT, TenBroek-Pastoor JMC, Feuth TB, Heijdra YF, Slenders JPL, et al. The predictive value of respiratory function tests for non-invasive ventilation in amyotrophic lateral sclerosis. Respir Res. 2017;18(1):144. Published 2017 Jul 25.

Infections

A 48-Year-Old Man With Recurrent Pneumonia

Ashley M. Egan, MD, and Andrew H. Limper, MD

Case Presentation

A 48-year-old Midwestern farmer with an unremarkable past medical history presented for evaluation of diffuse cutaneous lesions. He reported that he had difficulty hearing approximately 4 months earlier, so he cleaned his ears with hydrogen peroxide, but he said that he overused it and caused a chemical burn on his face.

His primary provider prescribed a 5-day course of prednisone, but after 2 days of prednisone, cutaneous lesions developed along the patient's face and extremities (Figure 25.1). A course of trimethoprim-sulfamethoxazole was prescribed, but the lesions did not improve. The patient stated that the lesions occasionally improved, but they always flared again. The lesions were not painful or pruritic.

Figure 25.1   Skin Lesions on Elbow and Forearm

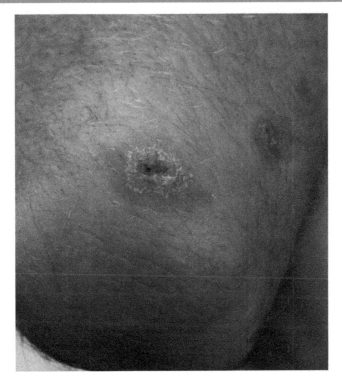

Figure 25.2   CT of the Chest (Lung Window)

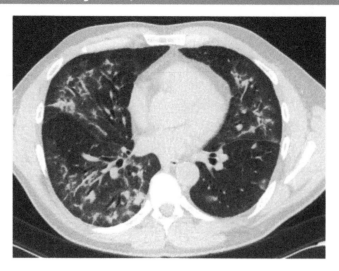

Earlier in the year, the patient had 2 episodes of pneumonia that were treated with azithromycin, but the symptoms did not completely resolve. In the preceding month, he had exertional shortness of breath, nonproductive cough, intermittent fevers, and night sweats. He did not have loss of appetite or weight loss. Given his symptoms, computed tomography (CT) of the chest was performed (Figure 25.2).

The patient was referred to the dermatology service for biopsy of a skin lesion. The biopsy showed pseudocarcinomatous hyperplasia with dermal mixed and granulomatous inflammation. With Gomori methenamine silver stain and periodic acid–Schiff stain in combination with diastase, fungal organisms with broad-based budding yeast forms were seen in the dermis.

Multiple Choice (choose the best answer)

25.1. When broad-based budding yeast cells are seen on microscopic examination of tissue or culture samples, which endemic mycosis is most likely?
a. Histoplasmosis
b. Cryptococcosis
c. Coccidioidomycosis
d. Paracoccidioidomycosis
e. Blastomycosis

25.2. What are the 2 most common sites of infection in disseminated blastomycosis?
a. Lung and brain
b. Bone and lung
c. Skin and bone
d. Lung and skin
e. Lung and urinary tract

25.3. Which statement correctly relates to the diagnosis of blastomycosis?
a. Diagnosis is often delayed because patients commonly receive a misdiagnosis of viral or bacterial pneumonia
b. Healthy patients can have colonization with *Blastomyces*, so growth on culture is not sufficient to make the diagnosis
c. Serologic testing can usually be used to make a definitive diagnosis of active blastomycosis
d. Yeast forms are often easy to identify with hematoxylin-eosin stain, so

additional staining of specimens is not necessary
e. Positive results on urine antigen testing always indicate active infection with *Blastomyces*

25.4. For treatment of blastomycosis, which of the following antimicrobials is correctly matched with disease severity?
a. Amphotericin B for moderate or severe disease
b. Itraconazole for moderate or severe disease
c. Fluconazole for moderate or severe disease
d. Caspofungin for mild or moderate disease
e. Micafungin for mild or moderate disease

25.5. Which of the following correctly describes treatment with azole antifungals?
a. Azole antifungals inhibit the enzyme necessary for conversion of ergosterol to lanosterol, which results in cell membrane damage
b. Itraconazole capsules require food intake and an acidic environment for absorption
c. The itraconazole oral solution should be administered with food
d. Because itraconazole has excellent bioavailability, checking the serum level is not necessary
e. Itraconazole is one of the few azoles that can be used safely in patients with heart disease

Case Follow-up and Outcome

The diagnosis of disseminated blastomycosis was confirmed with culture growth. Itraconazole therapy was initiated, and within 2 weeks the patient's skin lesions and respiratory symptoms improved. Results of an evaluation for an underlying immunocompromised state were negative. After 8 months of therapy, the symptoms and radiographic findings resolved.

Discussion

Blastomyces dermatitidis and *Blastomyces gilchristii* are endemic in North America, particularly in the northern and southeastern US and in areas bordering the Mississippi and Ohio river basins (1,2).

Inhalation of *Blastomyces* spores can result in infection (2,3), and patients can present with symptoms that are acute, subacute, or chronic (3). Infection commonly spreads to other organ systems besides the lungs. Skin is the second most common site of infection (2,3), but infections involving almost every organ system have been reported (2).

Of the several ways to diagnose blastomycosis infection, definitive diagnosis is established only with culture (2). In the appropriate clinical setting, diagnosis can be supported with serology, detection of antigen in urine and serum, and histopathology (2). Unlike the situation with other fungi, such as *Candida*, the identification or growth of *Blastomyces* indicates infection because colonization does not occur.

When blastomycosis is diagnosed, the treatment of choice generally includes amphotericin B for moderate or severe disease and itraconazole for mild or moderate disease (1-3). However, more aggressive treatment, such as amphotericin B, may be indicated if patients have less severe disease that involves certain organs or systems (eg, the central nervous system) or if the status of the immune system is a concern (eg, the patient is immunocompromised) (1-3). Therapy is generally continued for 6 to 12 months (3).

Summary

Although relatively rare, blastomycosis should be considered when patients present with pulmonary symptoms suggestive of pneumonia that have not responded to traditional treatment, especially if other organs are involved. Blastomycosis warrants treatment with antifungal therapy, usually itraconazole, although amphotericin B is appropriate in specific circumstances.

Answers

25.1. Answer e.

Endemic fungi can often be identified easily from their characteristic findings on microscopy. *Blastomyces* yeast cells have broad-based budding, while *Histoplasma* cells have narrow-based budding. The capsule of the *Cryptococcus* yeast form is easily identified with India ink staining. *Coccidioides* fungi classically show spherules, and *Paracoccidioides* have large, round cells with small, attached buds resembling the steering wheel of a ship. Additional information is available in the medical literature (4).

25.2. Answer d.

The point of entry for *Blastomyces* is generally the lungs, and thus the respiratory system is the most common site of infection. The skin is the second most common site of infection, and while direct inoculation can occur, involvement is generally due to dissemination. Published reports have described infection of virtually all organ systems, including bone, the urinary tract, and the central nervous system. Additional information is available in the medical literature (2,3).

25.3. Answer a.

Patients with blastomycosis usually present with symptoms of pneumonia, including fever, cough, and shortness of breath. Imaging often shows infiltrates that mimic pneumonia, so occasionally patients are treated with several courses of antibiotics before the correct diagnosis is determined. The diagnosis of *Blastomyces* is confirmed with culture or polymerase chain reaction because colonization without infection does not occur. Special stains, such as methenamine sliver stain or periodic acid–Schiff stain, are needed to identify yeast forms because hematoxylin-eosin stain is often insufficient. Serologic and urine antigen testing may help guide evaluation but should not be relied upon for a definitive diagnosis of blastomycosis because of the high potential for cross-reactivity with *Histoplasma*. Additional information is available in the medical literature (2).

25.4. Answer a.

Amphotericin B is the recommended antifungal agent for moderate or severe disease. For patients with mild to moderate disease, itraconazole is generally appropriate. While fluconazole has shown good activity against fungi such as *Cryptococcus*, its efficacy against *Blastomyces* has not been consistently demonstrated. Similarly, echinocandins such as caspofungin and micafungin do not have reliable activity. Additional information is available in the medical literature (3).

25.5. Answer b.

Azole antifungals inhibit the enzyme necessary for conversion of lanosterol to ergosterol, which results in increased permeability of the cell membrane and eventual cell damage. Absorption of itraconazole varies depending on its formulation. Adequate absorption of the capsule requires food intake and an acidic environment. Conversely, itraconazole solution should be administered on an empty stomach and is not dependent on gastric acidity. Because of the variable absorption, checking serum itraconazole levels is imperative to ensure therapeutic concentrations. Itraconazole can cause or exacerbate heart failure, so it should be used with caution in patients with cardiac dysfunction. Additional information is available in the medical literature (3,5).

References

1. Chapman SW, Bradsher RW Jr, Campbell GD Jr, Pappas PG, Kauffman CA; Infectious Diseases Society of America. Practice guidelines for the management of patients with blastomycosis. Clin Infect Dis. 2000 Apr;30(4):679–83.

2. McKinnell JA, Pappas PG. Blastomycosis: new insights into diagnosis, prevention, and treatment. Clin Chest Med. 2009 Jun;30(2):227–39.

3. Limper AH, Knox KS, Sarosi GA, Ampel NM, Bennett JE, Catanzaro A, et al; American Thoracic Society Fungal Working Group. An official American Thoracic Society statement: treatment of fungal infections in adult pulmonary and critical care patients. Am J Respir Crit Care Med. 2011 Jan 1;183(1):96–128.

4. Guarner J, Brandt ME. Histopathologic diagnosis of fungal infections in the 21st century. Clin Microbiol Rev. 2011 Apr;24(2):247–80.

5. Willems L, van der Geest R, de Beule K. Itraconazole oral solution and intravenous formulations: a review of pharmacokinetics and pharmacodynamics. J Clin Pharm Ther. 2001 Jun;26(3):159–69.

A 36-Year-Old Man With Recurrent Fevers, Dry Cough, and Weight Loss

Amjad N. Kanj, MD, MPH, and Kelly M. Pennington, MD

Case Presentation

A 36-year-old man presented to the hospital with a 2-month history of recurrent fevers, fatigue, night sweats, dry cough, and unintentional weight loss of 20 lb (9.1 kg). He had no known medical problems, he was not taking any medications, and he said that he did not smoke or use recreational drugs. He immigrated to the US from Southeast Asia 12 years earlier and worked at a glass manufacturing plant.

On physical examination, the patient was febrile (38.4 °C) and had sinus tachycardia (128 beats per minute). He had faint inspiratory crackles over both lung fields. Laboratory test results included normocytic anemia (hemoglobin, 8.1 g/dL) and mild leukocytosis (white blood cell count, 10.6×10^9/L; neutrophils, 98%).

Chest radiography showed right upper lobe paratracheal consolidation with intrinsic cavitation (Figure 26.1). Computed tomography (CT) of the chest showed numerous bilateral pulmonary nodules, bilateral patchy ground-glass opacities, and bilateral hilar and mediastinal lymphadenopathy; there was evidence of a small right-sided pleural effusion and a pericardial effusion (Figure 26.2). CT scans of the abdomen and pelvis were normal. The patient could not produce a sputum sample, so bronchoalveolar washings were collected from the right upper lobe. The washings were positive for acid-fast bacilli, and nucleic acid amplification testing was positive for *Mycobacterium tuberculosis* complex. Serologic testing for HIV was positive, with a viral load of 1.25 million copies/mL and an absolute CD4 count of 6 cells/μL.

Figure 26.1   Radiograph of the Chest, Anteroposterior View

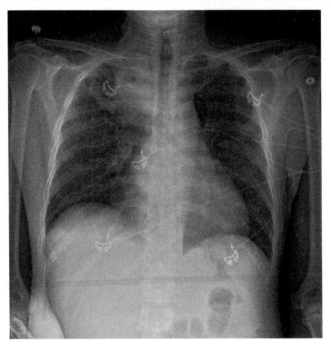

The radiograph shows right upper lobe paratracheal consolidation with intrinsic cavitation and diffuse interstitial thickening.

Figure 26.2   CT of the Chest, Axial Section

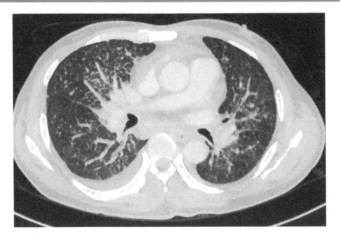

The CT image shows numerous bilateral pulmonary nodules with ground-glass opacities, a small right-sided pleural effusion, and a pericardial effusion.

Questions

Multiple Choice (choose the best answer)

26.1. Which of the following correctly describes antitubercular therapy for this patient?
   a. The continuation phase of therapy consists of isoniazid (INH) and ethambutol (EMB) administered for 2 months
   b. The intensive phase of therapy consists of INH and pyrazinamide (PZA) administered for 4 months
   c. Rifampin (RIF), a potent inhibitor of cytochrome P450 3A4 isozyme (CYP3A4), is preferred over rifabutin
   d. Rapid molecular drug-susceptibility testing for RIF should be performed if RIF is considered for empirical therapy
   e. The patient should be monitored for optic neuritis, an irreversible complication of EMB

26.2. When is the best time to initiate antiretroviral therapy (ART) for this patient?
   a. Before initiation of antitubercular therapy
   b. Within 2 weeks after initiation of antitubercular therapy
   c. Two months after initiation of antitubercular therapy
   d. Three months after initiation of antitubercular therapy
   e. After completion of antitubercular therapy

26.3. Which of the following describes the use of adjunctive corticosteroids in the management of tuberculosis (TB)?
   a. There is no use for adjunctive corticosteroids
   b. Adjunctive corticosteroids are used only if patients have tuberculous meningitis
   c. Use of adjunctive corticosteroids can be considered in patients with HIV and a low CD4 count to prevent immune reconstitution inflammatory syndrome (IRIS)
   d. Use of adjunctive corticosteroids should be considered in all patients with HIV regardless of immune status and CD4 count
   e. Use of adjunctive corticosteroids should be considered in a patient who has pericardial effusion

26.4. Which of the following best describes the imaging pattern and histopathologic features of pulmonary nodules in miliary TB?
   a. Perilymphatic distribution on high-resolution CT (HRCT); atypical spindle cells on histopathology
   b. Centrilobular distribution on HRCT; brown pigment–laden macrophages on histopathology
   c. Random distribution on HRCT; granulomatous inflammation on histopathology
   d. Centrilobular distribution on HRCT; eosinophilic proteinaceous material on histopathology
   e. Centrilobular distribution on HRCT; hyperplasia of cells expressing chromogranin A on histopathology

26.5. Which of the following statements is *not* true about pulmonary TB?
   a. Pulmonary TB is an airborne disease caused by infectious organisms of the *M tuberculosis* complex
   b. Atypical presentations of TB are common in patients with HIV infection
   c. Patients who have HIV infection and active TB infection are less likely to have granulomas on transbronchial biopsy compared to patients who are not infected with HIV
   d. HIV infection and anti–tumor necrosis factor α therapies increase the risk of reactivation of latent TB
   e. Most symptomatic pulmonary TB infections are primary TB, and only 10% are from reactivation of TB

Case Follow-up and Outcome

Miliary TB was diagnosed in this patient, and empirical antitubercular therapy was begun with INH, RIF, PZA, and EMB along with pyridoxine supplementation. INH and RIF rapid molecular drug-susceptibility testing was negative for *Mycobacterium tuberculosis* complex resistance factors for both agents. A few days later, the patient was administered HIV ART and prednisone to prevent IRIS. A case manager was closely involved in the patient's care, and directly observed therapy was planned before the patient was discharged to ensure continuity of care.

At 3-month follow-up, the patient's presenting symptoms had resolved, and CT of the chest showed a decrease in nodularity and in the consolidation size, indicating response to therapy. His CD4 count increased to 122 cells/µL, and the viral load was undetectable. RIF was switched to rifabutin, which is a much less potent CYP3A4 inducer, to allow for ART with a single-tablet combination.

Discussion

TB is an airborne disease caused by infectious organisms of the *M tuberculosis* complex. The disease is most common in resource-limited populations and affects around 10 million people worldwide every year (1).

When an individual is first exposed to *M tuberculosis*, the pathogen is either eliminated by the immune system or persists in a dormant state as a latent TB infection (LTBI). In a minority of patients, the immune system fails to control the primary infection, which results in primary TB (2).

In patients with LTBI, *M tuberculosis* organisms are contained within granulomas. These patients are asymptomatic but may well benefit from treatment aimed at preventing progression to active TB disease (2). In an estimated 10% of immunocompetent individuals, LTBI progresses to active TB at some point in life. Patients with active disease have various symptoms, such as fever, cough, and weight loss. Occasionally, the progression from the latent state to the active state is subtle, and patients present with abnormal findings on chest radiography without clinical symptoms. HIV infection and active use of tumor necrosis factor α inhibitors are both well-known risk factors for progression to active TB disease (2).

Chest imaging of patients who have active TB may show infiltrates and areas of consolidation and cavitation with a predilection to posterior segments of the upper lobes and superior segments of the lower lobes. Centrilobular nodules and a tree-in-bud pattern may also be seen with endobronchial spread (3). Miliary TB, which results from hematogenous dissemination of the disease, is characterized by innumerable tiny, randomly distributed nodules and often localized or diffuse ground-glass opacities (3).

Acid-fast bacilli smear microscopy, cultures, and nucleic acid amplification testing should be performed on respiratory samples of patients who may have active TB disease (4). When a sputum sample cannot be induced, or when TB is a high consideration despite negative findings with acid-fast bacilli smear microscopy, flexible bronchoscopy with sampling should be pursued. Sampling should include bronchoalveolar washings or either bronchial brushing or transbronchial biopsies (or both) if patients have miliary TB without draining lesions or cavities. If patients have HIV infection and active TB disease, granulomas are less likely to be seen on transbronchial biopsy than if patients do not have HIV infection (4).

All patients with active TB disease should be tested for HIV. HIV-infected patients are at increased risk for extrapulmonary TB. Adenosine deaminase and interferon-γ levels should be measured in fluid collected from patients with suspected pleural, pericardial, or peritoneal TB or TB meningitis (4).

First-line treatment of active TB disease with no known drug resistance consists of a 2-month *intensive phase* with INH, RIF, PZA, and EMB and then a 4-month *continuation phase* with INH and RIF, which can be extended further depending on disease response (5). Pyridoxine (vitamin B$_6$) is given in combination with INH to all patients who are at risk for neuropathy, including patients with HIV infection. INH, RIF, and PZA are associated with drug-induced liver injury. EMB can cause optic neuritis, which is usually reversible but requires prompt discontinuation of the drug. RIF is a potent CYP3A4 inducer that can increase the clearance of various drugs, including those used in management of HIV infection. In patients during pregnancy, PZA is occasionally excluded from the regimen, which then requires an extension of the continuation phase to 7 months (for a total treatment duration of 9 months) (5).

Rapid molecular drug-susceptibility testing for INH and RIF should be considered for select patients, including patients with HIV infection, patients with a history of treated TB, and patients with a risk for multidrug-resistant TB. Culture-based drug-susceptibility testing is the gold standard, but results may take much longer (4).

TB is a common cause of death among patients with HIV. The treatment of TB in HIV-infected patients is challenging because they are at increased risk for drug-drug interactions. For untreated HIV-infected patients who have TB, the prognosis is better with early initiation of ART, but early therapy increases the risk of IRIS. Ideally, ART should be initiated within the first 2 weeks of TB treatment if patients have a CD4 count of less than 50 cells/µL and within 8 to 12 weeks if patients have a CD4 count of at least 50 cells/µL (5). In a randomized placebo-controlled trial, administration of prednisone during the first 4 weeks after ART initiation resulted in a lower incidence of TB-associated IRIS in HIV-infected patients with a CD4 count of 100 cells/µL or less; no difference was observed in the risk of severe infections and malignancy (6). Adjunctive corticosteroids are not used for tuberculous pericarditis, but for tuberculous meningitis a long course of corticosteroids with a tapering dose should be considered (5).

Summary

TB is most common in resource-limited populations and has major public health implications. Usually the disease arises from reactivation of a latent focus in the lungs. Prompt diagnosis and effective treatment are essential. Adjunctive corticosteroids are important in the management of tuberculous meningitis and should be considered during the first 4 weeks after ART initiation in HIV-infected patients who have active TB disease and are at risk for TB-associated IRIS.

Answers

26.1. Answer d.

When RIF is considered for empirical therapy in patients with HIV, rapid molecular drug-susceptibility testing should be performed. Treatment of uncomplicated, culture-positive, active pulmonary TB disease with no known drug resistance consists of 6 months of multidrug therapy. The first 2 months of therapy are the intensive phase, which generally consists of treatment with INH, RIF, PZA, and EMB; the next 4 months are the continuation phase, which usually consists of treatment with INH and RIF. RIF is a more potent CYP3A4 inducer than rifabutin and can cause serious drug-drug interactions. EMB, commonly used in the intensive phase of therapy, is associated with optic neuritis, which is typically reversible with prompt discontinuation of therapy. Additional information is available in the medical literature (4).

26.2. Answer b.

This patient should receive ART during the first 2 weeks of his TB therapy. TB-associated IRIS is more common in patients with active TB and HIV infection, and early initiation of ART can reduce mortality. ART should be initiated during the first 2 weeks of TB treatment in patients with CD4 counts less than 50 cells/μL. In patients with CD4 counts of at least 50 cells/μL, ART should be initiated within the first 8 to 12 weeks of TB treatment. Additional information is available in the medical literature (5).

26.3. Answer c.

In a randomized trial, the incidence of TB-associated IRIS was lower when adjunctive corticosteroids were used during the first 4 weeks after initiation of ART in HIV-infected patients who had active TB disease and CD4 counts of 100 cells/μL or less. Corticosteroids are also used in patients with tuberculous meningitis and may provide a mortality benefit. Adjunctive corticosteroids are not used in patients who have TB and pericarditis. Additional information is available in the medical literature (5,6).

26.4. Answer c.

Nodules in miliary TB assume a random distribution and generally show granulomatous inflammation on histopathology. The other descriptions are more characteristic of nodules in other diseases of the lung, such as Kaposi sarcoma (perilymphatic distribution with atypical spindle cells), respiratory bronchiolitis (centrilobular distribution with brown pigment–laden macrophages), acute silicoproteinosis (centrilobular distribution with eosinophilic proteinaceous material), and diffuse idiopathic pulmonary neuroendocrine cell hyperplasia (hyperplasia of cells expressing chromogranin A). Additional information is available in the medical literature (3).

26.5. Answer e.

Among patients who are not immunocompromised, reactivation of TB accounts for 90% of the active TB infections. Additional information is available in the medical literature (2,4).

References

1. Furin J, Cox H, Pai M. Tuberculosis. Lancet. 2019;393(10181):1642–56.
2. Pai M, Behr MA, Dowdy D, Dheda K, Divangahi M, Boehme CC, et al. Tuberculosis. Nat Rev Dis Primers. 2016;2:16076.
3. Nachiappan AC, Rahbar K, Shi X, Guy ES, Mortani Barbosa EJ Jr, Shroff GS, et al. Pulmonary tuberculosis: role of radiology in diagnosis and management. Radiographics. 2017;37(1):52–72.
4. Lewinsohn DM, Leonard MK, LoBue PA, Cohn DL, Daley CL, Desmond E, et al. Official American Thoracic Society/Infectious Diseases Society of America/Centers for Disease Control and Prevention Clinical Practice Guidelines: Diagnosis of Tuberculosis in Adults and Children. Clin Infect Dis. 2017;64(2):111–5.
5. Nahid P, Dorman SE, Alipanah N, Barry PM, Brozek JL, Cattamanchi A, et al. Official American Thoracic Society/Centers for Disease Control and Prevention/Infectious Diseases Society of America Clinical Practice Guidelines: Treatment of Drug-Susceptible Tuberculosis. Clin Infect Dis. 2016;63(7):e147–e95.
6. Meintjes G, Stek C, Blumenthal L, Thienemann F, Schutz C, Buyze J, et al. Prednisone for the prevention of paradoxical tuberculosis-associated IRIS. N Engl J Med. 2018;379(20):1915–25.

A 37-Year-Old Man With Sudden Loss of Vision

Kathryn T. del Valle, MD, and Eric S. Edell, MD

Case Presentation

A 37-year-old man from northern Minnesota presented to the Department of Ophthalmology with sudden loss of vision in the left eye 2 weeks earlier. There was no ophthalmologic history, and he felt well otherwise without fevers, chills, headache, shortness of breath, or other new symptoms. His social history was notable for on-going tobacco use (he smoked 1 pack daily and had an approximately 20-pack-year history, and

he regularly used chewing tobacco). The patient's body mass index was 45 (calculated as weight in kilograms divided by height in meters squared). He worked as a truck driver, frequently traveling across the US. He was also a hunter and fisherman. The patient was not taking any prescribed or over-the-counter medications.

On funduscopic examination, the patient had a lesion in the left eye temporal to the macula that was most consistent with a subretinal abscess (Figure 27.1). Other findings on the initial

Figure 27.1   Funduscopic Examination

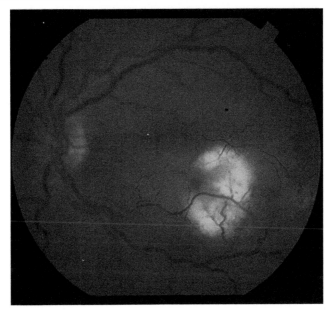

A lesion in the left eye temporal to the macula was most consistent with a subretinal abscess.

physical examination were unremarkable. He did not have a fever, and his vital signs were normal. Breath sounds were normal bilaterally without wheezes or crackles, and a cardiac murmur was not heard. Aside from loss of vision in the left eye, the neurologic examination findings were normal. Laboratory evaluation was notable for a mildly elevated white blood cell count (11.3×10^9/L); otherwise, the blood count results were normal, and the results for the electrolyte panel, liver function tests, C-reactive protein, and basic autoimmune testing (rheumatoid factor and antineutrophil cytoplasmic autoantibody screen) were within the reference ranges. Results for several infectious studies were pending. Given concern for an underlying infection, malignancy, or another systemic process, the patient underwent computed tomography (CT) of the chest, which showed a large mass (approximately 6×5 cm) in the left upper lobe with possible central necrosis and a slightly enlarged left hilar lymph node (Figure 27.2).

The patient was referred to the infectious diseases service, where serologic results were negative for HIV, cytomegalovirus, *Bartonella*, *Histoplasma*, and *Blastomyces*, and the interferon-gamma release assay was negative for *Mycobacterium tuberculosis*. The patient underwent bronchoscopy with fluoroscopic guidance with transbronchial biopsy of the left lung mass and bronchoalveolar lavage (BAL), and endobronchial ultrasonography (EBUS)-guided transbronchial needle aspiration of the station 11L hilar lymph node. Pathologic examination of the lung mass showed granulation tissue with fungal organisms and necrosis. Special stains (Grocott methenamine silver, periodic acid–Schiff with diastase, Gram, and mucicarmine) highlighted encapsulated yeast forms most consistent with *Cryptococcus*. Fungal culture from BAL ultimately grew *Cryptococcus gattii*, and EBUS sampling of the hilar node showed only lymphocytes consistent with lymph node sampling.

Figure 27.2   CT of the Chest

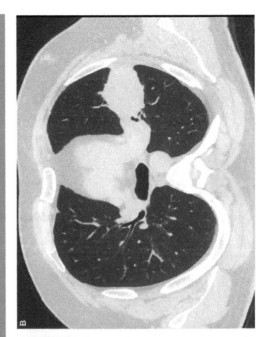

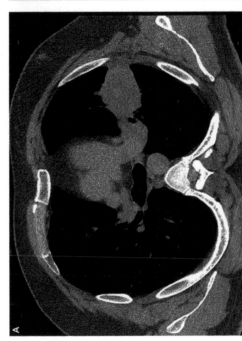

In the left upper lobe in these axial views, a large mass was present with possible central necrosis and a slightly enlarged left hilar lymph node. A, Mediastinal windows. B, Lung windows.

Questions

Multiple Choice (choose the best answer)

27.1. Which of the following do *not* typically cause pulmonary mass lesions?
   a. Fungal infections
   b. Mycobacterial infections
   c. Viral respiratory infections
   d. Bacterial infections
   e. Neoplasms

27.2. Which of the following sites is *least* commonly involved in disseminated *C gattii* infection?
   a. Eyes
   b. Joints
   c. Lungs
   d. Central nervous system
   e. Intra-abdominal sites

27.3. Which of the following aspects of the patient's history most likely increased his risk for *C gattii* infection?
   a. Obesity
   b. Fishing hobby
   c. Age
   d. Work as a truck driver traveling across the US
   e. Smoking

27.4. Which of the following should be performed if infection with *C gattii* is suspected?
   a. Lumbar puncture and chest imaging
   b. Electroencephalography and referral to a neurologist
   c. Echocardiography
   d. Contact tracing
   e. Referral to a dermatologist

27.5. Which of the following correctly describes the management of *C gattii* infections?
   a. Surgical intervention is the mainstay of treatment
   b. Antifungal therapy recommendations are generally similar to those for infections with *Cryptococcus neoformans*
   c. Use of amphotericin B should be avoided
   d. Duration of treatment is typically no more than 1 month
   e. Treatment typically should include only the best supportive care

Case Follow-up and Outcome

The patient's clinical presentation, pathology results, and imaging findings are consistent with a diagnosis of disseminated *C gattii* infection. Results for serum *Cryptococcus* antigen were positive, and the patient underwent lumbar puncture for evaluation for possible involvement of the central nervous system (CNS). The opening pressure was high (25.5 cm H_2O). Results of cerebrospinal fluid (CSF) analysis were notable for a high total nucleated cell count (272 cells/μL) with lymphocytic predominance (75%), high total protein (124 mg/dL), glucose concentration of 45 mg/dL, and positivity for *Cryptococcus* antigen. CT of the head without contrast material was negative for masses, hydrocephalus, hemorrhage, and other abnormalities. The patient was admitted to the hospital for induction antifungal therapy with amphotericin B and flucytosine. He was discharged with plans for long-term antifungal therapy, multiple intravitreal amphotericin B injections, and surgical drainage of the subretinal abscess.

Discussion

The differential diagnosis for lung nodules or masses is often broad, particularly for young, otherwise healthy patients. Malignancy should always be considered, but it is less likely in younger patients. Therefore, in addition to a thorough history and physical examination, evaluation should include tests for infection that are tailored to the patient's immune status and exposure history, autoimmune screening, and consideration of bronchoscopy or CT-guided lung biopsy to obtain pathology specimens. Infectious causes of pulmonary masses include fungal, mycobacterial, atypical, and bacterial pathogens. Noninfectious causes include autoimmune and other inflammatory disorders, such as vasculitis and sarcoidosis.

Patients who have infections with the fungal pathogen *C gattii* can present with pulmonary mass lesions or CNS manifestations (or both). The *C gattii* species complex includes 4 subspecies, each with a geographic preference; it was first identified as a pathogen in Australia and New Zealand, where it is considered endemic. An outbreak in British Columbia, Canada in the late 1990s led to its first recognition as an important fungal pathogen in North America, particularly in the Pacific Northwest (1). The patient described above, by driving a truck throughout the US, most likely had an increased exposure risk. Environmental sources of *C gattii* include *Eucalyptus* and other trees. Tree flowering, the presumed primary method of transmission, increases airborne dispersal of yeast or spores. Human-to-human transmission of *C gattii* does not occur (1,2).

A few key differences distinguish *C gattii* from its better-known relative, *C neoformans*: 1) *C gattii* often causes large masses (cryptococcomas) in the lungs or brain; 2) *C gattii* occurs more frequently in hosts who are immunocompetent rather than immunocompromised; 3) *C neoformans* classically presents in patients who have HIV infection, AIDS, or other forms of immune deficiency (3); and 4) although both species commonly cause neurologic disease, *C gattii* is more frequently associated with long-term neurologic sequelae (4). Only within the past several years has *C gattii* been classified as its own species; previously it was considered a species variant of *C neoformans* (5).

Typically the incubation period of *C gattii* in humans is prolonged (often 2-12 months or longer; median, 6-7 months) (6). Some patients may initially have a flulike syndrome within the first few weeks after exposure (7). Although the most frequently involved sites are the lungs, CNS, and eyes, constitutional symptoms and cutaneous manifestations may be present, but the majority of patients do not have them (1). In addition to pulmonary cryptococcomas, which are commonly asymptomatic, patients may have pneumonia symptoms, including dyspnea and cough. Patients with disease of the CNS usually have meningitis or mass lesions in the brain and typically present with headache and neck stiffness. Ophthalmologic involvement may include abscesses, as seen in this patient, and papilledema and optic disc swelling. Although immunocompetent patients are more often affected by *C gattii*, infection also occurs in those with immune compromise, particularly in those with HIV infection (1,3).

Diagnosis of suspected cryptococcal infection—with either *C gattii* or *C neoformans*—can be challenging and often requires complex, multisystem evaluation. Lumbar puncture should be performed in all patients with suspected or confirmed cryptococcal infection. Patients with cryptococcal meningitis typically have elevated opening pressure, which is a surrogate marker for elevated intracranial pressure (1). Evaluation of the CSF should include *Cryptococcus* antigen testing, India ink staining, and fungal culture. Additionally, CT of the head should be performed to rule out mass lesions or hydrocephalus. Funduscopic examination to assess for ophthalmologic lesions is also universally recommended. Serologic testing for *Cryptococcus* antigen can be helpful, especially for confirmation of disseminated disease, but typically additional pathologic or CSF studies are needed to finalize the diagnosis (8). If infection with *C gattii* is particularly suspected, lung imaging should be performed to screen for a cryptococcoma or other pulmonary involvement. As with this patient, pathology findings from lung masses can be extremely useful in confirming the diagnosis.

Treatment of *C gattii* infections varies and depends on a patient's particular disease manifestations. Generally, though, treatment requires prolonged antifungal therapy, similar to the treatment of *C neoformans* infections. Current guidelines from the Infectious Diseases Society of America and the American Thoracic Society recommend induction antifungal therapy with amphotericin B and flucytosine for patients who have *C gattii* or *C neoformans* meningoencephalitis. A similar regimen is recommended for those with large pulmonary cryptococcomas. For nearly all *C gattii* infections, regardless of the involved sites or degree of severity, long-term maintenance therapy (for ≥6-18 months) with antifungals such as fluconazole is recommended (9,10). In certain circumstances, surgical or other procedural interventions may be considered if the response to antifungal therapy is inadequate.

Summary

The fungal pathogen *C gattii* commonly occurs in the Pacific Northwest and most often affects the lungs, CNS, and eyes. Unlike its better-known relative, *C neoformans*, *C gattii* occurs more often in immunocompetent rather than immunocompromised hosts and is notably more likely to cause large pulmonary and brain mass lesions known as cryptococcomas. If a diagnosis of *C gattii* infection is strongly suspected, lumbar puncture, funduscopic examination, and head and chest imaging should be routinely performed. Standard treatment typically includes induction antifungal therapy with amphotericin B and flucytosine with subsequent prolonged treatment with fluconazole.

Answers

27.1. Answer c.

Unlike the other answer choices, viral infections do not typically cause pulmonary mass lesions. Additional information is available in the medical literature (11).

27.2. Answer e.

The eyes, joints, lungs, and central nervous system are commonly involved in *C gattii* infections. Intra-abdominal infection is relatively uncommon. Additional information is available in the medical literature (1).

27.3. Answer d.

The patient's work as a truck driver who traveled across the US most likely increased his risk for *C gattii* infection, which is generally more common in the Northwest. The other answer choices are not well-established risk factors. Additional information is available in the medical literature (7,12).

27.4. Answer a.

Lumbar puncture should be done to screen for CNS involvement given its high prevalence in *C gattii* disease, and chest imaging should be done to evaluate for pulmonary involvement. Electroencephalography and referral to a neurologist are not indicated in the initial evaluation stage. Cardiac involvement and serious dermatologic disease are relatively rare, so echocardiography and referral to a dermatologist are not routinely indicated. Human-to-human transmission is exceedingly rare, so contact tracing is not necessary. Additional information is available in the medical literature (1,7-9).

27.5. Answer b.

Antifungal therapy recommendations are generally similar to those for infections with *Cryptococcus neoformans*. The other choices are not accurate for the treatment of *Cryptococcus* infection. Additional information is available in the medical literature (9,10).

References

1. Chen SC, Meyer W, Sorrell TC. *Cryptococcus gattii* infections. Clin Microbiol Rev. 2014 Oct;27(4):980–1024.
2. Centers for Disease Control and Prevention. *C. gattii* infection [Internet]. [Cited 3-17-21]. c2021. Available from: https://www.cdc.gov/fungal/diseases/cryptococcosis-gattii/index.html.
3. Chen S, Sorrell T, Nimmo G, Speed B, Currie B, Ellis D, et al; Australasian Cryptococcal Study Group. Epidemiology and host- and variety-dependent characteristics of infection due to *Cryptococcus neoformans* in Australia and New Zealand. Clin Infect Dis. 2000 Aug;31(2):499–508. Epub 2000 Sep 7.
4. Speed B, Dunt D. Clinical and host differences between infections with the two varieties of *Cryptococcus neoformans*. Clin Infect Dis. 1995 Jul;21(1):28–34.
5. Chaturvedi V, Chaturvedi S. *Cryptococcus gattii*: a resurgent fungal pathogen. Trends Microbiol. 2011 Nov;19(11):564–71. Epub 2011 Aug 29.
6. MacDougall L, Fyfe M. Emergence of *Cryptococcus gattii* in a novel environment provides clues to its incubation period. J Clin Microbiol. 2006 May;44(5):1851–2.
7. Diaz JH. The disease ecology, epidemiology, clinical manifestations, and management of emerging *Cryptococcus gattii* complex infections. Wilderness Environ Med. 2020 Mar;31(1):101–9. Epub 2019 Dec 6.
8. Johannson KA, Huston SM, Mody CH, Davidson W. *Cryptococcus gattii* pneumonia. CMAJ. 2012 Sep 4;184(12):1387–90. Epub 2012 Aug 13.
9. Perfect JR, Dismukes WE, Dromer F, Goldman DL, Graybill JR, Hamill RJ, et al. Clinical practice guidelines for the management of cryptococcal disease: 2010 update by the Infectious Diseases Society of America. Clin Infect Dis. 2010 Feb 1;50(3):291–322.
10. Limper AH, Knox KS, Sarosi GA, Ampel NM, Bennett JE, Catanzaro A, et al; American Thoracic Society Fungal Working Group. An official American Thoracic Society statement: treatment of fungal infections in adult pulmonary and critical care patients. Am J Respir Crit Care Med. 2011 Jan 1;183(1):96–128.
11. Snoeckx A, Dendooven A, Carp L, Desbuquoit D, Spinhoven MJ, Lauwers P, et al. Wolf in sheep's clothing: primary lung cancer mimicking benign entities. Lung Cancer. 2017 Oct;112:109–117. Epub 2017 Aug 5.
12. MacDougall L, Fyfe M, Romney M, Starr M, Galanis E. Risk factors for *Cryptococcus gattii* infection, British Columbia, Canada. Emerg Infect Dis. 2011 Feb;17(2):193–9.

A 71-Year-Old Woman With Diarrhea and Recurrent Fever[a]

Swathi S. Sangli, MD, John C. O'Horo, MD,
and Paul D. Scanlon, MD

Case Presentation

A 71-year-old woman was admitted to the hospital with a history of diarrhea and recurrent fever for 4 weeks. Her medical history included obesity, peripheral arterial disease, coronary artery disease, hyperlipidemia, rheumatoid arthritis (RA), and diabetes. Her medications included aspirin, atorvastatin, metoprolol, methotrexate, hydroxychloroquine, and infliximab. She recently traveled to South Dakota and Missouri, where she was exposed to mosquitoes and "exotic birds." Her recent medical history included knee injections for RA.

The patient did not have any localizing symptoms. Laboratory test results indicated anemia, thrombocytopenia, and elevated levels of aspartate aminotransferase, bilirubin, lactic acid, and creatinine. After blood was drawn for cultures, treatment was started with vancomycin, cefepime, and doxycycline. Antibody titers were negative for tickborne illnesses, including anaplasmosis, Rocky Mountain spotted fever, babesiosis, ehrlichiosis, bartonellosis, and Lyme disease. Titers were also negative for viral hepatitis, Epstein-Barr virus, and HIV. Findings from ultrasonography of the liver were consistent with hepatic steatosis. Computed tomography of the abdomen and pelvis showed severe atherosclerosis with possible high-grade stenosis of the superior mesenteric artery. Acute deep vein thrombosis was ruled out after Doppler ultrasonography of the patient's lower extremities.

---

[a] Presented at the American Thoracic Society, San Diego, California, May 18–23, 2018.

Questions

Multiple Choice (choose the best answer)

28.1. With the information available so far, what diagnostic study would most likely confirm the correct diagnosis?
   a. Lumbar puncture
   b. Fungal antigen testing
   c. Bone marrow biopsy
   d. Peripheral smear
   e. Stool studies

28.2. Which of the following is *not* a cause of primary adrenal insufficiency?
   a. *Mycobacterium tuberculosis*
   b. Adrenal hemorrhage
   c. Autoimmune adrenalitis
   d. Histoplasmosis
   e. Sheehan syndrome

28.3. If the patient has high ferritin levels, what should be the next step?
   a. Magnetic resonance imaging of the hip
   b. Liver biopsy
   c. Bone marrow biopsy
   d. Further management
   e. Genetic testing

28.4. Which of the following is *not* a diagnostic criterion for hemophagocytic lymphohistiocytosis (HLH)?
   a. Increased levels of CD25
   b. Increased levels of interleukin 6
   c. Low or absent NK cell activity
   d. Peripheral blood cytopenia
   e. Splenomegaly

28.5. What is the first step in the management of a clinically stable infection associated with HLH?
   a. Administration of etoposide
   b. Treatment with hematopoietic stem cell transplant
   c. Treatment of underlying sepsis
   d. Administration of cyclosporine
   e. Administration of methotrexate

Case Follow-up and Outcome

Fungal studies were performed because the patient had a recent history of immunocompromising therapy, travel, and recurrent fever, and the recent test results indicated peripheral blood cytopenia (involving erythrocytes and platelets) and liver dysfunction. *Histoplasma* antigen was present in urine (3.41 ng/mL) and serum (16.57 ng/mL). Blood cultures grew *Histoplasma capsulatum* after 5 days. Therapy was promptly started with amphotericin B liposomal complex (4 mg/kg) and itraconazole.

The patient was transferred to the intensive care unit (ICU) because she had episodes of hypoglycemia over a 24-hour period despite dextrose administration and continued oral intake. Her condition suggested adrenal involvement, so she was given hydrocortisone therapy for several days. When her medical condition stabilized, she was transferred from the ICU, but her hemodynamic status became unstable, so she was readmitted to the ICU.

On laboratory evaluation, the fibrinogen level was low (170 mg/L), which was consistent with disseminated intravascular coagulation. Further testing showed high levels of inflammatory markers, including C-reactive protein (94.2 mg/L) and serum ferritin (which peaked at 13,850 µg/L). The markedly high ferritin level prompted consideration of secondary HLH. Bone marrow biopsy results were consistent with HLH (Figure 28.1). The patient was successfully treated with antifungal therapy for disseminated histoplasmosis and ruxolitinib for HLH. When her condition was stable, she was transferred out of ICU and was subsequently discharged home to continue antifungal therapy. She continued to have follow-up evaluations with the rheumatology and infectious diseases services.

Discussion

When an immunocompromised patient has sepsis, multiorgan dysfunction, and thrombocytopenia, the differential diagnosis can be broad. A patient with a history of recent travel and immunosuppression should prompt consideration of fungal infections that reflect their geographic distribution. Immunosuppression alone is a strong risk factor for histoplasmosis and may predispose a patient to dissemination in several organs. Dissemination often occurs in patients who are especially young or old, who have AIDS or primary immunodeficiency, or who have received immunosuppressive medications (like the patient described above). The immunosuppressive medications include systemic corticosteroids (with prolonged exposure), antirejection therapies in solid organ transplant recipients, and tumor necrosis factor α (TNF-α) inhibitors. Disseminated histoplasmosis can be diagnosed after microscopic identification of *Histoplasma* from bronchoalveolar lavage, tissue culture, blood culture, or bone marrow biopsy.

A point that must be emphasized is that histoplasmosis can be an important complication in patients who are receiving TNF-α inhibitors, especially infliximab. Some clinicians who work with immune-modulating biologic agents screen for histoplasmosis before immunosuppression is begun because of the concern for reactivation. Although this practice is controversial, the care of such vulnerable patients must be accompanied by a high level of vigilance.

The treatment and the duration of therapy for histoplasmosis depends on the severity of the disease. In patients with moderate to severe disease, antifungal therapy with amphotericin B liposomal complex must be initiated promptly. The total duration of therapy is usually 12 months, with a transition to azole-based therapy when the patient shows marked clinical improvement.

Furthermore, when a patient is receiving antifungal therapy, a high degree of awareness for secondary HLH is necessary if the patient's clinical condition decompensates and the patient has risk factors such as an immunosuppressed state, underlying systemic infections, and rheumatologic disease. Serum ferritin levels should be checked initially. The patient described above had disseminated histoplasmosis and secondary HLH, which is rare. Features that should prompt the diagnosis are fever, splenomegaly,

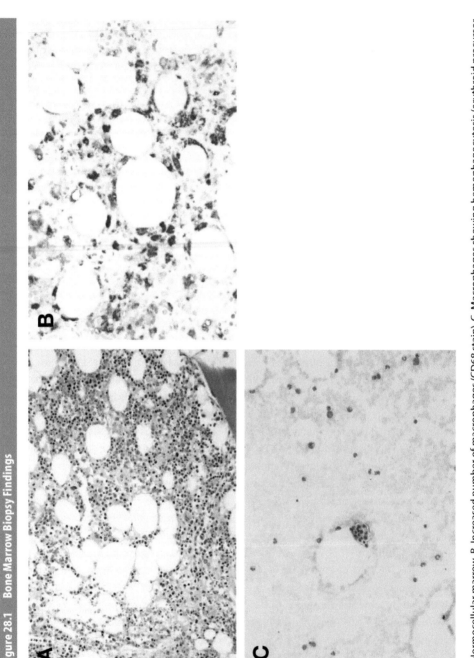

Figure 28.1   Bone Marrow Biopsy Findings

A, Normocellular marrow. B, Increased number of macrophages (CD68 stain). C, Macrophages showing hemophagocytosis (erythroid precursor and neutrophils).

and cytopenia in an immunocompromised host. Although all those features may overlap in patients who have disseminated histoplasmosis with liver involvement, bone marrow involvement, or adrenal involvement, decompensation in a patient receiving antifungal therapy should prompt measurement of serum ferritin levels. Ferritin levels greater than 10,000 µg/L have high sensitivity and specificity for HLH (1).

HLH is a life-threatening immune-activation syndrome that causes an uncontrolled inflammatory response and a cytokine storm resulting in multiorgan failure and death. HLH can occur in patients of any age without identified familial associations. Fewer than 30 cases of histoplasmosis-induced HLH have been described, and most of those involved patients who had HIV as a dominant risk factor and a high mortality rate (2,3). Resolution of HLH requires prompt treatment of the underlying inciting infection. For secondary HLH,

concurrent immunosuppressive therapy is recommended, especially for patients who do not have a response to targeted antimicrobial therapy alone. The clinical response can be monitored with complete blood cell counts, ferritin and fibrinogen levels, international normalized ratio, and liver function tests.

Summary

Histoplasmosis is an important complication in patients receiving TNF-α inhibitors, especially infliximab. If patients have risk factors such as an immunosuppressed state, certain infections, or rheumatologic disease, a high degree of awareness for secondary HLH is essential to secure the diagnosis. Prompt treatment of the underlying cause is critical for the resolution of HLH (1-3).

28.1. Answer b.

This immunocompromised patient, who has a recent travel history, presented with sepsis with recurrent fevers, which has worsened and resulted in multiorgan dysfunction and thrombocytopenia. Immunosuppression alone is a strong risk factor for fungal infections that may disseminate systemically and result in multiorgan failure. Diagnostic evaluation of a severely ill patient must include testing for *Aspergillus* antigen and the use of *Histoplasma* antigen enzyme immunoassay for rapid diagnosis. Lumbar puncture would be warranted if an immunocompromised host had signs of meningoencephalitis, such as fever, neck rigidity, and altered mental status. Bone marrow biopsy and further evaluation of thrombocytopenia would be indicated if the thrombocytopenia did not improve with resolution of the sepsis. Results of stool studies would not confirm the diagnosis. Additional information is available in the medical literature (4).

28.2. Answer e.

Postpartum pituitary infarction or Sheehan syndrome occurs after postpartum hemorrhage and leads to hypopituitarism, which interferes with corticotropin secretion and results in secondary adrenal insufficiency. Primary adrenal insufficiency, however, occurs as a result of adrenal cortex injury from underlying causes such as autoimmune or infectious disease, adrenal infarction, adrenal metastases, and drugs that accelerate cortisol metabolism. This process subsequently leads to glucocorticoid deficiency with or without other concurrent adrenal hormone deficiencies. The most common cause of primary adrenal insufficiency is autoimmune adrenalitis. Adrenalitis due to infections occurs frequently in patients who

are at risk for tuberculosis and disseminated fungal infections, especially histoplasmosis and paracoccidioidomycosis. Additional information is available in the medical literature (5).

28.3. Answer c.

If a patient has cytopenia, including anemia and thrombocytopenia, and markedly high ferritin levels, the possibility of a hyperinflammatory syndrome, such as HLH, should be considered. In addition to clinical judgment, the HLH-2004 diagnostic criteria are essential for establishing a diagnosis if HLH is a strong consideration. Bone marrow biopsy should be performed to evaluate the cytopenia and to look for hemophagocytosis, which is known to occur in more than 25% of patients who have HLH. Genetic testing is performed to identify HLH gene mutations in patients who meet the diagnostic criteria, but these genetic abnormalities rarely occur in adults. The utility of genetic testing is primarily to identify the risk of familial HLH and to risk stratify patients for recurrence of HLH, so genetic testing is not the best next diagnostic step for this patient. Increased levels of serum ferritin, a nonspecific inflammatory marker, are also present with other clinical syndromes, including renal disease, malignancies, HIV infections, and sickle cell disease. If HLH is ruled out as the cause of the high ferritin levels, other causes of inflammatory processes should be considered (which might involve imaging of the hip and further management). While ferritin levels can be elevated in patients with iron overload, this patient does not have clinical features that would suggest the need for liver biopsy. Additional information is available in the medical literature (6).

28.4. Answer b.

If HLH is a strong consideration upon initial evaluation of a patient, the HLH-2004 diagnostic criteria require fulfillment of 5 of the

8 diagnostic criteria (fever ≥38.5 °C; ferritin level >500 µg/L; peripheral blood cytopenia in >1 cell lineage; hypertriglyceridemia and/or hypofibrinogenemia; elevated soluble CD25; low or absent NK cell activity; hemophagocytosis in bone marrow, liver, spleen, or lymph nodes; and splenomegaly). Additional information is available in the medical literature (7,8).

28.5. Answer c.

HLH is a life-threatening condition that can be primary or secondary. When a clinically stable patient has been given a diagnosis of secondary HLH due to an infection, the next step should be to identify and treat the underlying sepsis responsible for triggering HLH. Patients who have progressive disease or clinical deterioration usually require specific therapy that includes chemotherapy in addition to high doses of corticosteroids. Induction chemotherapy includes an 8-week course of etoposide, which is typically administered in addition to dexamethasone, the preferred corticosteroid. Additional information is available in the medical literature (7,9).

References

1. Allen CE, Yu X, Kozinetz CA, McClain KL. Highly elevated ferritin levels and the diagnosis of hemophagocytic lymphohistiocytosis. Pediatr Blood Cancer. 2008 Jun;50(6):1227–35.

2. Townsend JL, Shanbhag S, Hancock J, Bowman K, Nijhawan AE. Histoplasmosis-induced hemophagocytic syndrome: a case series and review of the literature. Open Forum Infect Dis. 2015 Apr 15;2(2):ofv055.

3. Karthik Bommanan BK, Naseem S, Varma N. Hemophagocytic lymphohistiocytosis secondary to histoplasmosis. Blood Res. 2017 Jun;52(2):83.

4. Linden PK. Approach to the immunocompromised host with infection in the intensive care unit. Infect Dis Clin North Am. 2009 Sep;23(3):535–56.

5. Chabre O, Goichot B, Zenaty D, Bertherat J. Group 1. Epidemiology of primary and secondary adrenal insufficiency: prevalence and incidence, acute adrenal insufficiency, long-term morbidity and mortality. Ann Endocrinol (Paris). 2017 Dec;78(6):490–4. Epub 2017 Nov 27.

6. Jordan MB, Allen CE, Weitzman S, Filipovich AH, McClain KL. How I treat hemophagocytic lymphohistiocytosis. Blood. 2011 Oct 13;118(15):4041–52. Epub 2011 Aug 9.

7. Imashuku S. Advances in the management of hemophagocytic lymphohistiocytosis. Int J Hematol. 2000 Jul;72(1):1–11.

8. Henter JI, Horne A, Arico M, Egeler RM, Filipovich AH, Imashuku S, et al. HLH-2004: Diagnostic and therapeutic guidelines for hemophagocytic lymphohistiocytosis. Pediatr Blood Cancer. 2007 Feb;48(2): 124–31.

9. Berliner N, Kurra C, Chou D. Case records of the Massachusetts General Hospital. Case 1-2016: an 18-year-old man with fever, abdominal pain, and thrombocytopenia. N Engl J Med. 2016 Jan 14;374(2):165–73.

A 51-Year-Old Woman With Fever and Cough

Harsha V. Mudrakola, MD, MS, and Joseph H. Skalski, MD

Case Presentation

A 51-year-old woman presented with a 4-day history of fever and dry cough. Her medical history included chronic lymphocytic leukemia with transformation to diffuse, large B-cell lymphoma; hepatitis B; and hypothyroidism. The current fever was occurring daily and had been as high as 39 °C, and the cough was nonproductive. The patient also had fatigue, myalgias, and a bitemporal headache. She had received 2 cycles of cyclophosphamide, doxorubicin, vincristine, and prednisone (CHOP) at another facility, with the most recent cycle administered 3 weeks before the current presentation. Her medications at presentation included levothyroxine, entecavir, and a multivitamin. She reported that she did not have contact with anyone who was sick, and she did not have chest pain, hemoptysis, rashes, or other symptoms. She was living in Saudi Arabia and traveled to the US to receive care 2 weeks before this presentation.

At her initial visit in the emergency department, her vital signs were normal except for a fever. She was discharged with doxycycline and oseltamivir (which was discontinued the next day after a nasal swab sample was negative for influenza virus). She continued taking doxycycline, but she returned 5 days later because the fever and cough were persisting. She was febrile (38.5 °C), but the other vital signs were normal, and oxygen saturation with room air was normal. Physical examination findings were unremarkable, including the absence of crackles, rhonchi, or wheezes on pulmonary examination. The complete blood cell count was normal except for a lymphocytic predominance (50% lymphocytes). Results were normal for a basic metabolic panel, liver function tests, and lactate level. A screening test for HIV was negative.

An electrocardiogram showed normal sinus rhythm without any abnormalities. Chest radiography was notable for mild diffuse interstitial infiltrate (Figure 29.1). Computed tomography (CT) of the chest showed bulky lymphadenopathy in the lower neck and mediastinum consistent with lymphoma and diffuse ground-glass opacities with mosaic attenuation of the lung parenchyma (Figure 29.2). Findings from transthoracic echocardiography were normal with a left ventricular ejection fraction of 52% and normal right ventricular size and systolic function.

Figure 29.1   Radiography of the Chest

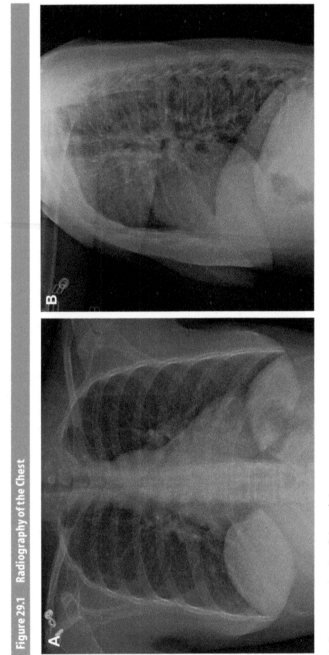

A, Anteroposterior view. B, Lateral view.

Figure 29.2   CT of the Chest

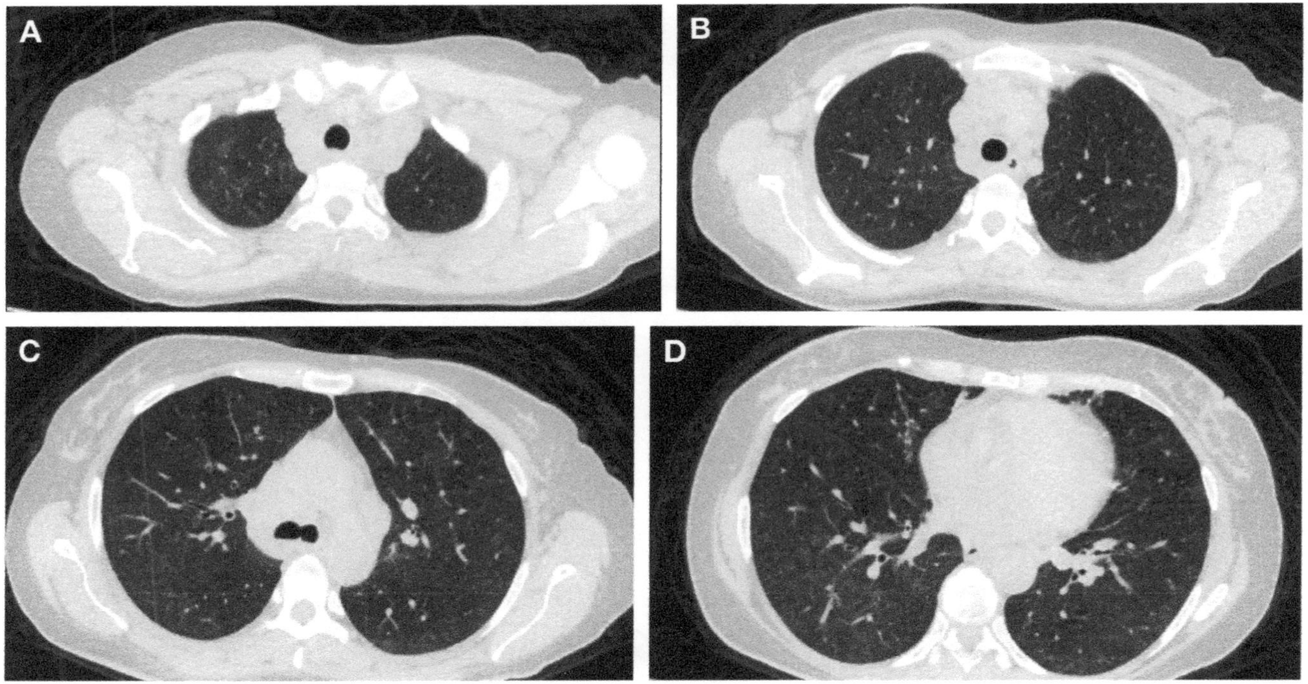

A-D, Axial views.

Multiple Choice (choose the best answer)

29.1. Which of the following would be *least* likely in the differential diagnosis for this patient's clinical presentation and radiologic findings?
   a. Cyclophosphamide toxicity
   b. *Pneumocystis jirovecii* pneumonia (PCP)
   c. Pulmonary edema
   d. Early lymphocytic carcinomatosis
   e. Lung infarct from pulmonary embolism

29.2. In patients without evidence of HIV, what is the most common underlying condition predisposing them to PCP?
   a. Hematologic malignancies
   b. Solid tumors
   c. Inflammatory or rheumatologic disease
   d. Vasculitis
   e. Solid organ transplant

29.3. Which of the following is an indication for adjunctive glucocorticoid treatment in patients with PCP?

   a. Alveolar-arterial oxygen gradient of 35 mm Hg or more
   b. Hemoptysis
   c. Pneumothorax
   d. Pao_2 less than 100 mm Hg
   e. Persistent dyspnea and cough

29.4. In patients with PCP who do not have HIV infection (in contrast to patients who have AIDS), which CT finding predominates?
   a. Lung nodules
   b. Ground-glass opacities
   c. Cystic lesions
   d. Pneumothorax
   e. Tree-in-bud pattern

29.5. If a patient requires prophylaxis for PCP but has had an anaphylactic reaction to trimethoprim-sulfamethoxazole (TMP-SMX) and has glucose-6-phosphate dehydrogenase deficiency, what is the preferred agent?
   a. Dapsone
   b. Intramuscular pentamidine
   c. Pyrimethamine
   d. Atovaquone
   e. Clindamycin

Case Follow-up and Outcome

Results from nasopharyngeal swab sampling were negative for influenza A virus, influenza B virus, respiratory syncytial virus, and several other viral respiratory pathogens. The patient could not produce any sputum. Because she had persistent symptoms and continued daily fevers, bronchoscopy and bronchoalveolar lavage were performed. The lavage fluid was clear and did not indicate diffuse alveolar hemorrhage. Results from all tests for an infectious cause were negative except for positive results from polymerase chain reaction for *P jirovecii*. Therapy was begun with TMP-SMX but without adjunctive glucocorticoids because the patient did not have hypoxia.

Discussion

Patients with hematologic malignancies are at risk for various acute pulmonary complications. When these patients have new radiologic and clinical pulmonary findings, the differential diagnosis is broad and includes both infectious and noninfectious causes. Noninfectious complications may result from the underlying malignancy itself or from the antineoplastic therapy. These complications include pulmonary embolism, pulmonary edema (cardiogenic and noncardiogenic), acute respiratory distress syndrome, pleural effusion, diffuse interstitial lung disease, pulmonary hypertension, diffuse alveolar hemorrhage, leukostasis, and drug toxicity. Patients may also have therapy-specific complications, including retinoic acid syndrome, tyrosine kinase inhibitor–related complications, and engraftment syndrome after stem cell transplant.

Pulmonary infection is the most common complication and a main cause of death among patients with hematologic malignancies. Patients are prone to various bacterial and fungal infections during the neutropenic phase after chemotherapy. T-cell defects are common in patients with lymphomas and lymphoblastic leukemias and in patients receiving corticosteroid therapy, hematopoietic stem cell transplant, or targeted monoclonal antibody therapy. These defects result in a higher incidence of pneumonia, including cytomegalovirus pneumonia and pneumonia from fungi such as *P jirovecii* and *Aspergillus* species (1).

In patients without HIV infection or AIDS, hematologic malignancies appear to convey the greatest risk of PCP (2). Among these patients, administration of glucocorticoids within the previous month portends additional risk (3). Cytotoxic chemotherapeutic agents and glucocorticoids increase the risk of PCP by suppression of cell-mediated immunity and alteration of lung surfactant. Clinical manifestations of PCP in patients with cancer range from mild disease to fulminant respiratory failure. In 1 series, the majority of cancer patients with PCP presented with a subacute febrile illness with cough and dyspnea. The median time to diagnosis was 7 days compared to 3 days for similar patients with bacterial pneumonia. The median Pao_2 was lower in those with PCP, and 20% needed to be in the intensive care unit (4).

The radiologic presentation of PCP in patients with cancer is also different from that in patients with AIDS. Bilateral interstitial infiltrates on plain radiographs are common to both patient groups, but most patients who have cancer and PCP have diffuse ground-glass opacities. Cystic lesions are seen in half the patients who have AIDS and PCP but are almost never seen in patients who have cancer and PCP (5).

Laboratory confirmation of the PCP diagnosis relies on the detection of organisms either microscopically or by molecular techniques. Given the lack of specificity of clinical and radiologic signs, a PCP diagnosis should not be based on clinical criteria alone. Since the 1990s, the gold standard has been microscopic visualization of the organisms with an immunofluorescence assay, but in recent years quantitative polymerase chain reaction (qPCR) has been shown to have nearly 100% sensitivity and specificity for PCP. Measurement of β-D-glucan, a major cell wall component of *Pneumocystis*, has a sensitivity of nearly 95% for PCP, but the specificity is less. Immunofluorescence or qPCR can be performed on sputum samples. However, if a patient cannot produce sputum or the diagnosis is not confirmed with sputum samples and the pretest probability is moderate to high, bronchoscopy and bronchoalveolar lavage should be performed (6).

TMP-SMX is the cornerstone of treatment of PCP. For patients with severe sulfa allergies that preclude desensitization, alternative agents are atovaquone, clindamycin in combination with primaquine, or trimethoprim in combination with dapsone. The use of adjunctive glucocorticoids is extrapolated from their use in patients with HIV infection. The criteria are the same: Pao_2 less than 70 mm Hg with room air or an arterial-alveolar oxygen gradient of 35 mm Hg or more.

Summary

When patients have isolated ground-glass opacities on radiography, the differential diagnosis is broad. PCP must be considered if a patient is immunosuppressed. In patients without HIV infection, hematologic malignancies and their therapy-related immunosuppression portend the greatest risk for PCP. The treatment algorithm is similar for patients with HIV infection and for patients without HIV infection.

Answers

29.1. Answer e.

The differential diagnosis for diffuse ground-glass opacities on CT is broad, particularly for this patient who is immunocompromised. Pulmonary infarction, however, has a distinct clinical and radiographic presentation that often includes sudden-onset dyspnea and subsequent pleuritic chest pain. A pleural friction rub or hemoptysis (or both) may also be present. The other possible choices are all reasonable and fit this patient's clinical and radiographic presentation. Additional information is available in the medical literature (7,8).

29.2. Answer a.

Although all the answer choices increase the risk of PCP to some degree, several studies in the past 2 decades have found that among patients without HIV infection, hematologic malignancies portend a high risk of PCP. Patients without AIDS who have PCP tend to have more severe illness, higher rates of mechanical ventilation, and higher mortality. Additional information is available in the medical literature (9,10).

29.3. Answer a.

The treatment algorithm for PCP is similar for patients without HIV infection and for patients with AIDS-related PCP. TMP-SMX is the preferred medication with a usual duration of therapy of 21 days. Adjunctive glucocorticoids are indicated for patients with a partial pressure of oxygen less than 70 mm Hg on arterial blood gas analysis, an alveolar-arterial oxygen gradient of at least 35 mm Hg, or room air oxygen saturation less than 92% on pulse oximetry. Additional information is available in the medical literature (11,12).

29.4. Answer b.

Although the radiographic presentation of PCP can be diverse, the presence of patchy or nodular ground-glass attenuation is a common finding. In a series of patients with cancer but without HIV infection, the presence of ground-glass opacities on CT was associated with an odds ratio of 14.24 for PCP compared to bacterial pneumonia. Additional information is available in the medical literature (4,13).

29.5. Answer d.

TMP-SMX is the agent of choice for prophylaxis against PCP because of its superior efficacy compared to the other agents listed and its broad spectrum of activity against other infectious agents, including *Nocardia*, *Toxoplasma*, and *Plasmodium*. If a patient cannot take TMP-SMX, alternative drugs include dapsone, atovaquone, and inhaled pentamidine. Dapsone is known to be associated with hemolysis in patients with glucose-6-phosphate dehydrogenase deficiency. Atovaquone is an oral drug that should be taken with fatty meals and is as efficacious as inhaled pentamidine. Additional information is available in the medical literature (11,14).

References

1. Choi MH, Jung JI, Chung WD, Kim YJ, Lee SE, Han DH, et al. Acute pulmonary complications in patients with hematologic malignancies. Radiographics. 2014 Oct;34(6):1755–68.

2. Yale SH, Limper AH. *Pneumocystis carinii* pneumonia in patients without acquired immunodeficiency syndrome: associated illness and prior corticosteroid therapy. Mayo Clin Proc. 1996 Jan;71(1):5–13.

3. Sepkowitz KA, Brown AE, Telzak EE, Gottlieb S, Armstrong D. *Pneumocystis carinii* pneumonia among patients without AIDS at a cancer hospital. JAMA. 1992 Feb 12;267(6):832–7.

4. Bollee G, Sarfati C, Thiery G, Bergeron A, de Miranda S, Menotti J, et al. Clinical picture of *Pneumocystis jiroveci* pneumonia in cancer patients. Chest. 2007 Oct;132(4):1305–10.

5. Hardak E, Brook O, Yigla M. Radiological features of *Pneumocystis jirovecii* pneumonia in immunocompromised patients with and without AIDS. Lung. 2010 Apr;188(2):159–63.

6. Alanio A, Hauser PM, Lagrou K, Melchers WJ, Helweg-Larsen J, Matos O, et al; 5th European Conference on Infections in Leukemia (ECIL-5), a joint venture of The European Group for Blood and Marrow Transplantation (EBMT), The European Organization for Research and Treatment of Cancer (EORTC), the Immunocompromised Host Society (ICHS) and The European LeukemiaNet (ELN). ECIL guidelines for the diagnosis of *Pneumocystis jirovecii* pneumonia in patients with haematological malignancies and stem cell transplant recipients. J Antimicrob Chemother. 2016 Sep;71(9):2386–96.

7. Miller WT Jr, Shah RM. Isolated diffuse ground-glass opacity in thoracic CT: causes and clinical presentations. AJR Am J Roentgenol. 2005 Feb;184(2): 613–22.

8. Miniati M. Pulmonary infarction: an often unrecognized clinical entity. Semin Thromb Hemost. 2016 Nov;42(8):865–9. Epub 2016 Oct 15.

9. Fillatre P, Decaux O, Jouneau S, Revest M, Gacouin A, Robert-Gangneux F, et al. Incidence of *Pneumocystis jiroveci* pneumonia among groups at risk in HIV-negative patients. Am J Med. 2014 Dec;127(12):1242. e11–7. Epub 2014 Jul 21.

10. Roux A, Canet E, Valade S, Gangneux-Robert F, Hamane S, Lafabrie A, et al. *Pneumocystis jirovecii* pneumonia in patients with or without AIDS, France. Emerg Infect Dis. 2014 Sep;20(9):1490–7.

11. Limper AH, Knox KS, Sarosi GA, Ampel NM, Bennett JE, Catanzaro A, et al; American Thoracic Society Fungal Working Group. An official American Thoracic Society statement: treatment of fungal infections in adult pulmonary and critical care patients. Am J Respir Crit Care Med. 2011 Jan 1;183(1):96–128.

12. Tomblyn M, Chiller T, Einsele H, Gress R, Sepkowitz K, Storek J, et al; Center for International Blood and Marrow Research; National Marrow Donor program; European Blood and MarrowTransplant Group; American Society of Blood and Marrow Transplantation; Canadian Blood and Marrow Transplant Group; Infectious Diseases Society of America; Society for Healthcare Epidemiology of America; Association of Medical Microbiology and Infectious Disease Canada; Centers for Disease Control and Prevention. Guidelines for preventing infectious complications among hematopoietic cell transplantation recipients: a global perspective. Biol Blood Marrow Transplant. 2009 Oct;15(10): 1143–238. Erratum in: Biol Blood Marrow Transplant. 2010 Feb;16(2):294.

13. Crans CA Jr, Boiselle PM. Imaging features of *Pneumocystis carinii* pneumonia. Crit Rev Diagn Imaging. 1999 Aug;40(4):251–84.

14. Chan C, Montaner J, Lefebvre EA, Morey G, Dohn M, McIvor RA, et al. Atovaquone suspension compared with aerosolized pentamidine for prevention of *Pneumocystis carinii* pneumonia in human immunodeficiency virus-infected subjects intolerant of trimethoprim or sulfonamides. J Infect Dis. 1999 Aug;180(2):369–76.

Neoplasia

A 54-Year-Old Woman With Chronic Hoarseness and Cough

A 54-Year-Old Woman With Chronic Hoarseness and Cough

30

Sarah J. Chalmers, MD, and Charles F. Thomas Jr, MD

Case Presentation

A 54-year-old woman presented to the otorhinolaryngology service for hoarse voice and cough of insidious onset over several years. She reported that she had undergone rhinolaryngoscopy in the past, at which time she was told that a nodule was present on her vocal cords. She did not know whether the nodule had been biopsied, but she did remember being told that follow-up was not required.

During the current visit, the patient underwent rhinolaryngoscopy, which showed a central exophytic, round, smooth, and edematous mass in the nasopharynx, with supraglottic and hypopharynx edema and erythema. Computed tomography (CT) of the soft tissue of the neck was ordered for further evaluation of the nasopharyngeal mass, and direct laryngoscopy with biopsy was scheduled. CT of the neck showed a 1.5-cm mass in the posterior portion of the nasopharynx, consistent with adenoid hypertrophy, which was confirmed on biopsy. An incidental finding was mediastinal lymphadenopathy with some lymph nodes as large as 1.5 cm. CT of the chest showed bilateral noncalcified hilar and mediastinal lymphadenopathy and multiple nodules (<6 mm) bilaterally and predominantly in the upper lobe (Figure 30.1). The patient was referred to the pulmonology service for further evaluation.

In the pulmonary clinic, the patient reported worsening of the hoarseness over the past several weeks such that sometimes her voice was nearly a whisper. The cough had worsened and

was associated with an abnormal sensation in her throat. She also had chronic stable exertional dyspnea that did not interfere with her daily activities. Her past medical history included obstructive sleep apnea, for which she had recently been prescribed continuous positive airway pressure therapy. She had morbid obesity (body mass index, 51.6; calculated as weight in kilograms divided by height in meters squared), and she was a current smoker with an 80-pack-year smoking history. She had been adopted, and her family history was unknown. She had no previous surgical history, and she worked for a construction company as a waste management truck driver.

On physical examination, she appeared to be well but with obesity and in no acute distress. Her oxygen saturation was 96% while breathing room air. There was no palpable cervical, supraclavicular, axillary, or femoral adenopathy. Heart examination findings were normal. Her respiratory effort was unlabored, and her lungs were clear on auscultation. Her abdomen was obese but soft and nontender. Her extremities were warm and without edema or cyanosis. Pulmonary function tests showed a borderline obstructive pattern (the ratio of forced expiratory volume in the first second of expiration [FEV_1] to forced vital capacity was slightly less than the lower limit of the reference range) and a concave expiratory loop. FEV_1 was 79% of the predicted value, and the adjusted diffusing capacity of lung for carbon monoxide was mildly reduced (74% of the predicted value). Results were negative for *Mycobacterium tuberculosis*

Figure 30.1   CT of the Chest at Initial Presentation

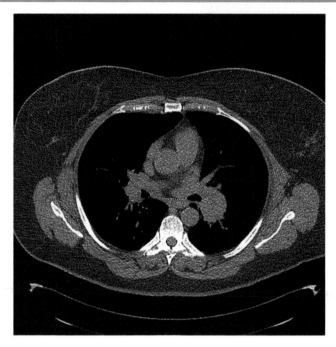

Axial view shows bilateral lymphadenopathy and nodules.

(according to quantification of interferon-γ in whole blood) and for antibodies for *Histoplasma*, *Blastomyces*, and *Coccidioides*. Blood test results were within the reference ranges for a complete blood cell count, electrolytes (including calcium), and liver and kidney function. C-reactive protein was mildly elevated (15 mg/L; reference range <8.0 mg/L). Results were negative for HIV antigen and antibody.

Findings were normal from flexible bronchoscopy and inspection. Endobronchial ultrasonography-guided transbronchial needle aspiration (EBUS-TBNA) was performed at lymph node stations 4R, 7, and 11L. Biopsy of station 4L was attempted, but an appropriate window for sampling was not identified. Rapid onsite cytology showed lymphocytes that were not diagnostic at each station; final cytology was negative for malignancy, but granulomatous inflammation was identified from station 11L. Bronchial washings were submitted for bacterial and fungal cultures. The presumptive diagnosis

was sarcoidosis. Given the relatively benign lung parenchyma findings, immunosuppressive therapy was not initiated and follow-up was scheduled.

Approximately 6 weeks later, the patient reported that the cough and dyspnea were worse. The dyspnea was worse with exertion and was associated with a wheeze. The cough was mildly productive, with episodes lasting 10 to 20 minutes, and was associated with posttussive emesis. She was prescribed tiotropium and albuterol inhalers, but she had no improvement. After the symptoms progressed over the next 2 weeks, she presented to the emergency department.

At the emergency department, the patient was in moderate respiratory distress. She reported progressive worsening of her cough and dyspnea and new-onset left-sided pleuritic chest pain. Her oxygen saturation was 84% while breathing room air, and it improved to more than 90% with 2 L of oxygen delivered through a nasal cannula. Rhonchi were present over the posterior portion

Axial view shows new left hilar mass.

of the left lung field, and breath sounds were diminished at the left base. Results from initial testing included normal serum pH and Pco_2 but low Po_2 (65 mm Hg) on arterial blood gas analysis; elevated blood glucose; and normal results for troponin, electrocardiography, electrolytes, and kidney and liver function tests. On CT angiography of the chest, the pulmonary nodules were unchanged, mediastinal and hilar lymphadenopathy was still present, the left-sided adenopathy was larger, a new left hilar mass (maximum dimension, 6.4×7.2×6.1 cm) was compressing the basilar left lower lobe segmental bronchus, and postobstructive consolidation and an adjacent small pleural effusion were present (Figure 30.2). The patient was referred to the general medicine team, and the pulmonology team was consulted. She underwent follow-up bronchoscopy with EBUS-TBNA at stations 4R, 11R, 7, and 4L and biopsy of the left hilar mass. Rapid onsite cytology of the sample showed sheets of small, round-to-spindled cells with indistinct nuclei, scant cytoplasm, and finely dispersed nuclear chromatin. Immunoperoxidase stains were positive for cytokeratin AE1/AE3, thyroid transcription factor (TTF)-1, synaptophysin, and chromogranin A (Figure 30.3). All biopsied lymph nodes were negative for malignancy.

Figure 30.3   Cytology of Samples From Bronchoscopy and EBUS-TBNA

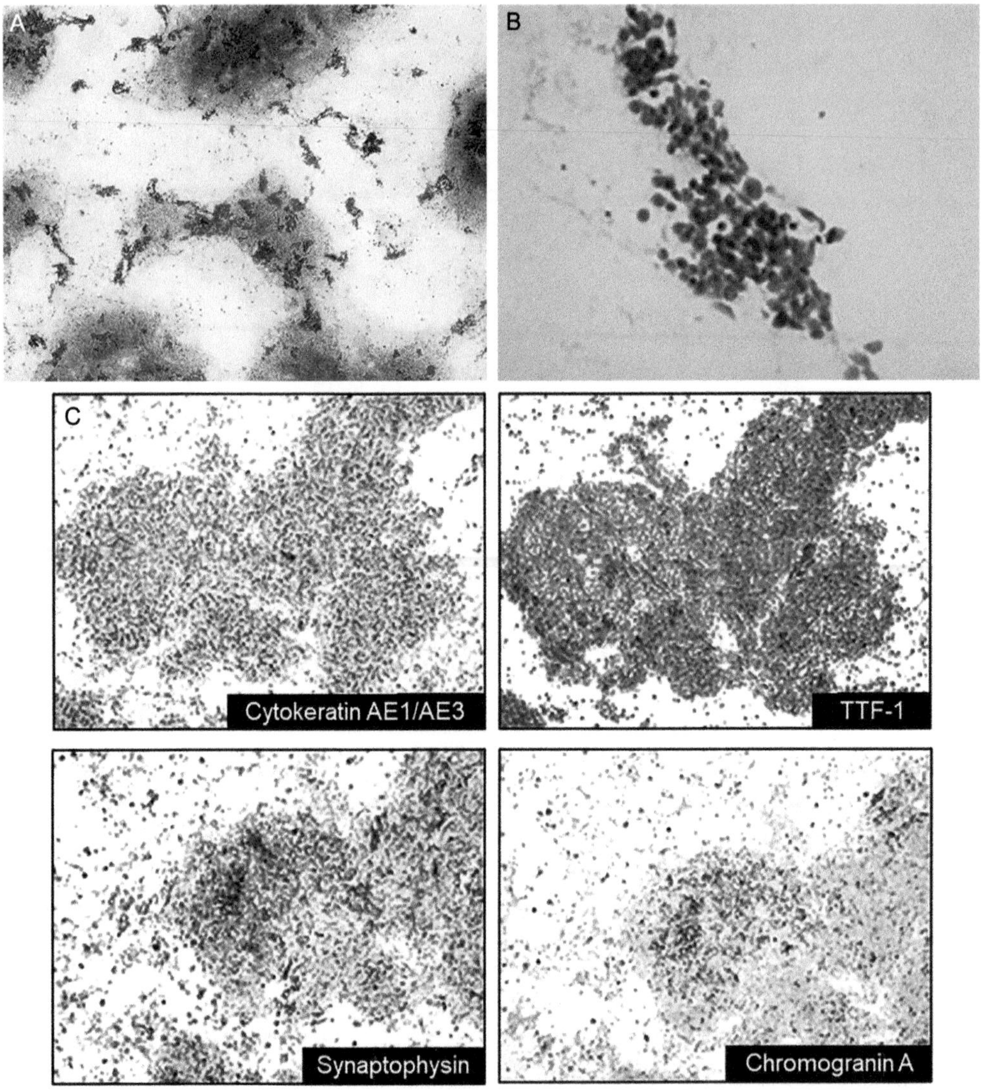

A, Clusters of blue cells with various shapes, from spindle to round, are present in the lung parenchyma. B, Small, blue spindle-shaped cells with scant cytoplasm are shown. C, Immunoperoxidase stains were positive for cytokeratin AE1/AE3 (upper left), TTF-1 (upper right), synaptophysin (lower left), and chromogranin A (lower right).

Questions

Multiple Choice (choose the best answer)

30.1. Which diagnostic test *cannot* be used to establish a diagnosis of small cell lung cancer (SCLC)?
   a. Sputum cytology
   b. Pleural fluid cytology
   c. CT-guided fine-needle aspiration
   d. EBUS-TBNA
   e. Serum α-fetoprotein tumor marker

30.2. Which risk factor is most strongly associated with SCLC?
   a. Previous radiotherapy
   b. Tobacco smoking
   c. Talc exposure
   d. Occupational exposure
   e. Marijuana smoke

30.3. Which immunohistochemical marker can be used to help differentiate SCLC from other neuroendocrine tumors?
   a. TTF-1
   b. Synaptophysin
   c. Chromogranin A
   d. p53
   e. Cytokeratins CK7/CK20

30.4. A 67-year-old woman who is a current smoker presents with cough and weight loss over the past several months. A 4-cm right hilar mass is identified as SCLC on CT-guided biopsy. Fluorodeoxyglucose F 18 (FDG) avidity is noted at stations 11R and 7. No other FDG-avid lesions are seen, and magnetic resonance imaging (MRI) of the brain is negative for lesions. What is the best initial therapy for this patient?
   a. Chemotherapy in combination with immunomodulator therapy
   b. Radiotherapy only
   c. Surgical resection only
   d. Chemotherapy in combination with radiotherapy
   e. Immunomodulator therapy only

30.5. A 70-year-old man with a 60-pack-year smoking history presented with a 4-cm left lower lobe mass consistent with SCLC on CT-guided biopsy. Positron emission tomography (PET) showed FDG avidity in the left hilar lymph nodes. MRI of the brain was negative for metastatic disease. What is the clinical stage of this malignancy?
   a. Limited-stage disease
   b. Extensive-stage disease
   c. Stage IV disease
   d. Stage III disease
   e. Stage IIIB disease

Case Follow-up and Outcome

Pathology results confirmed SCLC. MRI of the brain was negative for metastatic lesions, and PET findings were consistent with limited-stage disease. Treatment was initiated with chemotherapy (cisplatin and etoposide) and radiotherapy.

Discussion

The broad differential diagnosis for mediastinal and hilar lymphadenopathy includes infectious, malignant, and inflammatory causes. Mediastinoscopy has been considered the gold standard for tissue diagnosis in isolated mediastinal and hilar lymphadenopathy; however, other less-invasive modalities have essentially replaced mediastinoscopy. EBUS-TBNA is a less invasive technique for obtaining cytologic or histologic samples from lymph nodes at stations 1, 2R and 2L, 4R and 4L, 7, 10, and 11 and from a centrally located parenchymal lung mass. The specificity is nearly 98%, and the sensitivity is 92% (1). In addition, for patients who ultimately receive a diagnosis of lung cancer, EBUS-TBNA has shortened the time to reach a treatment decision as compared to mediastinoscopy (2). However, as with the patient described in this case, false-negative results are possible, and if a diagnosis is not made, alternative diagnostic methods should be pursued. For this patient, the finding of granulomatous change in the presence of isolated mediastinal and hilar lymphadenopathy was thought to be consistent with sarcoidosis; therefore, an alternative diagnostic method was not thought to be necessary. This case highlights the need for close follow-up and a high degree of clinical awareness of an alternative diagnosis if symptoms change or progress.

SCLC is a neuroendocrine malignancy characterized by its rapidly progressive nature, which leads to metastatic disease on presentation in approximately 70% of patients. The most common initial presentation is a centrally located mass with submucosal spread and associated hilar and mediastinal lymphadenopathy. Compression of the airway or adjacent nerves, such as the recurrent laryngeal nerve, can lead to cough, dyspnea, and hoarseness. Owing to the neuroendocrine origin of SCLC, patients occasionally present with paraneoplastic syndromes such as those involving hypercalcemia and parathyroid hormone–related protein, syndrome of inappropriate antidiuretic hormone secretion, Lambert-Eaton syndrome, and ectopic corticotropin syndrome. Patients have a poor prognosis (5-year survival rate, 5%-10%) (3). The predominant risk factor for SCLC is a history of smoking, and nearly all patients with SCLC have a smoking history (3,4). Other risk factors include working in a uranium mine and radon exposure. Histopathology findings include rapidly proliferative spindle-shaped, round, or oval small cells with scant cytoplasm, finely dispersed chromatin, an absence of nuclei, and a high mitotic index (5).

Guidelines recommend that the diagnosis should be made in the least invasive manner, and, if possible, the diagnostic evaluation should aid in staging the disease (6). For instance, biopsy of a peripheral, easily accessible lesion would be useful for diagnosing and staging the disease (as *extensive-stage disease*, as described below). Because SCLC is often centrally located, bronchoscopy is frequently used to obtain a tissue diagnosis (5). Other potential diagnostic methods include pleural fluid cytology, fine-needle aspiration biopsy, EBUS-TBNA, and mediastinoscopy if required (6). Sensitivity and specificity of these methods vary, and false-negative results are possible, so if clinical suspicion is high, further tissue diagnosis should be pursued (6). SCLC metastasizes by hematogenous spread and often involves the brain or bone (or both) and other organs. Therefore, additional evaluation for staging the disease may include CT of the chest, abdomen, and pelvis; MRI of the brain; bone scan; or PET (6). Although not necessary for diagnosis, immunohistochemistry may be useful in differentiating SCLC. In SCLC, staining is positive with synaptophysin, chromogranin A, CD56, TTF-1, and MIB-1 (5).

The 2 methods for staging SCLC are from the Veterans Administration Lung Study Group (VALG) and the International Association for the Study of Lung Cancer (IASLC). The modified staging criteria from the VALG categorize SCLC into limited-stage and extensive-stage disease. *Limited-stage disease* is confined to a single hemithorax or a single safe radiation field. All other disease not meeting limited-stage criteria is considered *extensive-stage disease*. The IASLC criteria use TNM staging.

Currently, treatment is largely based on VALG staging, although TNM staging is used to assist in identification of a small number of patients who would benefit from surgical resection (stage T1N0M0 or T2N0M0) and is also used for research purposes (3-5,7). Treatment largely consists of platinum-based chemotherapy and radiotherapy. SCLC is highly responsive to treatment with chemotherapy and radiotherapy (response rates are as high as 80%), and prophylactic cranial radiotherapy is often recommended also. In addition, smoking cessation reduces mortality and should be encouraged for all current smokers who have a diagnosis of SCLC. Reoccurrence is common and is often refractory to treatment (3-5).

Summary

The differential diagnosis for mediastinal and hilar lymphadenopathy is broad and includes malignancy. SCLC accounts for approximately 15% of all lung cancers and most commonly presents as a medially located pulmonary mass with associated mediastinal and hilar lymphadenopathy. SCLC is characterized by its rapidly progressive nature and often presents with widely metastatic disease. Diagnosis and staging should be made by the least invasive method. If results from initial diagnostic evaluations are negative and clinical suspicion is high, further tissue diagnosis should be pursued. Treatment of SCLC consists of chemotherapy, which is often given with radiotherapy and prophylactic cranial radiotherapy. Reoccurrence is common.

Answers

30.1. Answer e.

Sputum cytology, pleural fluid cytology, CT-guided fine-needle aspiration, and EBUS-TBNA can be used to make the diagnosis of SCLC. Mediastinoscopy could also provide a diagnosis. Current guidelines recommend use of the least invasive method that is needed to make the diagnosis. Unlike the staging of non-SCLC, the staging of SCLC can be confined to limited-stage disease and extensive-stage disease, and staging and diagnosis may be determined more easily. Serum α-fetoprotein tumor marker is not used in the diagnosis of SCLC. Additional information is available in the medical literature (6).

30.2. Answer b.

At least 98% of patients who receive a diagnosis of SCLC have a history of smoking. Radiotherapy of the chest and occupational or environmental exposure (eg, uranium mining, arsenic inhalation, and radon exposure) are risk factors, but smoking poses a much greater risk. Talc exposure and marijuana smoke may be associated with lung cancer, but a clear correlation has not been identified. Additional information is available in the medical literature (8).

30.3. Answer a.

Immunohistochemical stains can be useful to help differentiate between different types of primary and metastatic lung malignancies. Immunohistochemical stains such as chromogranin A, CD56, and synaptophysin can be used to identify neuroendocrine tumors of the lung such as SCLC. TTF-1 is positive in up to 90% of cases of SCLC and large cell neuroendocrine carcinoma and can be used to help differentiate SCLC from other neuroendocrine tumors such as carcinoid. For the identification of SCLC, p53 and CK7/CK20 are not usually used as markers. Additional information is available in the medical literature (6).

30.4. Answer d.

The mainstay of treatment of patients with limited-stage disease is concurrent chemoradiotherapy. Surgical resection can be considered for certain patients who have limited disease without nodal involvement. Although SCLC often has a robust response to initial therapy, the recurrence rate is high. Additional information is available in the medical literature (9).

30.5. Answer a.

The use of *limited-stage* and *extensive-stage* is the predominant method of describing the staging of SCLC. This method has been shown to correlate with prognosis and is useful in guiding treatment decisions. Limited-stage disease corresponds to TNM stages I through IIIB and is defined as tumor burden confined to the hemithorax with nodal involvement that can be reached in a single radiotherapy field. More recently, TNM staging was recommended for research purposes. Additional information is available in the medical literature (7).

References

1. Chandra S, Nehra M, Agarwal D, Mohan A. Diagnostic accuracy of endobronchial ultrasound-guided transbronchial needle biopsy in mediastinal lymphadenopathy: a systematic review and meta-analysis. Respir Care. 2012 Mar;57(3):384–91.

2. Navani N, Nankivell M, Lawrence DR, Lock S, Makker H, Baldwin DR, et al; Lung-BOOST trial investigators. Lung cancer diagnosis and staging with endobronchial ultrasound-guided transbronchial needle aspiration compared with conventional approaches: an open-label, pragmatic, randomised controlled trial. Lancet Respir Med. 2015 Apr;3(4):282–9.

3. Kalemkerian GP, Loo BW, Akerley W, Attia A, Bassetti M, Boumber Y, et al. NCCN Guidelines Insights: Small Cell Lung Cancer, Version 2.2018. J Natl Compr Canc Netw. 2018 Oct;16(10):1171–82.

4. National Cancer Institute. Small cell lung cancer treatment (PDQ): health professional version. Cited 2020 Nov 4; Updated: 2020 Mar 24. Available from https://www.cancer.gov/types/lung/hp/small-cell-lung-treatment-pdq#section/_1.Updated.

5. Fruh M, De Ruysscher D, Popat S, Crino L, Peters S, Felip E; ESMO Guidelines Working Group. Small-cell lung cancer (SCLC): ESMO clinical practice guidelines for diagnosis, treatment and follow-up. Ann Oncol. 2013 Oct;24 Suppl 6:vi99–105. Epub 2013 Jun 27.

6. Detterbeck FC, Boffa DJ, Kim AW, Tanoue LT. The eighth edition lung cancer stage classification. Chest. 2017 Jan;151(1):193–203. Epub 2016 Oct 22.

7. Shepherd FA, Crowley J, Van Houtte P, Postmus PE, Carney D, Chansky K, et al; International Association for the Study of Lung Cancer International Staging Committee and Participating Institutions. The International Association for the Study of Lung Cancer lung cancer staging project: proposals regarding the clinical staging of small cell lung cancer in the forthcoming (seventh) edition of the tumor, node, metastasis classification for lung cancer. J Thorac Oncol. 2007 Dec;2(12):1067–77.

8. Health USSGsACoSa. General USPHSOotS. Smoking and Health. United States. Public Health Service. Office of the Surgeon General [Internet]. Bethesda (MD): U.S. National Library of Medicine. c1964. [cited 2021 Oct 28]. Available from: https://profiles.nlm.nih.gov/spotlight/nn/catalog/nlm:nlmuid-101584932X202-doc.

9. Jett JR, Schild SE, Kesler KA, Kalemkerian GP. Treatment of small cell lung cancer: diagnosis and management of lung cancer, 3rd ed: American College of Chest Physicians evidence-based clinical practice guidelines. Chest. 2013 May;143(5 Suppl):e400S–e19S.

A 56-Year-Old Man With Persistent Pneumonia

Cameron M. Long, MD, MS, and Sumedh S. Hoskote, MBBS

Case Presentation

A 56-year-old man presented for a second opinion for persistent right lower lobe pneumonia. He was a nonsmoker with ischemic cardiomyopathy (ejection fraction, 35%), coronary artery disease (stents were inserted), and gastroesophageal reflux disease. His respiratory symptoms began 6 years earlier with 2 weeks of nonproductive cough, fever, and chills. Laboratory test results were notable for a white blood cell count of 13.8×10^9/L with a predominance of neutrophils; results were negative for antinuclear antibody, antineutrophil cytoplasmic autoantibody, fungal serologies, and sputum smear microscopy for acid-fast bacilli. Computed tomography (CT) of the chest showed an 8-cm cystic lesion with an air-fluid level in

the right lower lobe, scattered bilateral pulmonary nodules (all <1 cm), and mediastinal lymphadenopathy (Figure 31.1). Bronchoscopy with bronchoalveolar lavage showed lymphocyte predominance but no growth on bacterial, fungal, and mycobacterial cultures. The patient was discharged and treated with amoxicillin-clavulanic acid for 6 weeks. His symptoms resolved, and the size of the cystic lesion decreased to 5 cm. Three months later, CT-guided biopsy was negative for malignancy. The patient was followed for the next 3 years with CT of the chest; during that time, the lesion grew minimally.

Nine months before the patient's current presentation, he had fevers, chills, and a cough. CT of the chest showed that the lesion in the right lower lobe had enlarged to 8 cm and had mixed

Figure 31.1   CT Imaging of the Chest Over Nearly 19 Years

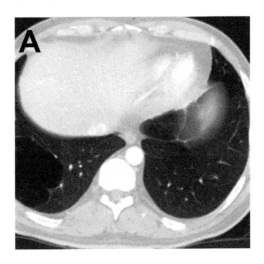

Figure 31.1   Continued

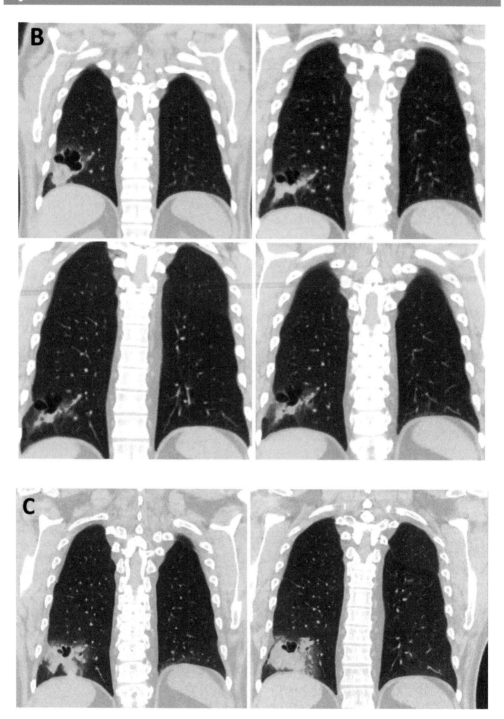

A, Initial axial view shows a cystic lesion in the right lower lobe that is most likely a congenital pulmonary airway malformation or possibly congenital emphysema. B, Subsequent coronal views show the lesion 13 years later (volume, 25 cm^3) (upper left); 13 years and 3 months later (upper right); 14 years and 5 months later (lower left); and 15 years and 5 months later (volume, 30 cm^3) (lower right). C, Coronal views show the lesion at 18 years and 3 months after the initial CT (volume, 66 cm^3) (left) and at 18 years and 9 months after the initial CT (right).

cavitary and solid components. The patient was treated with another course of antibiotics, and the symptoms resolved; however, the lesion was larger on imaging immediately before the current presentation. Results of fungal serologic testing and blood cultures were negative. Fluorine 18–labeled fluorodeoxyglucose positron emission tomography (PET) showed a heterogeneously enhancing mass (standardized uptake value, 3.2).

Questions

Multiple Choice (choose the best answer)

31.1. What is the most appropriate next step in management for this patient?
a. Follow-up CT-guided lung biopsy
b. Continued monitoring
c. Prolonged course of antibiotics
d. Bronchoscopy with bronchoalveolar lavage
e. Thoracic surgery referral

31.2. What is the negative predictive value of a CT-guided lung biopsy?
a. 25%
b. 50%
c. 75%
d. 90%
e. 99%

31.3. If the patient has a 7.5-cm adenocarcinoma without lymph node involvement, what stage of cancer would he have (according to the eighth edition of the American Joint Committee on Cancer [AJCC] TNM staging system for non–small cell lung cancer)?
a. Stage IIIA (T3N0M0)
b. Stage IIIB (T3N0M0)
c. Stage IIIA (T4N0M0)
d. Stage IVA (T4N0M0)
e. Stage IVA (T5N0M0)

31.4. The patient is deemed to have unresectable stage IIIA disease and undergoes electromagnetic navigational bronchoscopy. The diagnosis is adenocarcinoma. What would be the best next management step?
a. Next-generation sequencing of tissue for tumor markers
b. Initiation of chemotherapy
c. Surgical resection
d. Consultation for palliative care
e. Radiotherapy

31.5. A 74-year-old man undergoes CT of the chest, which shows a spiculated 2-cm nodule in the left upper lobe without mediastinal lymphadenopathy. CT-guided biopsy is positive for adenocarcinoma. He has a smoking history of 60 pack-years and chronic obstructive pulmonary disease (Global Initiative for Chronic Obstructive Lung Disease risk group C); forced expiratory volume in the first second of expiration, 40%; Medical Research Council dyspnea grade 2; and heart failure with reduced ejection fraction. What would be the best next option in the management of the malignancy?
a. Observation
b. Surgical resection
c. Stereotactic body radiotherapy
d. Chemotherapy
e. Immunotherapy

Case Follow-up and Outcome

The patient was referred to the thoracic surgery service, and he underwent a right lower lobectomy with hilar nodal dissection. The diagnosis was stage IIIA (T4N0M0) mucinous adenocarcinoma. He received adjuvant chemotherapy with carboplatin and pemetrexed because he had a prior history of sensorineural hearing loss and neuropathy.

Discussion

This case illustrates the clinical entity of unresolving pneumonia that is diagnosed as primary lung adenocarcinoma. Pneumonia visualized on chest radiography would be expected to resolve by 6 weeks in patients with healthy lungs. In patients with fibrotic or obstructive lung disease, the duration may be up to 16 weeks (1). This patient's clinical improvement without radiographic improvement would be concerning. The patient appropriately underwent further testing when the lesion did not resolve; however, the negative findings with CT-guided biopsy provided false reassurance. In a large cohort of 203 patients, 49% of the "nonmalignant or negative" transthoracic needle biopsy specimens were found to have false-negative results for malignancy after further investigations (2).

Malignancy is a relatively uncommon cause of unresolving pneumonia; the incidence is 1% to 2%, and the majority of cases are diagnosed within 3 months after the initial presentation (3). The risk of malignancy is increased with underlying lung disease, such as emphysema, idiopathic fibrosis, and type 1 CCAM (3,4). Sarcoidosis is characterized by noncaseating granulomas involving lymph nodes and organs but is not associated with lung cancer.

The incidence of lung cancer in the US was a little more than 220,000 in 2019 and has been decreasing the past 10 years (5). Adenocarcinoma,

the most common histologic type, accounts for 40% of all lung cancers (6). The greatest risk factor is tobacco exposure, but asbestos, diesel fuel, heavy metals, and radon gas have been associated with increased cancer risk (6).

Lung lesions that are localized to the lung parenchyma without hilar or mediastinal involvement should undergo curative resection in patients who have good functional status (7). If the pathologic margins are positive, local radiotherapy is recommended. With hilar involvement, adjuvant chemotherapy is recommended. Any lung cancer in category N2 (mediastinal nodal) is advanced (stage III or IV), and chemotherapy with or without radiotherapy is recommended. However, cases like the one described above that have large tumors (>7 cm) without lymph node involvement are stage III, and chemotherapy would be recommended (8).

If a patient has poor functional status, if the cancer is limited to the lung parenchyma, and if the patient is not a good candidate for surgery, stereotactic body radiotherapy is an alternative with nearly equivalent outcomes (9). Oligometastatic disease (solitary pulmonary metastasis in addition to primary lung cancer) should be treated as 2 separate entities with the metastatic lesion undergoing resection or radiotherapy for local control (10).

Systemic chemotherapy for nonresectable disease or any nodal disease is based on cisplatin or carboplatin, and either pemetrexed or paclitaxel is typically included. In addition to systemic therapy, the potential for biomarker-directed therapy should also be evaluated by testing for oncogenes *EGFR*, *ALK*, *KRAS*, and *ROS-1* and immune histochemical staining for PD-L1 (6). If the tumor has both oncogene and PD-L1 receptor positivity, the recommendation is to first use oncogene-targeted therapy with osimertinib (*EGFR* inhibitor) (11), alectinib (*ALK* inhibitor) (12), or crizotinib (*ROS-1* inhibitor) (13) and then use the immune checkpoint inhibitor durvalumab (PD-L1 inhibitor) (14) or pembrolizumab (PD-L1 receptor inhibitor) (15). Disease-free and total survival have improved with gene-targeted and immune checkpoint inhibitor therapies alone or in addition to cytotoxic chemotherapy.

Summary

Unresolving pneumonia, characterized by a lack of radiographic clearance in normal lungs by 6 weeks, has a broad differential diagnosis. Malignancy occurs in 1% to 2% of patients and requires vigilance to ensure timely diagnosis. Early-stage non–small cell lung cancer is curable, and surgical resection is recommended. Advanced-stage adenocarcinoma is treatable, and life expectancy is improving, but survival is still poor (40% survival at 5 years) for patients with stage III or IV disease (6).

Answers

31.1. Answer e.

The patient has a nonresolving cystic and cavitary mass (>3 cm) with a partly solid component after multiple rounds of antibiotics. CT shows growth over a 5-year follow-up period, and PET-CT shows FDG uptake. All these clinical and radiographic findings suggest a neoproliferative process. For clinically staged lung masses (stage ≤2 and local advanced stage 3), resection with total or partial lobectomy would be appropriate and would provide a diagnosis and possibly a cure by American College of Chest Physicians (ACCP) guidelines (grade 1B). The ACCP 2013 guidelines have not been updated to the new staging guidelines (eighth edition of TNM classification) by the International Association for the Study of Lung Cancer. Additional information is available in the medical literature (1,3,16).

31.2. Answer b.

When the possibility of a mass is a concern, a negative or nondiagnostic result from CT-guided lung biopsy should not lead to a conclusion that the lung mass is not a cancer. In a series of 204 patients 50% of the false-negative biopsies proved to be cancer after subsequent testing. Additional information is available in the medical literature (4).

31.3. Answer c.

According the eighth edition of the AJCC TNM staging system for non–small cell lung cancer, the cancer would be stage IIIA (T4N0M0). Additional information is available in the medical literature (8).

31.4. Answer a.

The potential for biomarker-directed therapy should be evaluated in advanced disease (stage III or IV) by testing for oncogenes *EGFR, ALK, KRAS,* and *ROS-1* and immune histochemical staining for PD-L1. Disease-free and total survival have improved with gene-targeted and immune checkpoint inhibitor therapies alone or in addition to cytotoxic chemotherapy. Additional information is available in the medical literature (6).

31.5. Answer c.

If a patient has poor functional status, if the cancer is limited to the lung parenchyma, and if the patient is not a good surgical candidate, stereotactic body radiotherapy is an alternative with nearly equivalent outcomes. Surgical morbidity outweighs the benefit of a resection. Immunotherapy and chemotherapy are used in more advanced disease. Additional information is available in the medical literature (9).

References

1. Jay SJ, Johanson WG Jr, Pierce AK. The radiographic resolution of *Streptococcus pneumoniae* pneumonia. N Engl J Med. 1975 Oct 16;293(16):798–801.
2. Fontaine-Delaruelle C, Souquet PJ, Gamondes D, Pradat E, De Leusse A, Ferretti GR, et al. Negative predictive value of transthoracic core-needle biopsy: a multicenter study. Chest. 2015 Aug;148(2):472–80.
3. Soyseth V, Benth JS, Stavem K. The association between hospitalisation for pneumonia and the diagnosis of lung cancer. Lung Cancer. 2007 Aug;57(2):152–8.
4. Kuru T, Lynch JP 3rd. Nonresolving or slowly resolving pneumonia. Clin Chest Med. 1999 Sep;20(3):623–51.
5. Siegel RL, Miller KD, Jemal A. Cancer statistics, 2019. CA Cancer J Clin. 2019 Jan;69(1):7–34.
6. Ettinger DS, Wood DE, Aggarwal C, Aisner DL, Akerley W, Bauman JR, et al. NCCN guidelines insights: non-small cell lung cancer, version 1.2020. J Natl Compr Canc Netw. 2019 Dec;17(12):1464–72.
7. Howington JA, Blum MG, Chang AC, Balekian AA, Murthy SC. Treatment of stage I and II non-small cell lung cancer: diagnosis and management of lung cancer, 3rd ed: American College of Chest Physicians evidence-based clinical practice guidelines. Chest. 2013 May;143(5 Suppl):e278S–e313S.
8. Goldstraw P, Chansky K, Crowley J, Rami-Porta R, Asamura H, Eberhardt WE, et al; International Association for the Study of Lung Cancer Staging and Prognostic Factors Committee, Advisory Boards, and Participating Institutions; International Association for the Study of Lung Cancer Staging and Prognostic Factors Committee Advisory Boards and Participating Institutions. The IASLC Lung Cancer Staging Project: proposals for revision of the TNM stage groupings in the forthcoming (eighth) edition of the TNM Classification for Lung Cancer. J Thorac Oncol. 2016 Jan;11(1):39–51.
9. Videtic GMM, Donington J, Giuliani M, Heinzerling J, Karas TZ, Kelsey CR, et al. Stereotactic body radiation therapy for early-stage non-small cell lung cancer: executive summary of an ASTRO evidence-based guideline. Pract Radiat Oncol. 2017 Sep-Oct;7(5):295–301.
10. Endo C, Hasumi T, Matsumura Y, Sato N, Deguchi H, Oizumi H, et al. A prospective study of surgical procedures for patients with oligometastatic non-small cell lung cancer. Ann Thorac Surg. 2014 Jul;98(1):258–64.
11. Soria JC, Ohe Y, Vansteenkiste J, Reungwetwattana T, Chewaskulyong B, Lee KH, et al; FLAURA Investigators. Osimertinib in untreated EGFR-mutated advanced non-small-cell lung cancer. N Engl J Med. 2018 Jan 11;378(2):113–25.
12. Peters S, Camidge DR, Shaw AT, Gadgeel S, Ahn JS, Kim DW, et al; ALEX Trial Investigators. Alectinib versus Crizotinib in untreated ALK-positive non-small-cell lung cancer. N Engl J Med. 2017 Aug 31;377(9):829–38.
13. Shaw AT, Ou SH, Bang YJ, Camidge DR, Solomon BJ, Salgia R, et al. Crizotinib in ROS1-rearranged non-small-cell lung cancer. N Engl J Med. 2014 Nov 20;371(21):1963–71.
14. Antonia SJ, Villegas A, Daniel D, Vicente D, Murakami S, Hui R, et al; PACIFIC Investigators. Overall survival with Durvalumab after chemoradiotherapy in stage III NSCLC. N Engl J Med. 2018 Dec 13;379(24):2342–50.
15. Gandhi L, Rodriguez-Abreu D, Gadgeel S, Esteban E, Felip E, De Angelis F, et al; KEYNOTE-189 Investigators. Pembrolizumab plus chemotherapy in metastatic non-small-cell lung cancer. N Engl J Med. 2018 May 31;378(22):2078–92.
16. Detterbeck FC, Lewis SZ, Diekemper R, Addrizzo-Harris D, Alberts WM. Executive Summary: Diagnosis and management of lung cancer, 3rd ed: American College of Chest Physicians evidence-based clinical practice guidelines. Chest. 2013 May;143(5 Suppl):7S–37S.

A 74-Year-Old Man With a Pulmonary Nodule and Neck Pain

32

Richard D. Koubek, MD, and Sumedh S. Hoskote, MBBS

Case Presentation

A 74-year-old man with obesity and a cigarette smoking history of 45 pack-years smoking 17 years ago) presented for a pulmonary nodule that was incidentally discovered on computed tomography (CT) during an evaluation of the patient's neck pain. He stated that he did not have any respiratory symptoms, and he had never received a diagnosis of chronic obstructive pulmonary disease, asthma, or any other lung condition. CT showed a nodule, which was in the anterior left upper lobe, that was 17×24 mm, irregular, solid, and noncalcified (Figure 32.1). Mediastinal and left hilar lymphadenopathy was also present on CT. Further imaging with fluorine 18–labeled fluorodeoxyglucose (FDG)–positron emission tomography (PET) showed a maximum standardized uptake value (SUVmax) of 2.5 in the lung nodule and FDG avidity in mediastinal and left hilar nodes with an SUVmax up to 7.5 (Figure 32.2).

On physical examination, his vital signs were normal, including oxygen saturation as measured by pulse oximetry (97% while breathing room air). On pulmonary examination, he had

Figure 32.1   CT of the Chest

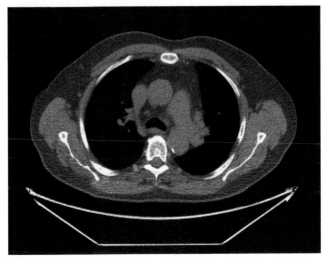

Axial view shows an irregular, solid, noncalcified 17×24-mm nodule in the anterior left upper lobe and mediastinal and left hilar lymphadenopathy.

Figure 32.2   FDG-PET of the Chest

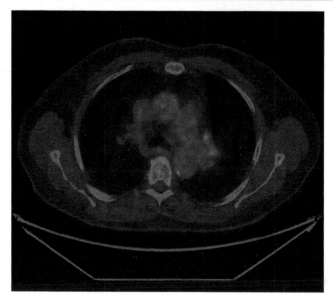

Axial view shows FDG avidity in the mediastinal and left hilar lymph nodes, which have an SUVmax up to 7.5. The lung nodule has an SUVmax of 2.5.

good air entry bilaterally with clear lung sounds on auscultation and no respiratory distress. The remainder of the examination findings were unremarkable.

After discussion with the patient about the risks and benefits of further diagnostic evaluation, bronchoscopy was performed with endobronchial ultrasonography-guided transbronchial needle aspiration and bronchoalveolar lavage (BAL). Lymph node stations 7 and 11L were sampled, and BAL samples were sent for cytology, bacterial, mycobacterial, and fungal testing. Serologic testing, staining, and cultures were negative for *Histoplasma*, *Blastomyces*, and *Coccidioides*. The pathology results from the station 11L lymph node were consistent with lung adenocarcinoma. Expression of programmed death ligand 1 (PD-L1) in the samples was 1% to 10%. The station 7 nodal sample showed atypical cells, so a reactive or degenerative cause was suspected.

Questions

Multiple Choice (choose the best answer)

32.1. Which of the following is most predictive of benign disease when lung nodules are evaluated for malignancy on PET-CT?
   a. Draining lymph nodes with an SUVmax that equals or exceeds the value for the associated lung nodule
   b. Solid lung nodule that measures 9 mm and has an SUVmax of 1.2 in a patient with emphysema
   c. Subsolid pulmonary nodule that measures 15 mm and has a 6-mm solid component with an SUVmax of 1.2
   d. Ground-glass nodule that measures 20 mm with an SUVmax of 1.2
   e. Upper lobe 9-mm spiculated nodule with an SUVmax of 3.0

32.2. For patients with non–small cell lung cancer (NSCLC), which of the following is true regarding mediastinal and extrathoracic staging?
   a. If patients have extensive mediastinal infiltration and no distinct metastases, invasive confirmation is required in addition to radiographic assessment
   b. For patients with clinical stage III or IV NSCLC, routine imaging of the head is not required if the clinical evaluation findings are negative
   c. For patients with peripheral tumors with negative nodal involvement on CT and PET (clinical stage IA), invasive preoperative evaluation of mediastinal nodes is not required
   d. If patients have mediastinal lymph node enlagement on CT without PET uptake, invasive staging of the mediastinum is not recommended

   e. If patients have mediastinal lymph node PET uptake, but nodes appear normal on CT without distant metastases, invasive staging of the mediastinum is not required

32.3. Which of the following is the best predictor of survival for patients with NSCLC?
   a. Adenocarcinoma compared to other subtypes
   b. Cancer stage
   c. SUVmax less than 5 in the primary tumor
   d. Smoking cessation
   e. Tumor grade

32.4. During evaluation for surgical resection of the primary nodule in a patient with stage II NSCLC, pulmonary function testing showed that the predicted postoperative (ppo) forced expiratory volume in the first second of expiration (FEV_1) was 53% of the predicted value, and the ppo diffusing capacity of lung for carbon monoxide (D_{LCO}) was 52% of the predicted value. With these findings, what should be recommended?
   a. Proceed with resection
   b. Perform shuttle-walk test
   c. Perform cardiopulmonary exercise testing (CPET) with assessment of maximum oxygen consumption ($\dot{V}o_2$max)
   d. Avoid resection (it is contraindicated)
   e. Refer the patient to the radiation oncology service for stereotactic beam radiotherapy before resection

32.5. With the information available for the patient described above in the Case Presentation, in addition to resection, what would be the most appropriate therapy?
   a. Erlotinib
   b. Crizotinib
   c. Pembrolizumab
   d. Platinum-based chemotherapy with prophylactic cranial radiotherapy
   e. Platinum-based chemotherapy

Case Follow-up and Outcome

The patient was referred to the thoracic surgery service for further evaluation for mediastinal sampling and possible left upper lobectomy because of the location of the nodule and concern for nodal spread. On pulmonary function testing, FEV$_1$ was 89% of the predicted value and D$_{LCO}$ was 79% of the predicted value. On tissue sampling during mediastinoscopy, the station 4L lymph node was positive, so lobectomy was not performed, and T1cN2M0 (stage IIIA) disease was confirmed. Molecular testing results were negative for sequence variations in *ALK*, *BRAF*, *EGFR*, *KRAS*, and *NRAS*. The patient was no longer a candidate for surgical resection, so he was assessed by the oncology service and plans were made to initiate a platinum-based chemotherapy regimen of carboplatin and paclitaxel in combination with radiotherapy, which was consistent with published guidelines.

Discussion

The finding of FDG-avid pulmonary nodules with mediastinal or hilar lymph node FDG uptake on PET nearly always prompts concern for malignancy. Recognition of imaging patterns that suggest a malignant or benign cause can be beneficial for an initial assessment. The characteristics of nodules observed on CT that correlate to increased risk of malignancy, as described by the Fleischner Society and others, include the following: increase in nodule diameter, subsolid nodules (ground-glass or partly solid appearance), spiculated nodules, and upper lobe location (1,2).

Typically on PET, an SUVmax of 2.5 or more is accepted as being associated with an increased risk of malignancy (3). A second PET indicator suggestive of a malignant pulmonary nodule is when the observed FDG uptake in the lesion is greater than that in the mediastinum (3).

PET-CT has a higher sensitivity and specificity compared to conventional CT, but studies can have false-positive findings, particularly with fungal pulmonary infections or other causes of granulomatous inflammation. These conditions can cause increased FDG uptake in lung nodules and mediastinal or hilar lymph nodes.

One study described the "flip-flop fungus" sign, which can aid in distinguishing benign granulomatous processes from malignancy (4). That study found that in benign processes, lymph nodes often have FDG avidity that is at least as much as in the associated pulmonary nodule. In contrast, in the pattern of uptake more commonly observed in lung cancer, the nodule has greater FDG avidity than the draining lymph nodes. The accuracy of the flip-flop fungus sign is increased when results are known for fungal serologies and CT imaging. Overall, a positive flip-flop fungus sign in combination with positive fungal serologies has 100% specificity for benign disease (4).

Another novel method of evaluating the likelihood of malignancy of lung nodules on PET-CT is through dual-time-point imaging, in which PET images are obtained at baseline and at 100-minute time points. Increasing or stable FDG nodule avidity at the 100-minute time point correlates with increased risk of malignancy (5).

Ideally diagnosis and staging of lung cancer should be accomplished simultaneously by performing the fewest procedures. Typically, this involves PET-CT with subsequent tissue sampling of the FDG-avid site that may represent the highest stage of disease. Accurate cancer staging is important for prognostication and for guiding management. If a solitary nodule is of concern in the absence of lymphadenopathy, direct surgical resection can be performed for diagnosis and cure.

As a general rule, the mainstay of therapy for stage I or stage II NSCLC is surgical resection with a minimally invasive technique such as video-assisted thoracoscopic surgery (6). When surgical resection is considered for a patient, the ppo values for D$_{LCO}$ and FEV$_1$ should be at least 60% of the predicted value. If the ppo values are

30% to 60% of the predicted values, stair-climb or shuttle-walk testing is recommended; if the predicted ppo values are less than 30% of the predicted values, CPET should be performed. Adjuvant chemotherapy is recommended for stage II disease but not for stage I disease. Adjuvant radiotherapy has been beneficial for completely resected stage I or stage II NSCLC.

Management guidelines for stage III NSCLC, as in the patient described above, are less clear owing to the broad spectrum of disease burden and nodal involvement with this stage (7). In summary, for patients who have appropriate performance status and are being considered for treatment with curative intent, the recommendation is platinum-based chemotherapy in combination with radiotherapy. Prophylactic cranial radiotherapy is not recommended (unlike for patients with small cell lung cancer). Either definitive chemoradiotherapy or induction therapy with subsequent surgery can be appropriate for patients with stage IIIA disease (in patients with discrete N2 involvement). A multidisciplinary team approach is necessary when patients have stage III NSCLC.

Management of stage IV disease can produce benefits in quality of life and duration of survival, even though disease at this stage is not considered curable. Platinum-based chemotherapy was the usual therapy for stage IV NSCLC, but current standards incorporate molecular pathology (eg, *EGFR* mutation, *ALK* translocation, and PD-L1 expression) and use specific targeted agents with or without traditional chemotherapy. Patients with oligometastatic disease (ie, 1 extrathoracic metastasis) may benefit from surgical resection (6).

Summary

FDG-avid pulmonary nodules with mediastinal or hilar lymph nodes on PET-CT can have malignant or benign origins. Certain characteristics of the nodule appearance and FDG uptake patterns can help guide consideration for a malignant basis in the appropriate clinical context. NSCLC with ipsilateral mediastinal lymph node involvement is considered N2 disease and indicates NSCLC that is at least stage IIIA. Treatment of stage III disease is best coordinated with a multidisciplinary team because of the complexity of the decisions involved and the broad spectrum of clinical severity within this stage, but management generally involves platinum-based chemotherapy in combination with radiotherapy.

Answers

32.1. Answer a.

Characteristics of pulmonary nodules predictive of malignancy have been studied well to avoid the risks of unrecognized malignancy and to avoid referring patients for invasive testing if nodules can be recognized as benign noninvasively. The data have shown that the following imaging findings are predictive of malignant causes: SUVmax of 2.5 or more, spiculation, upper lobe location, increasing nodule size larger than 6 mm, multiple nodules (total count ≤4; decreased malignancy risk with ≥5 nodules), and underlying emphysema or pulmonary fibrosis.

Thoracic adenopathy is also evaluated on CT and PET-CT. The finding of a pulmonary nodule with FDG-avid hilar or mediastinal adenopathy raises concern for a malignant cause of the pulmonary nodule. However, nodules with an FDG-avid adenopathy can have both malignant and benign causes (eg, granulomatous disease and infection). Studies have also defined features of this adenopathy that may predict benign causes, such as an SUVmax of the draining lymph node that is equal to or greater than the SUVmax of the nodule itself. This finding suggests that the nodule and the adenopathy are more likely due to fungal disease rather than malignancy. The other answer choices include features concerning for primary lung malignancy, including patient risk factors (7-mm nodule and SUVmax of 1.2), nodule size (a 15-mm subsolid nodule with a 6-mm solid component or a 20-mm ground-glass nodule), or a spiculated nodule with an SUVmax of 2.5 or more.

Additional information is available in the medical literature (1-3).

32.2. Answer c.

Appropriate staging of NSCLC is essential for the selection of therapy. This involves assessment for sites of additional pulmonary, nodal, and extrapulmonary involvement. In many patients, staging requires invasive sampling of thoracic lymph nodes with endobronchial ultrasonography and transbronchial needle biopsy. For mediastinal staging (in the absence of distant metastases), invasive staging is recommended to assess for potential nodal spread if there is either discrete lymph node enlargement or PET activity. However, if imaging shows extensive mediastinal infiltration with distant metastases, this finding is typically sufficient for staging without the need for invasive confirmation. Mediastinal infiltration would indicate T4 disease by TNM classification and would therefore be classified as stage III NSCLC.

Further, if stage IA disease has been determined from a peripheral tumor and negative nodal involvement on CT and PET, the incidence of nodal involvement is sufficiently low that preoperative evaluation of mediastinal nodes is not required. Routine imaging for distant metastases is not required for all patients with NSCLC. However, when focal signs or symptoms are present, imaging may be targeted to specific sites for further evaluation. An exception to this practice is patients with clinical stage III or IV disease, which carries an increased risk of occult metastasis. For these patients, magnetic resonance imaging (MRI) of the brain (or CT if MRI is unavailable) is recommended. If a patient has clinical stage I or II disease, though, routine imaging of the brain is not indicated.

Additional information is available in the medical literature (6).

32.3. Answer b.

Numerous prognostic factors have been identified in NSCLC, including extent or stage of disease, performance status, younger age, absence of weight loss, smoking cessation, and SUVmax. Of these, TNM stage at presentation is the most important for prognosis, and the purpose of the TNM system is to group the features of the malignancy into stages that correlate with prognosis and treatment.

SUVmax does appear to have prognostic value in NSCLC, with a high SUVmax indicating a poorer prognosis. However, there is no consensus on a specific SUVmax threshold that indicates poor prognosis. Current literature cites a broad range of thresholds, from 2.5 to 20. Smoking cessation is associated with a better prognosis, although not as strongly as TNM stage. Notably, the histologic subtype (adenocarcinoma compared to squamous cell carcinoma) and histopathology of NSCLC are not considered to be widely accepted predictors of survival because clinical studies have had conflicting results.

Additional information is available in the medical literature (8,9).

32.4. Answer b.

For patients who have stage I NSCLC and are candidates for surgery, surgical resection is curative. Patients who are not interested in pursuing surgery or are not candidates for resection owing to a nonfavorable risk-benefit ratio may be referred for stereotactic beam radiotherapy. Resection is often indicated also for patients with stage II disease and for certain patients with stage III disease.

When a patient's risk-benfit profile for surgical resection is evaluated, the physiologic risk of the procedure and the ppo lung function should be assessed. Patient risk may ultimately be classified as low, moderate, or high. For all patients, the first step is to determine the ppo values for D_{LCO} and FEV_1.

Those values are evaluated as percentages of the predicted values as follows: if both

are greater than 60%, the risk is low; if both are in the range of 30% to 60%, the patient should undergo shuttle-walk or stair-climb testing; if either ppo is greater than 60%, CPET should be performed. If patients have shuttle-walk results greater than 400 m or stair-climbing results greater than 22 m, they are classified as low risk. If patients have shuttle-walk results less than 400 m or stair-climb results less than 22 m, they should undergo CPET.

CPET results may then be used to categorize patients as having low risk (VO_2max >20 mL/kg/min or >75% of the predicted value); moderate risk (VO_2max, 10-20 mL/kg/min or 35%-75% of the predicted value); or high risk (VO_2max <10 mL/kg/min or <35% of the predicted value).

For the patient in the question, both the $ppoFEV_1$ and the $ppoD_{LCO}$ are between 30% and 60%, so further evaluation should be performed with either shuttle-walk or stair-climb testing. To proceed directly to resection would not be recommended because the risk profile is insufficiently characterized. CPET could be performed next, but shuttle-walk or stair-climb testing is a more efficient, cost-effective method of risk stratification. On the basis of the ppo values alone, surgery is not contraindicated, but not enough information has been obtained to accurately determine the risk profile, and further testing should be performed to evaluate for possible curative surgery before considering alternative therapies.

Additional information is available in the medical literature (6).

32.5. Answer e.

Adjuvant therapies are important for preventing disease recurrence and progression of NSCLC. These therapies can be categorized as radiotherapy, cytotoxic chemotherapy, targeted therapies, and immunotherapies. Cytotoxic chemotherapy includes agents that nonspecifically prevent cell proliferation. In NSCLC, the preferred regimen typically entails platinum-based chemotherapy. Increasingly, however, specific gene sequence variations are identified in the pathogenesis of NSCLC, and targeted agents can then be directed at specific cell signaling pathways. For example, driver mutations are found in approximately 64% of patients with lung adenocarcinoma.

When driver mutations are found with a specific targeted agent, median survival time is improved. Genes with sequence variations that have US Food and Drug Administration (FDA)-approved therapies include *EGFR* (erlotinib), *ALK* (crizotinib), *ROS1*, and *BRAF*. One of the most common sequence variations in NSCLC, *KRAS*, does not have a targeted therapy.

For patients with stage II (N1 nodal) disease and good performance status, current guidelines suggest the use of postoperative platinum-based chemotherapy. Tissue should be submitted for mutation analysis so that targeted agents may be used, although this testing may not be immediately available at all facilities, but platinum-based therapies may be used when this information is not available. Trial targeted therapy would not be appropriate without confirmation of a specific sequence variation.

Pembrolizumab is an immunotherapy agent that inhibits PD-L1. Blocking the PD-L1 pathway inhibits the immune downregluation by tumor cells and induces an antitumor response. An assessment for PD-L1 expression from NSCLC tissue samples is recommended. Pembrolizumab has FDA approval for use in stage III and stage IV NSCLC.

Unlike in small cell lung cancer, prophylactic cranial radiotherapy is not typically indicated for use in patients with NSCLC. Additional information is available in the medical literature (6,10).

References

1. MacMahon H, Naidich DP, Goo JM, Lee KS, Leung ANC, Mayo JR, et al. Guidelines for management of incidental pulmonary nodules detected on CT images: from the Fleischner Society 2017. Radiology. 2017 Jul;284(1):228–43.
2. Swensen SJ, Silverstein MD, Ilstrup DM, Schleck CD, Edell ES. The probability of malignancy in solitary pulmonary nodules. Application to small radiologically indeterminate nodules. Arch Intern Med. 1997 Apr 28;157(8):849–55.
3. Chundru S, Wong CY, Wu D, Balon H, Palka J, Chang CY, et al. Granulomatous disease: is it a nuisance or an asset during PET/computed tomography evaluation of lung cancers? Nucl Med Commun. 2008 Jul;29(7):623–7.
4. Nagelschneider AA, Broski SM, Holland WP, Midthun DE, Sykes AM, Lowe VJ, et al. The flip-flop fungus sign: an FDG PET/CT sign of benignity. Am J Nucl Med Mol Imaging. 2017 Nov 1;7(5):212–7.
5. Alkhawaldeh K, Bural G, Kumar R, Alavi A. Impact of dual-time-point (18)F-FDG PET imaging and partial volume correction in the assessment of solitary pulmonary nodules. Eur J Nucl Med Mol Imaging. 2008 Feb;35(2):246–52.
6. Detterbeck FC, Lewis SZ, Diekemper R, Addrizzo-Harris D, Alberts WM. Executive summary: diagnosis and management of lung cancer, 3rd ed: American College of Chest Physicians evidence-based clinical practice guidelines. Chest. 2013 May;143(5 Suppl):7S–37S.
7. Ramnath N, Dilling TJ, Harris LJ, Kim AW, Michaud GC, Balekian AA, et al. Treatment of stage III non-small cell lung cancer: diagnosis and management of lung cancer, 3rd ed: American College of Chest Physicians evidence-based clinical practice guidelines. Chest. 2013 May;143(5 Suppl):e314S–40S.
8. Berghmans T, Dusart M, Paesmans M, Hossein-Foucher C, Buvat I, Castaigne C, et al; European Lung Cancer Working Party for the IASLC Lung Cancer Staging Project. Primary tumor standardized uptake value (SUVmax) measured on fluorodeoxyglucose positron emission tomography (FDG-PET) is of prognostic value for survival in non-small cell lung cancer (NSCLC): a systematic review and meta-analysis (MA) by the European Lung Cancer Working Party for the IASLC Lung Cancer Staging Project. J Thorac Oncol. 2008 Jan;3(1):6–12.
9. Sculier JP, Chansky K, Crowley JJ, Van Meerbeeck J, Goldstraw P; International Staging Committee and Participating Institutions. The impact of additional prognostic factors on survival and their relationship with the anatomical extent of disease expressed by the 6th Edition of the TNM Classification of Malignant Tumors and the proposals for the 7th Edition. J Thorac Oncol. 2008 May;3(5):457–66.
10. Kris MG, Johnson BE, Berry LD, Kwiatkowski DJ, Iafrate AJ, Wistuba II, et al. Using multiplexed assays of oncogenic drivers in lung cancers to select targeted drugs. JAMA. 2014 May 21;311(19):1998–2006.

A 68-Year-Old Man With Dyspnea and Multiple Pulmonary Nodules

Scott M. Canepa, MD, Gregory R. Stroh, MD, and Jay H. Ryu, MD

Case Presentation

A 68-year-old man was referred to the pulmonary service from the thoracic surgery service for further evaluation of dyspnea and abnormal findings on computed tomography (CT) of the chest after he had been referred from another facility for surgical lung biopsy.

Three months before his evaluation at our clinic, he had been evaluated at his local facility for dyspnea. Radiography of the chest showed diffuse reticulonodular opacities, and COVID-19 test results were negative. He was treated with antibiotics for presumed atypical pneumonia, but his condition did not improve. Several weeks later, follow-up radiography of the chest showed persistent abnormalities. Those findings prompted CT of the chest, which showed diffuse, bilateral pulmonary nodules with mediastinal and hilar lymphadenopathy, patchy ground-glass opacities in the right lower lobe, a focal consolidation in the right upper lobe, and a small right-sided pleural effusion (Figures 33.1 and 33.2).

At the other facility, additional findings included a high antinuclear antibody titer (1:320; speckled pattern) and normal or negative results for complete blood cell count, comprehensive metabolic panel, rheumatoid factor, blood testing for tuberculosis (TB), erythrocyte sedimentation rate, histoplasma serology, and histoplasma urine antigen. Echocardiographic findings were normal.

At our institution, the patient reported that he did not have cough, fevers, arthralgias or myalgias, rash, or night sweats. He described an intentional weight loss of 20 lb (9 kg) over the past 3 months associated with modest dietary interventions. His past medical history included asthma, gastroesophageal reflux disease, migraines, and nonmelanomatous skin cancer. He had never smoked and he worked in pharmaceutical sales. His only relevant environmental or occupational exposure was owning 2 cockatiels for the preceding 2 decades. He reported that he did not have any TB exposures or risk factors, and he did not have a family history of pulmonary or rheumatologic disease.

His oxygen saturation was 94% while breathing room air. Physical examination findings were remarkable only for inspiratory crackles and decreased breath sounds at the right lung base. Specifically, he did not have a rash, palpable lymphadenopathy, or synovitis.

Pulmonary function testing showed moderate restriction and a moderate reduction in diffusing capacity of lung for carbon monoxide (D$_{LCO}$) (total lung capacity, 54% of the predicted value; ratio of forced expiratory volume in the first second of expiration to forced vital capacity, 66%; and D$_{LCO}$, 54% of the predicted value). Thoracic ultrasonography showed a modestly sized right-sided pleural effusion (Figure 33.3).

With thoracentesis, 650 mL of serous fluid was removed (protein, 3.7 g/dL; lactate dehydrogenase

Figure 33.1   Axial Section From the Patient's First Chest CT

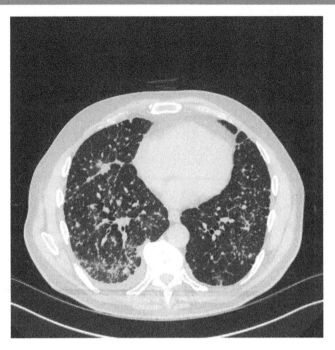

Figure 33.2   Coronal Section From the Patient's First Chest CT

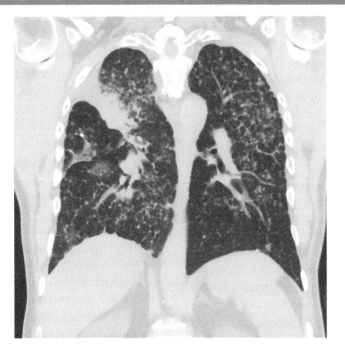

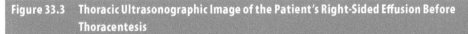

Figure 33.3   Thoracic Ultrasonographic Image of the Patient's Right-Sided Effusion Before Thoracentesis

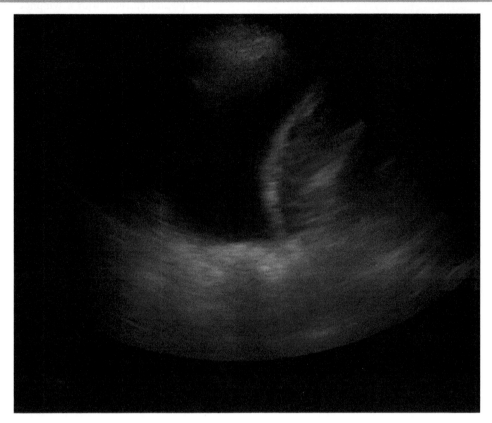

[LDH], 177 U/L [upper limit of reference range for serum, 222 U/L]). The fluid was exudative according to the Light criteria. (That is, the fluid met ≥1 of the following 3 criteria: ratio of pleural fluid protein to serum protein >0.5; ratio of pleural fluid LDH to serum LDH >0.6; or pleural fluid LDH exceeds two-thirds the upper limit of the reference range for serum LDH.) The fluid had a total nucleated cell count of 789/μL (87% lymphocytes).

Questions

Multiple Choice (choose the best answer)

33.1. Which of the following diseases is most likely to have multiple pulmonary nodules?
   a. Chronic eosinophilic pneumonia
   b. Birt-Hogg-Dube (BHD) syndrome
   c. Lymphangioleiomyomatosis (LAM)
   d. Rheumatoid arthritis
   e. Alveolar proteinosis

33.2. Which of the following diffuse lung diseases can present with cavitary pulmonary nodules?
   a. Granulomatosis with polyangiitis (GPA)
   b. Idiopathic pulmonary fibrosis (IPF)
   c. Fibrotic (chronic) hypersensitivity pneumonitis (HP)
   d. Lymphocytic interstitial pneumonia (LIP)
   e. Granulomatous-lymphocytic interstitial lung disease (GL-ILD)

33.3. Which of the following should be included in the differential diagnosis for an exudative pleural effusion with a lymphocytic predominance?
   a. Empyema
   b. Hepatic hydrothorax
   c. Malignancy
   d. Esophageal rupture
   e. Heart failure

33.4. What is the diagnostic yield of a single thoracentesis for a malignant pleural effusion?
   a. 15%
   b. 35%
   c. 50%
   d. 65%
   e. 90%

33.5. What type of malignant pleural effusion has the lowest diagnostic yield from thoracentesis?
   a. Ovarian adenocarcinoma
   b. Pancreatic adenocarcinoma
   c. Melanoma
   d. Prostate adenocarcinoma
   e. Mesothelioma

Case Follow-up and Outcome

Pleural fluid cytology findings were consistent with metastatic adenocarcinoma of pulmonary origin, and the patient was given a diagnosis of stage IV lung adenocarcinoma. The patient was referred to the medical oncology service and underwent positron emission tomography–CT and magnetic resonance imaging of the brain, which showed innumerable bony metastases throughout the skull and axial skeleton. Uptake of fluorodeoxyglucose F 18 was apparent in the consolidative opacity in the right upper lobe, and patchy uptake had occurred in both lungs and in the right hilar and mediastinal lymph nodes.

Discussion

Diffuse pulmonary nodules can be a diagnostic challenge because the pulmonologist must consider a wide range of potential diagnoses (both common and uncommon). Therefore, a structured approach is essential to secure the correct diagnosis. The history, physical examination, and chest CT are the foundations of the diagnostic approach to the patient with diffuse pulmonary nodules. To further refine the differential diagnosis, the clinician must incorporate other information, including the duration of disease, its temporal evolution, and other clinical features. The diagnostic approach to patients who have 1 or only a few pulmonary nodules differs from that for patients with diffuse nodularity, and the following discussion focuses on an initial interpretive approach to the chest CT and the clinical features of some of the more common diseases that present with diffuse pulmonary nodules.

First, however, further discussion of the secondary pulmonary lobule is warranted because familiarity with this anatomical unit of the lung is essential for describing the distribution of lesions on chest CT. A *secondary pulmonary lobule* contains alveolar sacs and is centered on terminal bronchioles and pulmonary arterioles. The boundaries are demarcated by connective tissue (interlobular septae) and pulmonary venules and lymphatics (Figure 33.4). The generation of a radiologic differential diagnosis requires recognition of the location of pulmonary nodules in relation to the structures of the secondary pulmonary lobule (perilymphatic, centrilobular, or

Figure 33.4   Diagram Showing the Components of a Secondary Pulmonary Lobule

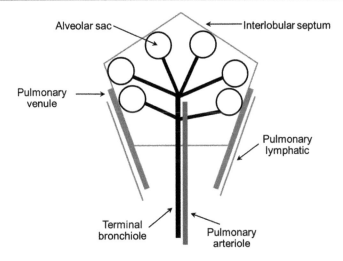

Categorization of Diffuse Pulmonary Nodules According to Their Appearance on Chest CT

Pleural surfaces or pulmonary fissures involved

Random distribution of nodules
  Metastases
  Miliary infection
Perilymphatic distribution of nodules
  Sarcoidosis
  Silicosis
  Coal workers' pneumoconiosis
  Lymphangitic carcinomatosis

Pleural surfaces and pulmonary fissures spared

Centrilobular nodularity
  HP
  RB-ILD
  Infection
  Vasculitis
Hemorrhage
  Tree-in-bud nodularity
  Mycobacterial infection
  Bacterial infection
  Fungal infection
  Airway disease (cystic fibrosis; bronchiectasis)

random) and recognition of the involvement of the pleural or fissural surfaces.

The first step in the radiologic evaluation is to identify whether the nodules involve the pleural surfaces or pulmonary fissures (or both). Next, the distribution of nodules must be identified (Box 33.1) (1,2).

In the case described above, the patient's nodules did involve the pleurae and pulmonary fissures, so important diagnostic considerations include sarcoidosis, silicosis, coal workers' pneumoconiosis, malignancy, and miliary infection (typically TB or fungal infection) (Box 33.1). The pattern of distribution should be identified as either perilymphatic or random. In this patient the distribution of

nodules was random, which indicates that a miliary infection or malignancy would be the most likely diagnosis (Figures 33.1 and 33.2). With the absence of fever, malaise, and cough, infection would be less likely but should not be excluded. The diagnosis of a malignant process is supported by the development of a new pleural effusion in a patient who had a recent echocardiogram with normal findings, who lacked infectious symptoms, and who had weight loss that was disproportionate to the reported dietary changes.

When miliary infection is suspected, a thorough evaluation for TB should include the tuberculin skin test or interferon-γ release assay in conjunction with sputum analysis with acid-fast bacilli smear microscopy, mycobacterial culture, and nucleic acid amplification testing. Extrapulmonary manifestations of TB should be considered, and adenosine deaminase testing should be performed on suspected tubercular pleural effusions (3,4). Evaluation for diffuse or disseminated endemic fungal infections (histoplasmosis, blastomycosis, and coccidioidomycosis) should be guided by the patient's exposure and travel history and may include serologic testing, antigen detection, and fungal culture and smear. Immunocompromised patients should be evaluated for opportunistic infections (eg, aspergillosis and mucormycosis), and these patients may have atypical imaging findings.

The presentation of the patient described above has some features that overlap clinically and radiographically with sarcoidosis, particularly given the calcified hilar and mediastinal lymphadenopathy. However, in sarcoidosis, the nodularity is perilymphatic and most prominent in the upper and mid lung zones. Pleural effusions and consolidations are uncommon radiologic findings. Scarring can be present in later stages of sarcoidosis (4). Patients often present with cough, dyspnea, fatigue, fever, and weight loss; however, extrathoracic involvement is common and further emphasizes the importance of a comprehensive review of systems and an evaluation to exclude alternative diagnoses.

Biopsy of involved tissues shows nonnecrotizing granulomas (4).

Similarly, silicosis and coal workers' pneumoconiosis may be considered if the nodules have a perilymphatic distribution (5). However, these diagnoses must be supported by the appropriate exposure history.

When nodules do not involve the surfaces of the pleurae or fissures, a distinction must be made between centrilobular nodules and tree-in-bud nodularity. For centrilobular nodules, important diagnostic considerations include acute or subacute HP, respiratory bronchiolitis–associated interstitial lung disease (RB-ILD), infection, vasculitis, and hemorrhage (Box 33.1) (1,6).

Salient features of HP include cough, dyspnea, and fatigue. Patients with acute or subacute (nonfibrotic) HP typically have ground-glass centrilobular nodules, but mosaic ground-glass opacities throughout the lung from air trapping are also commonly seen (7). Patients with fibrotic (chronic) HP have scarring and fibrosis, which may be confused with IPF. Other supportive features of HP include a lymphocyte predominance on bronchoalveolar lavage (BAL), specific immunoglobulin (Ig)G antibodies to sensitizing antigens, and histologic findings of poorly formed nonnecrotizing granulomas, cellular bronchiolitis, and organizing pneumonia (7).

RB-ILD occurs nearly exclusively in smokers who present with upper lobe–predominant centrilobular nodules and bronchial wall thickening. Pigmented macrophages are seen with BAL and lung biopsies, but these studies are most useful for the exclusion of other diagnoses. This condition frequently improves with smoking cessation (8).

Diffuse alveolar hemorrhage (DAH) often presents with diffuse ground-glass opacities, but it can present with centrilobular nodules (which are thought to represent intra-alveolar macrophages). DAH can be diagnosed with bronchoscopy and BAL showing 1 or both of the following: progressive bloody return of lavage fluid and hemosiderin-laden macrophages with Prussian blue staining (>20% of macrophages) (9).

DAH has numerous possible causes and requires a thorough evaluation. One cause is vasculitis, but *vasculitis* is a descriptive term that encompasses a broad spectrum of diseases, which may or may not involve the lungs. When patients have pulmonary involvement, the pulmonary imaging findings are quite diverse. Pulmonary involvement occurs in some forms of small-vessel vasculitis. Most cases of centrilobular nodularity due to vasculitis are secondary to DAH (eg, IgA vasculitis, cryoglobulinemia, systemic lupus erythematosus, and drug-induced vasculitis). Nonhemorrhagic centrilobular nodules are present in some patients with eosinophilic GPA, although patchy ground-glass opacities are the most common imaging abnormalities (10-13). Patients with GPA typically have cavitary nodules that are subpleural or perilymphatic, and only a minority of patients present with centrilobular nodules (14,15).

If the nodularity is associated with a tree-in-bud pattern, infectious causes and aspiration encompass the majority of identified causes (16). A clinical history of aspiration with predisposing risk factors, such as bulbar weakness and alcoholism, and a dependent distribution of nodules support a diagnosis of aspiration. This may be confirmed (although not excluded) with fluoroscopic visualization in a barium swallow study. Infectious causes include mycobacterial, bacterial, fungal, and viral diseases, and confirmation of a diagnosis usually requires additional testing (serology, nasopharyngeal swab, BAL, or biopsy). However, clinical clues such as the disease course may help direct initial investigations (eg, a prolonged disease course may suggest fungal or mycobacterial disease, while an abrupt onset frequently supports bacterial infections) (16). Rarely, some forms of vascular diseases (eg, intravenous talcosis) may also demonstrate the tree-in-bud pattern.

Summary

The differential diagnosis of pulmonary nodules is broad and encompasses various systemic and lung-limited diseases. An organized and algorithmic diagnostic approach is necessary to formulate and narrow an accurate differential diagnosis. The present case demonstrates how the use of such an approach with key features of the clinical history can direct a focused and successful diagnostic investigation.

Answers

33.1. Answer d.

Patients with rheumatoid arthritis may present with a broad spectrum of pulmonary findings, including multiple pulmonary nodules (rheumatoid lung nodules). Other pulmonary manifestations include airway diseases, pleural effusions, and rheumatoid arthritis–associated interstitial lung disease (RA-ILD). CT findings of RA-ILD include bronchiolitis, organizing pneumonia, and a nonspecific interstitial pneumonia or a usual interstitial pneumonia pattern. Pulmonary nodules are not characteristic features of LAM, BHD syndrome, chronic eosinophilic pneumonia, or alveolar proteinosis. LAM and BHD syndrome are rare diseases with characteristic findings of diffuse or multifocal cysts. The radiologic presentation of alveolar proteinosis is a diffuse or geographic pattern of ground-glass opacities with or without associated thickened interlobular structures. The presence of interlobular thickening with superimposed ground-glass opacities is typically described as the "crazy-paving" pattern. Common findings with chronic eosinophilic pneumonia include bilateral, predominantly peripheral consolidative and ground-glass opacities. Findings on radiography of the chest are usually described as the photographic negative shadow of pulmonary edema, but those findings are encountered in less than half the patients who have chronic eosinophilic pneumonia. Additional information is available in the medical literature (11,12,17-23).

33.2. Answer a.

Patients with GPA frequently present with multiple bilateral pulmonary nodules or masses that are subpleural or perilymphatic. Cavitary lesions may be seen in as many as 49% of patients who have nodules.

Additional common findings include consolidative or ground-glass opacities. Characteristic features of IPF include peripheral, predominantly basilar reticular opacities associated with honeycombing and traction bronchiectasis. Nodules are not a usual feature. Fibrotic (chronic) hypersensitivity pneumonitis, LIP, and GL-ILD are frequently characterized by nodules, but cavitation is not typical. Additional information is available in the medical literature (7,14,15,24-28).

33.3. Answer c.

An exudative pleural effusion with a lymphocytic predominance suggests malignancy, tuberculosis, rheumatoid arthritis, chylothorax, or yellow nail syndrome as the common causes. Patients with empyema or esophageal rupture may present with unilateral exudative effusions but typically with a neutrophilic predominance. Patients with hepatic hydrothorax or heart failure have transudative effusions. Additional information is available in the medical literature (29).

33.4. Answer d.

A single thoracentesis with pleural fluid cytology has a diagnostic yield of 65%. The sensitivity may increase with repeated sampling, but the additional yield decreases considerably beyond the second thoracentesis, and further diagnostic attempts are not recommended. The diagnostic yield does not, however, markedly change if the volume of fluid removed is increased. Additional factors that affect the yield include sample preparation, tumor burden (the number of cells per milliliter), and the tumor type. Additional information is available in the medical literature (30-33).

33.5. Answer e.

The diagnostic sensitivity of thoracentesis for malignant pleural effusions is highly dependent on the type of primary tumor. The sensitivity is lowest for mesothelioma, compared with the other malignancies listed, and usually mesothelioma cannot be diagnosed from cytology alone. In descending order, the reported sensitivities for the listed cancers are pancreatic adenocarcinoma, ovarian adenocarcinoma, melanoma, and prostate adenocarcinoma. Understanding the expected diagnostic yield on the basis of the most likely primary cancer may tailor the clinician's diagnostic approach. Additional information is available in the medical literature (31).

References

1. Gruden JF, Naidich DP, Machnicki SC, Cohen SL, Girvin F, Raoof S. An algorithmic approach to the interpretation of diffuse lung disease on chest CT imaging: a theory of almost everything. Chest. 2020;157(3):612–35.

2. Raoof S, Amchentsev A, Vlahos I, Goud A, Naidich DP. Pictorial essay: multinodular disease: a high-resolution CT scan diagnostic algorithm. Chest. 2006;129(3): 805–15.

3. Aggarwal AN, Agarwal R, Gupta D, Dhooria S, Behera D. Interferon gamma release assays for diagnosis of pleural tuberculosis: a systematic review and meta-analysis. J Clin Microbiol. 2015;53(8):2451–9.

4. Baughman RP, Teirstein AS, Judson MA, Rossman MD, Yeager H, Jr., Bresnitz EA, et al. Clinical characteristics of patients in a case control study of sarcoidosis. Am J Respir Crit Care Med. 2001;164(10 Pt 1):1885–9.

5. Ryu JH, Daniels CE, Hartman TE, Yi ES. Diagnosis of interstitial lung diseases. Mayo Clin Proc. 2007;82(8):976–86.

6. Okada F, Ando Y, Yoshitake S, Ono A, Tanoue S, Matsumoto S, et al. Clinical/pathologic correlations in 553 patients with primary centrilobular findings on high-resolution CT scan of the thorax. Chest. 2007;132(6):1939–48.

7. Vasakova M, Morell F, Walsh S, Leslie K, Raghu G. Hypersensitivity pneumonitis: perspectives in diagnosis and management. Am J Respir Crit Care Med. 2017;196(6):680–9.

8. Ryu JH, Myers JL, Capizzi SA, Douglas WW, Vassallo R, Decker PA. Desquamative interstitial pneumonia and respiratory bronchiolitis-associated interstitial lung disease. Chest. 2005;127(1):178–84.

9. De Lassence A, Fleury-Feith J, Escudier E, Beaune J, Bernaudin JF, Cordonnier C. Alveolar hemorrhage: diagnostic criteria and results in 194 immunocompromised hosts. Am J Respir Crit Care Med. 1995;151(1):157–63.

10. Silva CI, Muller NL, Fujimoto K, Johkoh T, Ajzen SA, Churg A. Churg-Strauss syndrome: high resolution CT and pathologic findings. J Thorac Imaging. 2005;20(2):74–80.

11. Johkoh T, Muller NL, Akira M, Ichikado K, Suga M, Ando M, et al. Eosinophilic lung diseases: diagnostic accuracy of thin-section CT in 111 patients. Radiology. 2000;216(3):773–80.

12. Jeong YJ, Kim KI, Seo IJ, Lee CH, Lee KN, Kim KN, et al. Eosinophilic lung diseases: a clinical, radiologic, and pathologic overview. Radiographics. 2007;27(3):617–37; discussion 37-9.

13. Chung MP, Yi CA, Lee HY, Han J, Lee KS. Imaging of pulmonary vasculitis. Radiology. 2010;255(2): 322–41.

14. Lee KS, Kim TS, Fujimoto K, Moriya H, Watanabe H, Tateishi U, et al. Thoracic manifestation of Wegener's granulomatosis: CT findings in 30 patients. Eur Radiol. 2003;13(1):43–51.

15. Ananthakrishnan L, Sharma N, Kanne JP. Wegener's granulomatosis in the chest: high-resolution CT findings. AJR Am J Roentgenol. 2009;192(3):676–82.

16. Miller WT Jr, Panosian JS. Causes and imaging patterns of tree-in-bud opacities. Chest. 2013;144(6):1883–92.

17. Lee HK, Kim DS, Yoo B, Seo JB, Rho JY, Colby TV, et al. Histopathologic pattern and clinical features of rheumatoid arthritis-associated interstitial lung disease. Chest. 2005;127(6):2019–27.

18. Tanaka N, Kim JS, Newell JD, Brown KK, Cool CD, Meehan R, et al. Rheumatoid arthritis-related lung diseases: CT findings. Radiology. 2004;232(1):81–91.

19. Raoof S, Bondalapati P, Vydyula R, Ryu JH, Gupta N, Raoof S, et al. Cystic lung diseases: algorithmic approach. Chest. 2016;150(4):945–65.

20. Holbert JM, Costello P, Li W, Hoffman RM, Rogers RM. CT features of pulmonary alveolar proteinosis. AJR Am J Roentgenol. 2001;176(5):1287–94.

21. Ishii H, Trapnell BC, Tazawa R, Inoue Y, Akira M, Kogure Y, et al. Comparative study of high-resolution CT findings between autoimmune and secondary pulmonary alveolar proteinosis. Chest. 2009;136(5):1348–55.

22. Koslow M, Young JR, Yi ES, Baqir M, Decker PA, Johnson GB, et al. Rheumatoid pulmonary nodules: clinical and imaging features compared with malignancy. Eur Radiol. 2019;29(4):1684–92.

23. Jederlinic PJ, Sicilian L, Gaensler EA. Chronic eosinophilic pneumonia: a report of 19 cases and a review of the literature. Medicine (Baltimore). 1988;67(3):154–62.

24. Panchabhai TS, Farver C, Highland KB. Lymphocytic interstitial pneumonia. Clin Chest Med. 2016;37(3):463–74.

25. Raghu G, Remy-Jardin M, Myers JL, Richeldi L, Ryerson CJ, Lederer DJ, et al. Diagnosis of idiopathic pulmonary fibrosis: an official ATS/ERS/JRS/ALAT Clinical Practice Guideline. Am J Respir Crit Care Med. 2018;198(5):e44–e68.

26. Mannina A, Chung JH, Swigris JJ, Solomon JJ, Huie TJ, Yunt ZX, et al. Clinical predictors of a diagnosis of common variable immunodeficiency-related granulomatous-lymphocytic interstitial lung disease. Ann Am Thorac Soc. 2016;13(7):1042–9.

27. Lohrmann C, Uhl M, Kotter E, Burger D, Ghanem N, Langer M. Pulmonary manifestations of wegener granulomatosis: CT findings in 57 patients and a review of the literature. Eur J Radiol. 2005;53(3): 471–7.

28. Cordier JF, Valeyre D, Guillevin L, Loire R, Brechot JM. Pulmonary Wegener's granulomatosis: a clinical and imaging study of 77 cases. Chest. 1990;97(4): 906–12.

29. Sahn SA HJ, San Jose E, Alvarez-Dobano JM, Valdes L. The art of pleural fluid analysis. Clin Pulm Med. 2013;20(2):77–96.

30. Rivera MP, Mehta AC, Wahidi MM. Establishing the diagnosis of lung cancer: diagnosis and management of lung cancer, 3rd ed: American College

of Chest Physicians evidence-based clinical practice guidelines. Chest. 2013;143(5 Suppl):e142S–e65S.

31. Grosu HB, Kazzaz F, Vakil E, Molina S, Ost D. Sensitivity of initial thoracentesis for malignant pleural effusion stratified by tumor type in patients with strong evidence of metastatic disease. Respiration. 2018;96(4):363–9.

32. Hooper C, Lee YC, Maskell N, Group BTSPG. Investigation of a unilateral pleural effusion in adults: British Thoracic Society Pleural Disease Guideline 2010. Thorax. 2010;65 Suppl 2:ii4–17.

33. Garcia LW, Ducatman BS, Wang HH. The value of multiple fluid specimens in the cytological diagnosis of malignancy. Mod Pathol. 1994;7(6):665–8.

A 49-Year-Old Man With Dizziness, Fatigue, Muscle Weakness, and Shortness of Breath

34

Catherine Wegner Wippel, Dante N. Schiavo, MD,
and Ryan M. Kern, MD

Case Presentation

A 49-year-old man presented to his physician because of dizziness, fatigue, muscle weakness, and shortness of breath on exertion. Past medical history was notable for recent-onset hypertension, for which he was taking lisinopril, and gastroesophageal reflux disease. He was recently hospitalized for pneumonia and sepsis and was treated with antibiotics for 5 days. He had never smoked, and his social history was unremarkable.

On echocardiography his ejection fraction was normal, but a nuclear stress test showed abnormal retrocardiac uptake. Further investigation with computed tomography (CT) of the chest showed a 33×35-mm left hilar mass (Figure 34.1). With bronchoscopy and biopsy, the mass was identified as an endobronchial carcinoid tumor. A nuclear medicine examination with an octreotide scan showed a single focus of abnormal uptake within the left hilar region that corresponded to the biopsy-proven carcinoid tumor. There was no evidence of metastatic disease.

The patient underwent a left upper lobe sleeve lobectomy and mediastinal lymphadenectomy. Pathologic findings included a 3.5×2.3×1.7-cm typical carcinoid tumor with free margins

(Figure 34.2), no malignant involvement of mediastinal lymph nodes, and nonnecrotizing granulomas in a lymphangitic distribution. Even though granulomatous inflammation can be present adjacent to resected neoplasms, sarcoidosis was considered in the differential diagnosis, but therapy was withheld until further investigation.

One week after the patient was discharged, progressive breathlessness and cough interfered with his activities of daily living. One month after he underwent surgery, flexible bronchoscopy showed stenosis and malacia of the distal left mainstem–left lower lobe bronchial anastomosis. He was treated with balloon dilation, but his symptoms did not improve.

The patient began a glucocorticoid trial because of the diagnosis of sarcoidosis, but he did not have a response to treatment. Subsequent bronchoscopy showed no change in the stenosis and malacia at the same area; he was treated with placement of a polytetrafluoroethylene (PTFE)-covered stainless steel stent in the left lower lobe with no complications. Nevertheless, the patient remained symptomatic and had a grade of 3 on the Modified Medical Research Council dyspnea scale. One month later, bronchoscopy showed distal migration of the stent, which was removed.

Figure 34.1   Chest CT

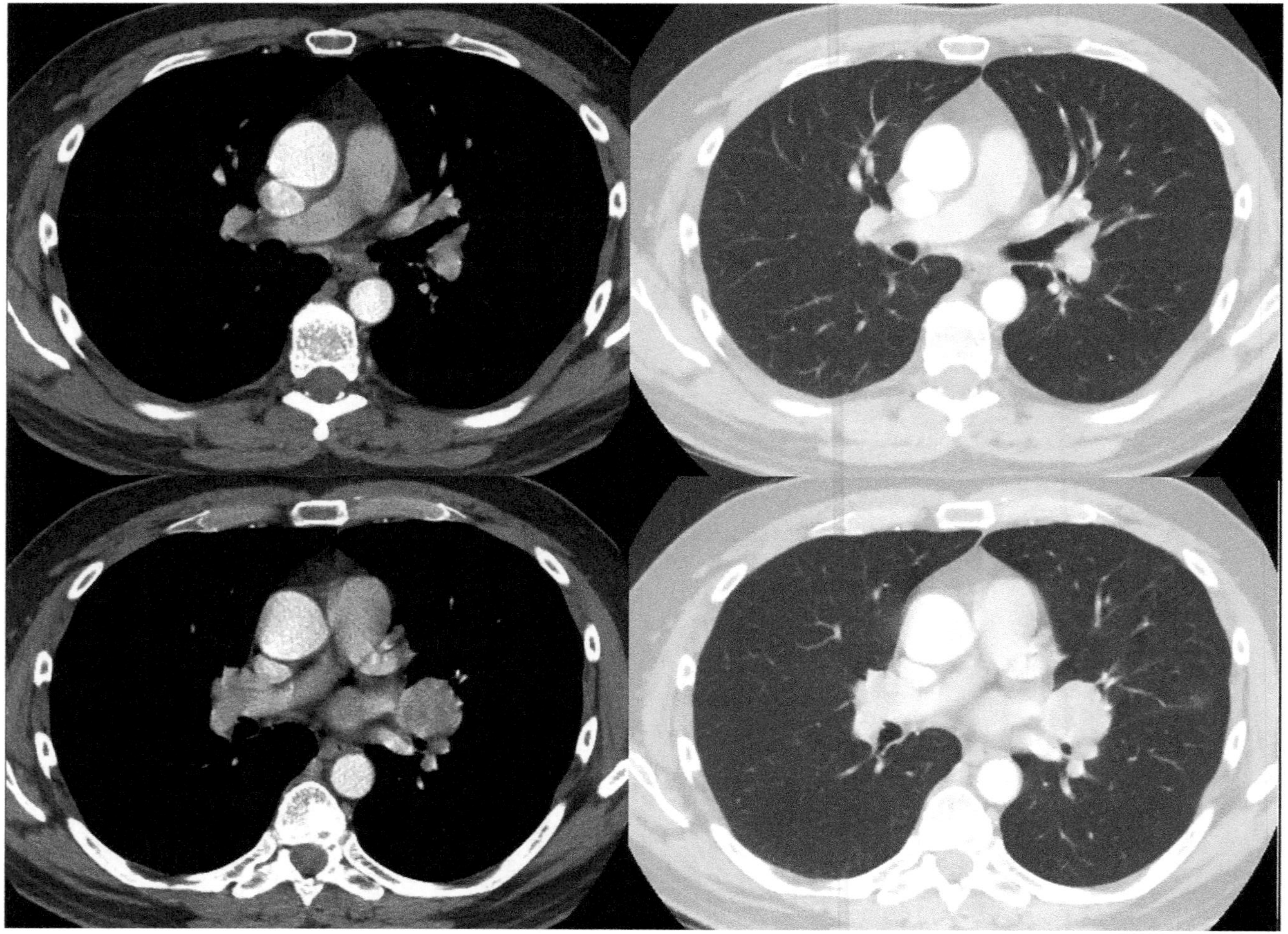

Axial sections show a 33×35-mm hypovascular left upper lobe hilar mass deforming the lingular bronchus. Left, Mediastinal window. Right, Lung window.

Figure 34.2   Gross Specimen of the Resected Tumor

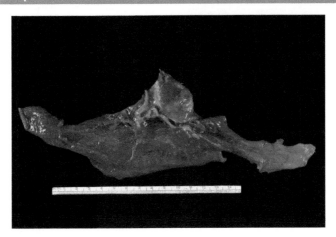

This 3.5×2.3×1.7-cm carcinoid was removed with the left upper lobe.

Questions

Multiple Choice (choose the best answer)

34.1. What is the most common cause of incidental pulmonary nodules?
   a. Hamartoma
   b. Infectious granuloma
   c. Arteriovenous malformation
   d. Adenocarcinoma
   e. Pleural pseudotumor

34.2. Which statement below correctly describes carcinoid syndrome in patients with lung neuroendocrine tumors (NETs)?
   a. Carcinoid syndrome is the most common initial presentation
   b. Carcinoid syndrome occurs only in patients with liver metastasis
   c. The prevalence of carcinoid syndrome is higher among patients with lung NETs than among patients with midgut NETs
   d. Carcinoid syndrome is uncommon in patients with lung NETs because they produce low amounts of serotonin and other bioactive amines

   e. Given the high rate of occurrence of carcinoid syndrome among patients with lung NETs, prophylactic treatment with octreotide is recommended

34.3. Which of the following features is shared by pulmonary NETs?
   a. Production of neuropeptides
   b. Low mitotic rate
   c. Presence of necrosis
   d. Cytologic atypia
   e. Fibrotic stroma

34.4. If a patient has dyspnea, which of the following features should *not* prompt further investigation for malignancy?
   a. Hemoptysis
   b. Recurrent postobstructive pneumonia
   c. Wheezing with no history of asthma
   d. Worsening of symptoms upon supine positioning
   e. New-onset cough

34.5. Which of the following is most strongly associated with a favorable prognosis?
   a. T stage
   b. Absence of residual disease
   c. Type of surgical procedure
   d. Laterality of disease
   e. Typical histologic findings

Case Follow-up and Outcome

The patient, who had no baseline dyspnea before the sleeve lobectomy, had fluctuating dyspnea and unsatisfying respirations for a year after resection. Given the patient's lack of clinical response and the complications with balloon dilations and PTFE-covered stainless steel stent placements, it was clear that standard care was ineffective for his clinical situation. After providing informed consent, the patient agreed to try a custom Y stent produced through 3-dimensional printing (Figure 34.3). With the use of rigid bronchoscopy, the stent was placed in the left lower lobe. Patency improved in the distal left mainstream bronchus and the basilar bronchus of the left lower lobe. The stent remained in place, and the patient's symptoms improved.

Discussion

Dyspnea is a common, distressing symptom attributed to diseases in various systems, including lung disease, cardiac dysfunction, anemia, and neuromuscular diseases (1). In the US, the complaint of shortness of breath accounts for 3 to 4 million emergency department visits annually (2,3). Dyspnea can be *acute* (lasting for hours to days) or *chronic* (lasting for more than 4 to 8 weeks) (1).

Various pathophysiologic mechanisms underlie dyspnea, but a thoughtful clinical evaluation should narrow the diagnostic possibilities. The presence of associated symptoms, the severity of dyspnea, and the temporal pattern and triggers are important considerations in the diagnostic approach. Clinical impression alone can be sufficient to determine a correct diagnosis in up to two-thirds of patients presenting with dyspnea (4).

The annual incidence of pulmonary carcinoids (PCs), an uncommon subtype of NETs, ranges from 0.2 to 2 per 100,000 in the US and Europe (5). Despite being grouped with the highly aggressive small cell lung cancer (SCLC), carcinoids usually have an indolent clinical progression, carry a better prognosis, and lack an association with smoking (6). PCs are divided into 2 main groups: *typical* (low grade) and *atypical* (intermediate grade) according to the number of mitotic figures and the presence or absence of necrosis (7).

Figure 34.3   Patient-Specific Design of Airway Stent

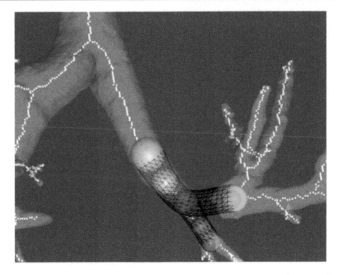

A custom Y stent was produced through 3-dimensional printing and placed in the left lower lobe.

Since most tumors arise in the proximal airways, the clinical presentation of symptomatic patients is usually related to obstruction or bleeding from the tumor (8). The most common symptoms and signs at presentation are persistent cough, hemoptysis, and recurrent or obstructive pneumonitis (9). Although a common feature of NETs is the production of bioactive amines and peptides, syndromes related to PCs occur in only 1% to 2% of patients.

Despite its name, carcinoid syndrome, which is caused by the systemic release of vasoactive substances, is uncommon in patients with NETs of the lungs, especially when compared with other primary sites (eg, small bowel) (10). PCs produce substantially less serotonin than midgut NETs. When symptoms such as cutaneous flushing, wheezing, and diarrhea are present, patients usually have larger tumors (>5 cm), which are uncommon (11).

Cushing syndrome due to ectopic corticotropin production can occur with NETs; 50% are caused by SCLC (12). Among patients with lung NETs, Cushing syndrome can be the main reason for initially seeking medical care (13).

High-resolution CT, the imaging method of choice for evaluation of a PC (14), can be used for accurate determination of tumor location and extension and for evaluation of the differential diagnosis (eg, postobstructive atelectasis) (15). Although CT of the chest is highly sensitive, the specificity for detection of hilar and mediastinal nodes is as low as 45%. Thus, other imaging modalities should confer complementary data for the assessment of tumor location and staging.

Although PCs are highly vascular, their metabolic activity is not high enough to be evaluated with fluorodeoxyglucose F 18 (FDG)–positron emission tomography (PET). Since somatostatin receptors are highly expressed in most PCs, imaging with somatostatin receptor scintigraphy (octreotide scan) or PET with gallium Ga 68 DOTATATE (or DOTATOC) can be used to assess for whole-body identification of metastatic disease (15).

About 75% of PCs are central and visible with bronchoscopy, so the procedure is a suitable approach for biopsy (15). For peripherally located tumors, CT-guided percutaneous needle aspiration is often the preferred method.

The preferred therapeutic approach for patients with localized disease is surgical resection with mediastinal lymph node sampling. Some data suggest that anatomical resections (eg, segmentectomies) confer a lower recurrence rate than wedge resections, even for low-grade tumors (16). However, some single-center studies and database reviews suggest that sublobar resection are noninferior to lobectomy for atypical PCs (17-20). For low-grade tumors affecting the mainstem bronchus, wedge or sleeve resection can be performed to preserve distal lung parenchyma (21).

For surgically unresectable tumors or for patients whose clinical condition is not suitable for surgery and who have disease that is not metastatic, radiotherapy (with or without chemotherapy) and palliative endobronchial resection are possible options (22). Because PCs are rare, and PCs with metastatic disease are even rarer, few data are available for recurrent or metastatic disease. The risk of metastasis is higher for atypical PCs, and the most common site of metastasis is the liver (9). Everolimus, an oral indirect inhibitor of mammalian target of rapamycin (mTOR), in a comparison with placebo, was shown to decrease the estimated risk of progression to death for 52% of patients in the RADIANT-4 trial (23). Comprehensive data are lacking for somatostatin analogues, so they are usually reserved for patients with carcinoid syndrome or positive findings on octreotide scans (22). Systemic cytotoxic chemotherapy has limited use, and it is usually recommended for aggressive atypical PCs (23).

Patients with typical carcinoids have an excellent prognosis; reported 5-year survival rates range from 87% to 100%, and 10-year survival rates range from 92% to 87%. Patients with atypical PCs usually have a poorer prognosis; 5-year survival rates range widely from 30% to 95%, and 10-year survival rates range from 35% to 56% (24,25). For patients who undergo surgical resection for typical or atypical carcinoids, survival rates are 93% with stage I disease, 85% with stage II, 75% with stage III, and 57% with stage IV (25).

Summary

PCs are a subgroup of well-differentiated lung NETs. Typical carcinoids have a more indolent course and carry a better prognosis than atypical carcinoids. Most tumors arise in the proximal airways, and patients present with cough, wheeze, hemoptysis, chest pain, and recurrent pneumonia. The preferred treatment is surgery. Radiotherapy with or without chemotherapy can be considered for patients who are not surgical candidates.

Answers

34.1. Answer b.

Screening studies suggest that most incidental pulmonary nodules are benign, even in high-risk populations. In the Pan-Canadian Early Detection of Lung Cancer Study and the British Columbia Cancer Agency studies, only 1% of the nodules were malignant. Among the benign nodules, about 80% are infectious granulomas. Additional information is available in the medical literature (26,27).

34.2. Answer d.

PCs produce minimal amounts of serotonin, and the occurrence of carcinoid syndrome is rare, even in patients with large tumors or disseminated disease. Additional information is available in the medical literature (10,28).

34.3. Answer a.

A common feature of NETs is the production of bioactive amines and peptides. The tumor mitotic rate, the presence of necrosis, and cytologic atypia are used to differentiate between typical and atypical NETs. Fibrotic stroma is found in a specific type of peripheral carcinoid called tumorlet. Additional information is available in the medical literature (10,29).

34.4. Answer d.

Hemoptysis, recurrent pneumonia, wheezing with no history of asthma, and cough are clinical symptoms associated with malignancy, especially in patients with risk factors for lung cancer. Worsening of symptoms upon supine positioning indicates a cardiac cause of dyspnea. Additional information is available in the medical literature (30).

34.5. Answer e.

Patients with typical (low-grade) PCs have an excellent prognosis, with reported 5-year survival rates of 87% to 100%. Patients with atypical (intermediate-grade) PCs have a worse prognosis than those with low-grade tumors, which have a greater tendency to metastasize and recur locally. Atypical tumor histology and nodal involvement are independent negative prognostic factors. Additional information is available in the medical literature (10,31).

References

1. Parshall MB, Schwartzstein RM, Adams L, Banzett RB, Manning HL, Bourbeau J, et al. An official American Thoracic Society statement: update on the mechanisms, assessment, and management of dyspnea. Am J Respir Crit Care Med. 2012;185(4):435–52.

2. Hammond EC. Some preliminary findings on physical complaints from a prospective study of 1,064,004 men and women. Am J Public Health Nations Health. 1964;54:11–23.

3. Kroenke K, Arrington ME, Mangelsdorff AD. The prevalence of symptoms in medical outpatients and the adequacy of therapy. Arch Intern Med. 1990;150(8):1685–9.

4. Pratter MR, Curley FJ, Dubois J, Irwin RS. Cause and evaluation of chronic dyspnea in a pulmonary disease clinic. Arch Intern Med. 1989;149(10):2277–82.

5. Caplin ME, Baudin E, Ferolla P, Filosso P, Garcia-Yuste M, Lim E, et al. Pulmonary neuroendocrine (carcinoid) tumors: European Neuroendocrine Tumor Society expert consensus and recommendations for best practice for typical and atypical pulmonary carcinoids. Ann Oncol. 2015;26(8):1604–20.

6. Travis WD, Brambilla E, Nicholson AG, Yatabe Y, Austin JHM, Beasley MB, et al. The 2015 World Health Organization Classification of Lung Tumors: impact of genetic, clinical and radiologic advances since the 2004 classification. J Thorac Oncol. 2015;10(9):1243–60.

7. Travis WD, Brambilla E, Burke A, Marx A, Nicholson AG, International Agency for Research on Cancer. WHO classification of tumours of the lung, pleura, thymus and heart. 412 p.

8. Skuladottir H, Hirsch FR, Hansen HH, Olsen JH. Pulmonary neuroendocrine tumors: incidence and prognosis of histological subtypes. a population-based study in Denmark. Lung Cancer. 2002;37(2):127–35.

9. Fink G, Krelbaum T, Yellin A, Bendayan D, Saute M, Glazer M, et al. Pulmonary carcinoid: presentation, diagnosis, and outcome in 142 cases in Israel and review of 640 cases from the literature. Chest. 2001;119(6):1647–51.

10. Gustafsson BI, Kidd M, Chan A, Malfertheiner MV, Modlin IM. Bronchopulmonary neuroendocrine tumors. Cancer. 2008;113(1):5–21.

11. Fischer S, Kruger M, McRae K, Merchant N, Tsao MS, Keshavjee S. Giant bronchial carcinoid tumors: a multidisciplinary approach. Ann Thorac Surg. 2001;71(1):386–93.

12. Limper AH, Carpenter PC, Scheithauer B, Staats BA. The Cushing syndrome induced by bronchial carcinoid tumors. Ann Intern Med. 1992;117(3):209–14.

13. Orth DN. Ectopic hormone production. In: Endocrinology and metabolism. Felig P, Baxter JD, Broadus AE, Frohman LA, editors. lst ed. New York (NY): McGraw-Hill; c1987. 1692 p.

14. Meisinger QC, Klein JS, Butnor KJ, Gentchos G, Leavitt BJ. CT features of peripheral pulmonary carcinoid tumors. AJR Am J Roentgenol. 2011;197(5):1073–80.

15. Hashmi H, Vanberkel V, Bade BC, Kloecker G. Clinical presentation, diagnosis, and management of typical and atypical bronchopulmonary carcinoid. JCSO. 2017;15(6):e303–8.

16. Filosso PL, Guerrera F, Falco NR, Thomas P, Garcia Yuste M, Rocco G, et al. Anatomical resections are superior to wedge resections for overall survival in patients with Stage 1 typical carcinoids. Eur J Cardiothorac Surg. 2019;55(2):273–9.

17. Ferguson MK, Landreneau RJ, Hazelrigg SR, Altorki NK, Naunheim KS, Zwischenberger JB, et al. Long-term outcome after resection for bronchial carcinoid tumors. Eur J Cardiothorac Surg. 2000;18(2):156–61.

18. Lucchi M, Melfi F, Ribechini A, Dini P, Duranti L, Fontanini G, et al. Sleeve and wedge parenchyma-sparing bronchial resections in low-grade neoplasms of the bronchial airway. J Thorac Cardiovasc Surg. 2007;134(2):373–7.

19. Yendamuri S, Gold D, Jayaprakash V, Dexter E, Nwogu C, Demmy T. Is sublobar resection sufficient for carcinoid tumors? Ann Thorac Surg. 2011;92(5):1774–8; discussion 8-9.

20. Fox M, Van Berkel V, Bousamra M 2nd, Sloan S, Martin RC 2nd. Surgical management of pulmonary carcinoid tumors: sublobar resection versus lobectomy. Am J Surg. 2013;205(2):200–8.

21. Cerfolio RJ, Deschamps C, Allen MS, Trastek VF, Pairolero PC. Mainstem bronchial sleeve resection with pulmonary preservation. Ann Thorac Surg. 1996;61(5):1458–62; discussion 62-3.

22. Kulke MH, Shah MH, Benson AB 3rd, Bergsland E, Berlin JD, Blaszkowsky LS, et al. Neuroendocrine tumors, version 1.2015. J Natl Compr Canc Netw. 2015;13(1):78–108.

23. Yao JC, Fazio N, Singh S, Buzzoni R, Carnaghi C, Wolin E, et al. Everolimus for the treatment of advanced, non-functional neuroendocrine tumours of the lung or gastrointestinal tract (RADIANT-4): a randomised, placebo-controlled, phase 3 study. Lancet. 2016;387(10022):968–77.

24. Cardillo G, Sera F, Di Martino M, Graziano P, Giunti R, Carbone L, et al. Bronchial carcinoid tumors: nodal status and long-term survival after resection. Ann Thorac Surg. 2004;77(5):1781–5.

25. Beasley MB, Thunnissen FB, Brambilla E, Hasleton P, Steele R, Hammar SP, et al. Pulmonary atypical carcinoid: predictors of survival in 106 cases. Hum Pathol. 2000;31(10):1255–65.

26. Trunk G, Gracey DR, Byrd RB. The management and evaluation of the solitary pulmonary nodule. Chest. 1974;66(3):236–9.

27. McWilliams A, Tammemagi MC, Mayo JR, Roberts H, Liu G, Soghrati K, et al. Probability of cancer in

pulmonary nodules detected on first screening CT. N Engl J Med. 2013;369(10):910–9.

28. Halperin DM, Shen C, Dasari A, Xu Y, Chu Y, Zhou S, et al. Frequency of carcinoid syndrome at neuroendocrine tumour diagnosis: a population-based study. Lancet Oncol. 2017;18(4):525–34.

29. Churg A, Warnock ML. Pulmonary tumorlet: a form of peripheral carcinoid. Cancer. 1976;37(3):1469–77.

30. Kocher F, Hilbe W, Seeber A, Pircher A, Schmid T, Greil R, et al. Longitudinal analysis of 2293 NSCLC patients: a comprehensive study from the TYROL registry. Lung Cancer. 2015;87(2):193–200.

31. Filosso PL, Oliaro A, Ruffini E, Bora G, Lyberis P, Asioli S, et al. Outcome and prognostic factors in bronchial carcinoids: a single-center experience. J Thorac Oncol. 2013;8(10):1282–8.

A 71-Year-Old Woman With a Nodule in the Right Lung

Naresh K. Veerabattini, MD, Catarina N. Aragon Pinto, MD, and Sumedh S. Hoskote, MBBS

Case Presentation

A 71-year-old woman presented for a second opinion after computed tomography (CT) of the chest showed a nodule in the right lung. She had a 40-pack-year smoking history and quit 4 years before presentation. Her past medical history included chronic obstructive pulmonary disease and cholelithiasis. Her family history included coronary artery disease and hypertension but no lung cancer. After undergoing cholecystectomy at another hospital, she had persistent postoperative pain. On CT of the abdomen at that hospital, an incidental finding was a right lower lobe lung nodule. She had no respiratory symptoms. After CT of the abdomen, fluorodeoxyglucose F 18 (FDG)–positron emission tomography (PET)/CT showed hypermetabolic activity within the lung nodule and within a lesion in the left femur.

A CT-guided biopsy of the left femur lesion at that time was negative for malignancy.

When the patient presented for a second opinion, subsequent biopsy of the left femur lesion showed metastatic adenocarcinoma consistent with primary tumor of the lung. As part of the staging process, magnetic resonance imaging of the brain showed no evidence of metastatic disease. Pulmonary function tests showed severe obstruction with air trapping (forced expiratory volume in the first second of expiration [FEV_1], 38% of the predicted value); severely reduced diffusion (diffusing capacity of lung for carbon monoxide [D_{LCO}], 39% of the predicted value); and exercise-induced desaturation. Molecular diagnostic testing did not identify any targetable sequence variations, and the cells showed 0% positivity for programmed cell death ligand 1 (PD-L1). The patient was given a diagnosis of oligometastatic lung adenocarcinoma (stage IVA).

Multiple Choice (choose the best answer)

35.1. Which statement does *not* correctly describe FDG-PET/CT in the management of pulmonary nodules?
  a. FDG-avid solid nodules larger than 8 mm are more likely to be malignant and should be biopsied
  b. Non–FDG-avid solid nodules are less likely to be malignant
  c. FDG-PET/CT can be used to evaluate for metastasis and to select the safest target for biopsy
  d. FDG-PET/CT can be helpful for identifying malignancy in patients with an indeterminate solitary pulmonary nodule
  e. Non–FDG-avid solid nodules are always benign

35.2. According to the latest edition of the TNM staging system, what would be the M classification for the tumor in the patient described above?
  a. M1a
  b. M1b
  c. M1c
  d. M0
  e. M2

35.3. Which of the following is *not* a poor prognostic factor for patients with oligometastatic non–small cell lung cancer (NSCLC)?
  a. Brain metastases
  b. Metastases to more than 1 organ

  c. Only intrapulmonary metastases
  d. Older age of patient
  e. Poor performance status

35.4. Which statement correctly describes therapy for patients with oligometastatic NSCLC?
  a. Patients with brain metastases should receive definitive therapy for only the primary site
  b. The primary site and the oligometastatic sites should be treated with surgery or ablation and then chemotherapy
  c. The primary site and the oligometastatic sites should be treated with surgery or ablation without chemotherapy
  d. Hepatic metastasis should never be resected
  e. Local consolidative therapy with surgery is superior to radiotherapy

35.5. If biopsy findings from a solitary pulmonary nodule indicate adenocarcinoma, which statement about immunohistochemical staining is accurate?
  a. Positivity for thyroid transcription factor 1 (TTF1) in an adenocarcinoma is consistent with a pulmonary origin
  b. Positivity for TTF1 in an adenocarcinoma is consistent with an intestinal origin for the adenocarcinoma
  c. Positivity for p40 is consistent with a uterine origin for the adenocarcinoma
  d. Positivity for PD-L1 is used in the decision of whether to include erlotinib in the treatment regimen
  e. PD-L1 has no role in predicting response to immune checkpoint inhibitors

Case Follow-up and Outcome

After oligometastatic adenocarcinoma of the lung was diagnosed, the case was discussed at an interdisciplinary tumor board meeting. Right lower lobectomy was not favored because the patient's pulmonary function was severely compromised. The patient was offered stereotactic body radiotherapy for the lung nodule in the right lower lobe and for the left femoral metastasis with subsequent systemic chemotherapy. An orthopedic consultation was prompted by the risk of pathologic fracture (as predicted from the patient's Mirels score), but prophylactic fixation was not recommended.

Discussion

The *AJCC Cancer Staging Manual,* 8th edition (1), which includes TNM classification of lung cancer, was published in 2017 and was adopted for use in the US in 2018. An extensive collection of data from diverse sources and validation with data from more than 70,000 patients served as the foundation for the revision with the purpose of improving the prognostic accuracy of each staging category and the TNM cutoff points (2). In the eighth edition, the classification of stage IV disease distinguishes between cancers that have a single extrathoracic metastasis and those that have multiple metastases (3). In patients with intrathoracic metastatic disease to the contralateral lung or with pleural or pericardial dissemination, the cancer is classified as M1a; cancers with only 1 extrathoracic metastasis are classified as M1b; and cancers with multiple extrathoracic metastases involving 1 or more organs are classified as M1c. The M1a and M1b cancers are now classified as stage IVA, and M1c cancer is classified as stage IVB. Patients who

have stage IVA cancer, compared with patients who have stage IVB cancer, have better survival at 24 months (23% vs 10%) and at 60 months (10% vs 0%) (3).

There is no uniform definition for how many metastases constitute *oligometastatic* disease. Published trials have used various cutoffs for the number of metastatic lesions (eg, ≤3 and ≤5). Patients who receive local consolidative therapy (ie, either high-dose radiotherapy or surgery) in addition to systemic chemotherapy or immunotherapy with monoclonal antibodies have longer disease-free survival than patients who receive only systemic therapy (4). Surgery has not been shown to be superior to radiotherapy for local treatment (5). Management should also include therapy for metastatic bone disease. Therapy with zoledronic acid or denosumab, to decrease the incidence of pathologic fractures, is recommended for stage IV metastatic bone disease (5). Prophylactic surgical intervention is indicated if the Mirels score is 9 or more (6). All patients who have metastatic lung cancer should also receive careful consideration for the involvement of palliative care according to the values, preferences, and expectations of the patient and caregivers.

Summary

Oligometastatic adenocarcinoma of the lung is a distinct subset of stage IV NSCLC that potentially carries a better prognosis. In the early course of the disease, surgery or radiotherapy for local control therapy should be considered before systemic therapy. Guidelines recommend performing molecular testing and PD-L1 testing for all patients with metastatic adenocarcinomas. The eighth edition of the *AJCC Cancer Staging Manual* (1) for TNM staging has been the standard of care since 2018 in the US.

Answers

35.1. Answer e.

FDG avidity and tracer activity cannot be reliably assessed if a solid nodule is less than 8 mm in size, so the diagnostic accuracy is limited. However, for solid nodules larger than 2 cm, the sensitivity is 91% and the specificity is 76%. Additional information is available in the medical literature (7,8).

35.2. Answer b.

According to the latest guidelines for TNM staging, cancers with intrathoracic metastatic disease in the contralateral lung or with pleural or pericardial dissemination are classified as M1a; cancers with only 1 extrathoracic metastasis are classified as M1b; and cancers with multiple extrathoracic metastases involving 1 or more organs are classified as M1c. Additional information is available in the medical literature (3).

35.3. Answer c.

The presence of only intrapulmonary metastases is not a poor prognostic factor for patients with oligometastatic NSCLC. Poor prognostic factors are the presence of extrapulmonary metastases, brain metastases, metastases to more than 1 organ, and older age of patient. Other poor prognostic factors are synchronous rather than metachronous lesions, involvement of several nodes, squamous cell histology, poor performance status, lack of epidermal growth factor receptor (EGFR) mutation, and shorter interval from initial diagnosis to metastatic development. Additional information is available in the medical literature (9-11).

35.4. Answer b.

For patients who have oligometastatic NSCLC, the primary site and all metastases should be treated with surgery or ablation and then systemic chemotherapy. For patients with an untreated primary NSCLC and newly diagnosed oligometastasis, there appears to be a benefit to treating all sites of malignancy with surgical or ablative therapies. Additional information is available in the medical literature (12,13).

35.5. Answer a.

TTF1 is expressed by lung adenocarcinomas and thyroid carcinomas but not by adenocarcinomas from other primary sites. It is a useful marker for pulmonary origin, especially to determine whether a pulmonary lesion is a primary lung adenocarcinoma (ie, TTF1 positive) or an adenocarcinoma that has metastasized to the lung from the colon, for example (ie, TTF1 negative). Positivity for p40 is a marker for squamous cell carcinoma. Positivity for PD-L1 can predict a response to immune checkpoint inhibitors such as pembrolizumab and nivolumab (but not erlotinib, a tyrosine kinase inhibitor that acts on the EGFR). Additional information is available in the medical literature (14).

References

1. Amin MB, Edge SB, American Joint Committee on Cancer. AJCC cancer staging manual. Eighth edition. xvii, 1024 pages p.
2. Detterbeck FC, Boffa DJ, Kim AW, Tanoue LT. The Eighth Edition Lung Cancer Stage Classification. Chest. 2017;151(1):193–203.
3. Goldstraw P, Chansky K, Crowley J, Rami-Porta R, Asamura H, Eberhardt WE, et al. The IASLC Lung Cancer Staging Project: proposals for revision of the TNM Stage Groupings in the forthcoming (Eighth) Edition of the TNM Classification for Lung Cancer. J Thorac Oncol. 2016;11(1):39–51.
4. Hu F, Xu J, Zhang B, Li C, Nie W, Gu P, et al. Efficacy of local consolidative therapy for oligometastatic lung adenocarcinoma patients harboring epidermal growth factor receptor mutations. Clin Lung Cancer. 2019;20(1):e81–e90.
5. Planchard D, Popat S, Kerr K, Novello S, Smit EF, Faivre-Finn C, et al. Metastatic non-small cell lung cancer: ESMO Clinical Practice Guidelines for diagnosis, treatment and follow-up. Ann Oncol. 2018; 29(Suppl 4):iv192–iv237.
6. Johnson SK, Knobf MT. Surgical interventions for cancer patients with impending or actual pathologic fractures. Orthop Nurs. 2008;27(3):160–71; quiz 72-3.
7. Deppen SA, Blume JD, Kensinger CD, Morgan AM, Aldrich MC, Massion PP, et al. Accuracy of FDG-PET to diagnose lung cancer in areas with infectious lung disease: a meta-analysis. JAMA. 2014 Sep 24;312(12):1227–36.
8. Gould MK, Donington J, Lynch WR, Mazzone PJ, Midthun DE, Naidich DP, et al. Evaluation of individuals with pulmonary nodules: when is it lung cancer? Diagnosis and management of lung cancer, 3rd ed: American College of Chest Physicians evidence-based clinical practice guidelines. Chest. 2013;143(5 Suppl):e93S–e120S.
9. Ashworth AB, Senan S, Palma DA, Riquet M, Ahn YC, Ricardi U, et al. An individual patient data metaanalysis of outcomes and prognostic factors after treatment of oligometastatic non-small-cell lung cancer. Clin Lung Cancer. 2014;15(5):346–55.
10. Hong JC, Ayala-Peacock DN, Lee J, Blackstock AW, Okunieff P, Sung MW, et al. Classification for long-term survival in oligometastatic patients treated with ablative radiotherapy: a multi-institutional pooled analysis. PLoS One. 2018;13(4):e0195149.
11. Lussier YA, Khodarev NN, Regan K, Corbin K, Li H, Ganai S, et al. Oligo- and polymetastatic progression in lung metastasis(es) patients is associated with specific microRNAs. PLoS One. 2012;7(12):e50141.
12. Lopez Guerra JL, Gomez D, Zhuang Y, Hong DS, Heymach JV, Swisher SG, et al. Prognostic impact of radiation therapy to the primary tumor in patients with non-small cell lung cancer and oligometastasis at diagnosis. Int J Radiat Oncol Biol Phys. 2012; 84(1):e61–7.
13. Ashworth A, Rodrigues G, Boldt G, Palma D. Is there an oligometastatic state in non-small cell lung cancer? A systematic review of the literature. Lung Cancer. 2013;82(2):197–203.
14. Travis WD, Brambilla E, Nicholson AG, Yatabe Y, Austin JHM, Beasley MB, et al. The 2015 World Health Organization Classification of Lung Tumors: impact of genetic, clinical and radiologic advances since the 2004 classification. J Thorac Oncol. 2015;10(9):1243–60.

A 65-Year-Old Man With Shoulder Pain, Cough, and Dyspnea[a]

Ann N. Vu, MD, Heyi Li, MD, and Ryan M. Kern, MD

Case Presentation

A 65-year-old man presented with pain in the right shoulder, productive cough with white sputum, and increasing dyspnea on exertion, which all began 3 weeks earlier. Initially he had gone to a local emergency department, where he was prescribed a 5-day course of antibiotics for presumed community-acquired pneumonia, but his symptoms progressed. The patient had been healthy previously and was not taking any long-term medications. He was a retired truck driver who did not have any known asbestos exposure. He had a smoking history of 40 pack-years, but he quit smoking 1 month before presentation.

On initial physical examination, the patient had decreased breath sounds over the right lung base with occasional expiratory wheezing. Laboratory data were notable for leukocytosis (leukocytes, 25.3×10^9/L; 96.8% neutrophils). The erythrocyte sedimentation rate was high (60 mm/h), and the C-reactive protein level was high (204 mg/L). After he was admitted, he underwent computed tomographic (CT) angiography of the chest, which showed a moderate, loculated pleural effusion with a rounded 9-mm density in the right middle lobe, diffuse ground-glass opacities that were most prominent in the right upper lobe, and marked subcarinal

lymphadenopathy (Figure 36.1A and B). Bedside ultrasonography showed a complex effusion with thin septations and loculations against the lateral chest wall. The patient underwent placement of a 14F pigtail chest tube, and pleural fluid analysis showed the following: pH 7.24; total nucleated cells, 972 cells/μL (20% neutrophils, 35% lymphocytes, and 2% eosinophils); lactate dehydrogenase, 475 U/L; and protein, 4.4 g/dL. Findings were negative on Gram staining and cultures. Pleural fluid cytology was negative for malignant cells.

The patient was initially treated for a complex pleural effusion with likely necrotizing pneumonia or pulmonary abscess. He completed a course of lytic therapy with intrapleural tissue plasminogen activator and deoxyribonuclease. The pleural fluid cultures continued to show no growth, and the patient had symptomatic improvement with decreased leukocytosis. He was discharged to complete an outpatient course of antibiotics.

Within 1 month, however, the patient returned to the emergency department with worsening dyspnea. CT angiography of the chest showed marked progression of the right pleural thickening, increased right lower lobe consolidation, and multiloculated pleural effusion (Figure 36.1C and D). Other findings included

[a] Portions of this case have been published in Baas P, Fennell D, Kerr KM, Van Schil PE, Haas RL, Peters S; ESMO Guidelines Committee. Malignant pleural mesothelioma: ESMO clinical practice guidelines for diagnosis, treatment and follow-up. Ann Oncol. 2015 Sep;26 Suppl 5:v31-9. Epub 2015 Jul 28; used with permission and Berzenji L, Van Schil P. Multimodality treatment of malignant pleural mesothelioma. F1000Res. 2018 Oct 22;7:F1000 Faculty Rev-1681; used under Creative Common Attribution License (https://creativecommons.org/licenses/by/4.0/).

Figure 36.1   CT Angiography of the Chest

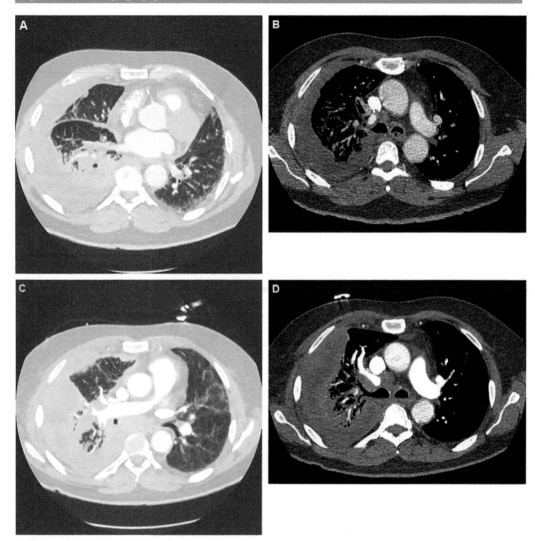

A and B, Axial sections show loculated pleural effusion with a round 9-mm density in the right middle lobe. C and D, Axial sections 1 month later show marked progression of the right pleural thickening with increased consolidation in the right lower lobe and multiloculated pleural effusion.

a lytic lesion of the right manubrium, several lucent foci in the ribs, and thoracic adenopathy. Empirical therapy with broad-spectrum antibiotics was begun again, and a 14F pigtail chest tube was placed anteriorly. Approximately 50 mL of purulent, caseous fluid was drained. The patient subsequently underwent right thoracotomy and decortication. Inflammatory tissue and rind completely encased the right lung, and frank pus was present in combination with fibrinous tissue that involved the lower lobe and the diaphragm.

Questions

Multiple Choice (choose the best answer)

36.1. If malignant mesothelioma is suspected, which diagnostic method is usually *not* sufficient for demonstrating malignancy?
   a. Surgical resection
   b. Thoracoscopic biopsy
   c. Open pleural biopsy
   d. Core needle biopsy of an accessible lesion
   e. Cytologic evaluation of pleural fluid alone

36.2. Which of the following is *not* part of the staging evaluation for malignant mesothelioma?
   a. CT scan of the chest and upper abdomen with intravenous (IV) contrast medium
   b. Fluorodeoxyglucose F 18–positron emission tomography/CT
   c. Magnetic resonance imaging with IV contrast medium
   d. Circulating carcinoembryonic antigen (CEA) level
   e. Thoracoscopy

36.3. Which of the following histologic subtypes of malignant pleural mesothelioma (MPM) is associated with the worst prognosis?
   a. Epithelioid
   b. Sarcomatoid
   c. Biphasic (mixed)
   d. Pleomorphic
   e. Histologic subtypes are not related to prognosis

36.4. Which statement correctly describes treatment of malignant mesothelioma?
   a. Radiotherapy alone improves survival and quality of life
   b. Select patients treated with checkpoint inhibitors have longer survival compared with patients who receive pemetrexed-based chemotherapy
   c. For asymptomatic patients, radical surgical therapy should be offered as early as possible
   d. Maximal surgical cytoreduction is usually adequate without chemotherapy or radiotherapy
   e. Extrapleural pneumonectomy offers a survival benefit over standard nonradical therapy

36.5. Which of the following is *not* an indication for radiotherapy for malignant mesothelioma?
   a. Prophylactic irradiation of the biopsy tract
   b. Palliation of symptoms
   c. Treatment of local recurrence after chemotherapy
   d. Adjuvant radiotherapy after cytoreductive surgery
   e. Component of multimodality treatment

Case Follow-up and Outcome

Surgical pathology showed a poorly differentiated neoplasm, which was most likely malignant mesothelioma or a poorly differentiated carcinoma. Immunohistochemical studies showed that the neoplastic cells were positive for cytokeratin (CK) 7, D2-40, and BAP1. Rare cells were positive for Wilms tumor 1 (WT1), Ber-EP4, and MOC-31. The neoplastic cells were negative for CK20, calretinin, thyroid transcription factor 1 (TTF1), CK5/6, and p40. The immunohistochemical profile was determined to be nonspecific. In the absence of radiographic evidence of extrathoracic disease, the diagnosis was presumed mesothelioma. The patient had a prolonged, complicated postoperative course. Multiorgan failure occurred with septic shock, persistent hypoxemic respiratory failure that required tracheostomy, and kidney failure that required prolonged kidney replacement therapy. He began receiving comfort care and died in the presence of his family.

Discussion

MPM is an aggressive, primary malignancy of the pleurae. According to National Cancer Database 2003-2014 data, the median survival for patients with MPM was 4.8 to 19.9 months (1). The Centers for Disease Control and Prevention identified 45,221 MPM-related deaths between 1999 and 2015 (2). Occupational exposure to asbestos accounts for more than 80% of the cases (3). The asbestos fibers enter the pleurae and signal a cascade of inflammation, which leads to activation of an oncogene. DNA damage and somatic mutations that cause loss of tumor suppressor genes also increase the risk for MPM (4). Owing to the long latency period between asbestos exposure and diagnosis, which can be up to 45 years, the incidence of MPM is expected to peak between the years 2020 and 2025

(5). However, no studies have recommended screening for patients who have an occupational history of asbestos exposure (3).

Most patients with MPM eventually have pleural effusions, which often cause symptoms, but pleural fluid cytology is often inadequate for identification of the histologic classification and is never adequate for assessment of invasion. Invasive biopsies are required for obtaining sufficient tissue for diagnosis, identification of histologic subtypes, and staging (1). Traditionally, thoracoscopy is recommended for adequate histologic studies, optimal staging, and evacuation of pleural fluid (with or without pleurodesis). In a retrospective study, percutaneous image-guided cutting needle biopsy for MPM was associated with acceptable sensitivity, an extremely low complication rate, and a negligible risk of tract seeding (6). Multiple passes may further improve the accuracy of cutting needle biopsy. Circulating tumor markers (CK-19 fragment [CYFRA 21-1], fibulin-3, and mesothelin) can be used to facilitate diagnosis of MPM, but none of them has good specificity. CEA is a negative marker and can be used to rule out MPM if cytohistologic analysis is inconclusive (7).

The use of immunohistochemistry is usually necessary for the diagnosis of MPM. Useful diagnostic mesothelial markers include calretinin, WT1, CK5/6, and D2-40 (which recognizes podoplanin). For adenocarcinoma, the most useful markers are TTF1, CEA, and Ber-EP4. The recommendation is to use at least 2 mesothelial markers and 2 carcinoma markers (with >80% sensitivity and specificity) for the diagnosis of mesothelioma when all clinical, radiologic, and histologic features are concordant (8).

The optimal treatment regimen for MPM is unclear (2). The first US Food and Drug Administration (FDA)-approved therapy for MPM was chemotherapy with pemetrexed plus cisplatin (2). Biologic agents are also being studied in the treatment of MPM. Bevacizumab was shown to increase survival by 2 months when added to cisplatin and pemetrexed therapy (9). In 2020, the FDA approved use of a PD-1 immune checkpoint inhibitor (nivolumab) in combination with a CTLA-4 inhibitor (ipilimumab), on the basis of its survival benefit compared to chemotherapy, for first-line treatment of adults who have unresectable MPM.

Various regimens with surgery in combination with radiotherapy have been investigated. However, the most effective multimodality treatment combinations for improving the prognosis with MPM have not been determined. Free resection margins are virtually impossible to obtain because of the intricate location and relation to normal tissue. Therefore, the aim is to obtain a macroscopic resection by removing as much visible tumor as possible. Surgical treatment of MPM with a curative intent includes extrapleural pneumonectomy (EPP) and extended pleurectomy-decortication (P/D). With EPP, the involved parietal and visceral pleurae are removed en bloc with the entire ipsilateral lung. The procedure is the same with extended P/D except that the lung remains in situ. In the Mesothelioma and Radical Surgery (MARS) randomized control trial, EPP in combination with postoperative hemithoracic radiotherapy, compared with standard (nonradical) therapy alone after platinum-based chemotherapy, offered no survival benefit. Furthermore, the EPP group also had higher morbidity and more serious adverse events than the non-EPP group (10). The MARS2 clinical trial (ClinicalTrials.gov identifier: NCT02040272) is a randomized

controlled trial that will compare outcomes between patients receiving platinum-based chemotherapy in combination with P/D and patients receiving chemotherapy alone.

Radiotherapy is sometimes used for palliation or as part of a multimodality treatment; however, the evidence to support its effectiveness is scarce, and some evidence suggests that it may not be useful. A systematic review suggested that there is no high-quality evidence to support the use of radiotherapy for the treatment of pain in MPM (11). Patients who have symptomatic pleural effusion should be offered palliative approaches, such as permanent placement of a tunneled catheter or thoracoscopic exploration with either partial resection or pleurodesis (or both) (12).

Summary

MPM is a rare but aggressive primary pleural malignancy. Diagnosis often requires invasive biopsy for acquisition of sufficient tissue. Despite decades of research and multimodality therapy, the optimal treatment regimen for MPM is unclear, and the prognosis is poor. In the future, though, the use of immunotherapy and biologic agents may revolutionize treatment guidelines and improve patient survival.

Answers

36.1. Answer e.

Pleural fluid cytology is often inadequate for identification of the histologic classification and is never adequate for assessment of invasion. Invasive biopsies are required for obtaining sufficient tissue for diagnosis. Additional information is available in the medical literature (1).

36.2. Answer d.

Circulating tumor markers can be used to facilitate diagnosis of MPM, but none of them has good specificity. CEA is a negative marker that can be used to rule out MPM if cytohistologic analysis is inconclusive, but it is not part of the staging evaluation. Additional information is available in the medical literature (7).

36.3. Answer b.

Patients with sarcomatoid mesothelioma have significantly shorter survival times than patients with other subtypes. Sarcomatoid mesothelioma is poorly responsive to chemotherapy and is associated with the worst prognosis. Additional information is available in the medical literature (3).

36.4. Answer b.

In 2020, the FDA approved use of a PD-1 immune checkpoint inhibitor (nivolumab) in combination with a CTLA-4 inhibitor (ipilimumab), on the basis of its survival benefit compared to chemotherapy, for first-line treatment of adults who have unresectable MPM. In the MARS randomized control trial, EPP in combination with postoperative hemithoracic radiotherapy offered no survival benefit when compared with standard (nonradical) therapy alone after platinum-based chemotherapy. Additional information is available in the medical literature (10).

36.5. Answer a.

Radiotherapy is sometimes used for palliation of symptoms or as part of multimodality treatment of mesothelioma or recurrence. However, radiotherapy is not used for prophylactic irradiation of the biopsy tract. Additional information is available in the medical literature (11).

References

1. Katzman D, Sterman DH. Updates in the diagnosis and treatment of malignant pleural mesothelioma. Curr Opin Pulm Med. 2018;24(4):319–26.

2. McCambridge AJ, Napolitano A, Mansfield AS, Fennell DA, Sekido Y, Nowak AK, et al. Progress in the management of malignant pleural mesothelioma in 2017. J Thorac Oncol. 2018;13(5):606–23.

3. van Zandwijk N, Clarke C, Henderson D, Musk AW, Fong K, Nowak A, et al. Guidelines for the diagnosis and treatment of malignant pleural mesothelioma. J Thorac Dis. 2013;5(6):E254–307.

4. Rossini M, Rizzo P, Bononi I, Clementz A, Ferrari R, Martini F, et al. New perspectives on diagnosis and therapy of malignant pleural mesothelioma. Front Oncol. 2018;8:91.

5. Odisio EG, Marom EM, Shroff GS, Wu CC, Benveniste APA, Truong MT, et al. Malignant pleural mesothelioma: diagnosis, staging, pitfalls and follow-up. Semin Ultrasound CT MR. 2017;38(6):559–70.

6. Welch BT, Eiken PW, Atwell TD, Peikert T, Yi ES, Nichols F, et al. A single-institution experience in percutaneous image-guided biopsy of malignant pleural mesothelioma. Cardiovasc Intervent Radiol. 2017;40(6):860–3.

7. van den Heuvel MM, Korse CM, Bonfrer JM, Baas P. Non-invasive diagnosis of pleural malignancies: the role of tumour markers. Lung Cancer. 2008;59(3): 350–4.

8. Arif Q, Husain AN. Malignant mesothelioma diagnosis. Arch Pathol Lab Med. 2015;139(8):978–80.

9. Lapidot M, Freyaldenhoven S, Bueno R. New concepts in the treatment of malignant pleural mesothelioma. J Thorac Dis. 2018;10(3):1283–5.

10. Treasure T, Lang-Lazdunski L, Waller D, Bliss JM, Tan C, Entwisle J, et al. Extra-pleural pneumonectomy versus no extra-pleural pneumonectomy for patients with malignant pleural mesothelioma: clinical outcomes of the Mesothelioma and Radical Surgery (MARS) randomised feasibility study. Lancet Oncol. 2011;12(8): 763–72.

11. Macleod N, Price A, O'Rourke N, Fallon M, Laird B. Radiotherapy for the treatment of pain in malignant pleural mesothelioma: a systematic review. Lung Cancer. 2014;83(2):133–8.

12. Kindler HL, Ismaila N, Armato SG 3rd, Bueno R, Hesdorffer M, Jahan T, et al. Treatment of malignant pleural mesothelioma: American Society of Clinical Oncology Clinical Practice Guideline. J Clin Oncol. 2018;36(13):1343–73.

Pleural Diseases

A 49-Year-Old Man With Cough, Dyspnea, and Right-Sided Chest Pain

Catarina N. Aragon Pinto, MD, Phanindra Antharam, MD,
and David E. Midthun, MD

Case Presentation

A 49-year-old man presented to the emergency department (ED) with a 1-week history of a nonproductive cough, dyspnea, and right-sided pleuritic chest pain. His history also included sour taste in his mouth, progressive shortness of breath, and a 7-lb (3.2-kg) weight loss over the past 2 to 3 months. He had not had fevers or chills.

Physical examination findings were unremarkable except for tachycardia, and laboratory test results were unremarkable except for leukocytosis (leukocyte count, 24.5×10^9/L). Chest radiography showed basilar atelectasis or consolidation on the right side and a small pleural effusion on the right side. The presence of a small, nonseptated effusion was confirmed with bedside ultrasonographic imaging of the chest.

When thoracentesis was performed on the right side, 700 mL of serous-appearing fluid was removed. Results of pleural fluid analysis indicated an exudate with the following characteristics: lactate dehydrogenase (LDH), 551 U/L (serum LDH 135 U/L); protein, 3.8 g/dL (serum protein 5.7 g/dL); glucose, 116 mg/dL (reference range, 79-160 mg/dL); total nucleated cells, 27,229/μL (reference range <500/μL); and pH, 7.38 (reference range, 7.35-7.45). Computed tomography (CT) of the chest showed consolidation and a cavity in the right lower lobe of the lung and a small residual pleural effusion. Pleural fluid cultures were negative for aerobic and anaerobic bacteria.

The patient was thought to have cavitary pneumonia and lung abscess with an uncomplicated pleural effusion; therapy was started with intravenous (IV) vancomycin and piperacillin-tazobactam. Aspiration related to poor dentition was thought to be the cause of the pneumonia and lung abscess. The leukocyte count decreased to 11.3×10^9/L within 2 days, and he was dismissed with a 6-week course of oral amoxicillin-clavulanic acid. At dismissal, chest radiography showed an unchanged, small right pleural effusion.

The patient returned to the ED 30 days after he was dismissed. He was still taking the antibiotics, but he described a recurrence of pleuritic chest pain. CT of the chest showed enlargement of the right-sided pleural effusion and the presence of loculations. Bedside ultrasonography showed a septated pleural effusion, and follow-up thoracentesis showed the following results: LDH, 1,192 U/L; protein, 4.8 g/dL; pH, 7.15; glucose, 27 mg/dL; and leukocyte count, 48.9×10^9/L, with 86% neutrophils. The fluid was confirmed as a recurrent (and now complicated) purulent pleural effusion (ie, empyema).

Multiple Choice (choose the best answer)

37.1. What is the appropriate next step in management for this patient?
a. Postponement of antibiotic therapy until culture and susceptibility results are available
b. Administration of broad-spectrum IV antibiotics with aerobic and anaerobic coverage
c. Insertion of a pigtail catheter for intrapleural lytic therapy
d. Insertion of a pigtail catheter for intrapleural antibiotic therapy
e. Administration of broad-spectrum IV antibiotics and insertion of a pigtail catheter for intrapleural lytic therapy

37.2. What is the recommended duration for intrapleural therapy?
a. Three days (3 doses)
b. Three days (≤6 doses)
c. Six days (6 doses)
d. Ten days (10 doses)
e. Daily until the effusion resolves radiologically

37.3. If intrapleural fibrinolytic therapy were administered and if the patient showed clinical improvement and chest radiography showed a much smaller pleural effusion, which of the following would be the most appropriate next step?
a. Continued administration of antibiotics alone
b. Thoracentesis
c. Administration of a second course of lytic therapy
d. Surgical decortication
e. No further intervention

37.4. A 54-year-old man presented with left-sided pleuritic chest pain for the past several

weeks. On radiography of the chest he had moderate pleural effusion with consolidation on the left side. Results from analysis of the fluid were consistent with an exudative effusion: LDH, 853 U/L (serum LDH, 244 U/L); protein, 4.2 g/dL (serum protein, 6.2 g/dL); and total nucleated cells, 55,000/μL. He had new leukocytosis (leukocyte count, 13.5×10^9/L). He began therapy with vancomycin and piperacillin-tazobactam. Which of the following would be the most helpful in guiding the next step in clinical decision making?
a. Sputum culture and susceptibility
b. Blood culture and susceptibility
c. Spirometry
d. CT of the chest
e. Ultrasonography of the chest

37.5. A 60-year-old woman was brought to the ED because of shortness of breath and fatigue for the past 2 weeks. She had a history of a broken tooth and sore gum for which she did not seek medical attention. Results of a complete blood cell count showed leukocytosis, and chest imaging showed right-sided consolidation with some fluid collection in the pleural space. Analysis of the pleural fluid showed an exudative effusion with a pH of 7.10; culture results were negative. She began antibiotic therapy, and a pleural drain was placed. Imaging showed continued signs of ongoing infection and incomplete drainage, so an intrapleural fibrinolytic agent and a mucolytic agent were administered. When should the intrapleural therapy be discontinued?
a. When radiologic imaging shows complete resolution
b. When the patient has clinical improvement
c. After 2 courses of lytic therapy
d. After 3 days and 6 courses of therapy
e. After 10 courses of lytic therapy

Case Follow-up and Outcome

After the intrapleural fibrinolytic therapy was completed, the patient improved clinically, and chest radiography showed that the pleural effusion was considerably smaller.

Discussion

Fluid accumulation in the pleural space requires an imbalance in the hydrostatic, oncotic, and pleural pressures (for a transudate) or a change in the microvascular permeability, lymphatic drainage, or peritoneal-to-pleural movement of fluid (for an exudate) (1-3). Parapneumonic effusions form in the pleural space adjacent to the site of bacterial pneumonia.

An effusion develops when interstitial fluid in the lung increases during pneumonia and moves to the pleural space, and the resorptive capacity of the pleural space is exceeded. This fluid is exudative because neutrophils also move into the pleural space (4). A complicated effusion develops when bacteria invade the pleural space. Usually the pH of the pleural fluid decreases because neutrophils and bacteria are undergoing anaerobic glycolysis. With lysis of the neutrophils, LDH concentration may increase to more than 1,000 U/L (2).

Presentation depends on many factors, including the immune competence of the patient and the organism causing the infection. Effusions from infection may also develop without the obvious radiographic presence of an adjacent pneumonia. Clinical features of a complicated parapneumonic effusion or empyema include cough, fever, pleuritic chest pain, dyspnea, and sputum production. Patients may have all or any of these symptoms. On physical examination, the presence of pleural fluid may be apparent from reduced expansion of the chest on respiration, decreased breath sounds, dullness on percussion, and reduced fremitus. The use of inhaled corticosteroid for either chronic obstructive pulmonary disease or asthma decreases the incidence of parapneumonic effusions (5).

Chest radiography and ultrasonography are essential for the evaluation and management of these patients (6). While chest radiographs show the extent of accumulation of pleural fluid, ultrasonography helps to quantify the accumulated fluid and identify the presence of loculations (7). Ultrasonography also facilitates differentiation of loculated effusions from lung consolidation or lung or pleural masses. CT of the chest is helpful for defining the extent and distribution of the abnormalities, particularly within fissures and along the mediastinum. While imaging is essential for diagnosis, thoracentesis with chemical analysis and culture of the pleural fluid are vital for guiding management with antibiotics and determining the need for tube drainage.

Therapeutic measures for parapneumonic effusions depend on whether the effusion is complicated or uncomplicated. Uncomplicated effusions are managed with thoracentesis and systemic antibiotic therapy alone; the goal is resolution of the effusion (8). Response to therapy is monitored with serial chest radiographs or ultrasonographic examinations and possibly follow-up thoracentesis. Complicated parapneumonic effusions of sufficient size do not respond adequately to antibiotic therapy alone. Few are managed with only antibiotics; the majority require early pleural fluid drainage with thoracentesis, and many require drainage of fluid with tube thoracostomy under ultrasonographic or CT guidance (8) or with placement of a surgical tube at the bedside. In general, indications for tube drainage of a parapneumonic effusion are pH less than 7.20, glucose less than 60 mg/dL, or LDH greater than 1,000 U/L (8,9). If loculations are present, intrapleural lytic therapy or multiple tubes (or both) may be necessary to facilitate adequate drainage. Intrapleural tPA-DNase therapy has been shown to improve fluid drainage in patients with pleural infection, reduce the need for surgical intervention, and shorten the duration of hospital stay (10). Video-assisted thoracoscopic surgery (VATS) is used to evacuate multiloculated or uniloculated empyema that does not resolve with the therapies mentioned above (11-13). VATS allows for minimally invasive access and for conversion to open thoracotomy if adequate pleural decortication and lung expansion are not achieved (14).

Summary

Clinical presentation, radiologic findings, and pleural fluid analysis are essential to differentiate a simple effusion from a complicated pleural effusion or empyema and can guide therapeutic management. Cultures from pleural fluid samples help guide antibiotic therapy but are not mandatory for initiation of antibiotic therapy. False-negative culture results may occur depending on which loculation in the pleural space is aspirated and analyzed. One loculation may be serous while a neighboring loculation may contain pus. Intrapleural fibrinolytic therapy is a highly valuable management option for patients concurrently treated with antibiotics. Pleural drainage and lytic therapy can be an alternative to surgical intervention and eliminate the need for surgery for the majority of patients.

Answers

37.1. Answer e.

The standard of care for this patient, who has pus in the pleural space, is thoracostomy for drainage and antibiotic therapy. In the Second Multicenter Intrapleural Sepsis Trial (MIST2) (a prospective double-blind placebo-controlled trial in the UK), when infection of the pleural space was treated with an intrapleural fibrinolytic agent and mucolytic agents concurrently with antibiotic therapy and thoracostomy drainage, the patients had shorter length of hospital stay, increased fluid drainage, and 70% fewer surgical referrals compared to patients treated with antibiotics and thoracostomy drainage alone. The patient described above had a pigtail catheter placed in the right pleural space during the second thoracocentesis, and he was given intrapleural fibrinolytic and mucolytic agents (tissue plasminogen [tPA] and deoxyribonuclease [DNase]), in accordance with the MIST2 protocol, in addition to broad-spectrum IV antibiotics (vancomycin and piperacillin-tazobactam). Direct intrapleural antibiotic therapy may seem to be useful, but according to the American Association for Thoracic Surgery guidelines, there is no evidence that direct administration of antibiotics into the pleural space (compared to use of systemic antibiotics alone) increases microbial clearance or outcomes, so it is not recommended. Additional information is available in the medical literature (8,10,12).

37.2. Answer b.

In the MIST2 trial, the intrapleural lytic therapy was administered twice daily for 3 days. However, effective pleural drainage and shorter median hospital stay have been achieved with fewer than 6 doses of intrapleural lytic therapy when the timing

for starting and discontinuing fibrinolytic therapy was determined from clinical and radiologic criteria. Additional information is available in the medical literature (10,15).

37.3. Answer a.

The continued administration of antibiotics alone would be most appropriate because this patient showed clinical improvement and the residual effusion was relatively small. The other answer choices could be appropriate depending on several factors, including whether infection had been controlled at the site, the extent of abnormality in the pleural space, whether the residual areas were appropriate for a second tube or thoracentesis, and whether the patient required surgery because drainage and control of the infection source were inadequate. A second course of lytic therapy would not be appropriate because complete radiologic resolution is not an indication for lytic therapy, and few data are available for determining when further lytic therapy is appropriate. Additional information is available in the medical literature (15).

37.4. Answer d.

Imaging is most important in the management of a complicated effusion or empyema. Ultrasonography shows the underlying loculations and facilitates therapeutic intervention, but it is less useful for identifying the extent of pleural involvement within fissures, in apices, and along the mediastinum. CT with an IV contrast agent is more sensitive and is recommended for optimal evaluation of adults who have empyema or loculated effusion. Use of a contrast agent gives a clearer picture of all the pleural surfaces and helps in delineating lung from fluid and pleural thickening from fluid. Spirometry is not indicated in the evaluation of a pleural effusion, and even though blood and sputum cultures are recommended, they will not guide clinical decision making on presentation. Additional information is available in the medical literature (7).

37.5. Answer b.

The use of intrapleural fibrinolytic agents facilitates drainage of loculated or complicated pleural effusions, shortens the hospital stay, and decreases the need for surgical intervention. The general tendency is to continue treatment until radiologic resolution of the empyema is complete or nearly complete; however, clinical improvement is a good indication to stop therapy for these patients, and many do not need 6 doses of intrapleural lytic therapy. Patients often feel better with tube placement if much of the fluid is removed with adequate fluid evacuation and if the source of the infection is controlled. Additional information is available in the medical literature (15-17).

References

1. Sahn SA. The pathophysiology of pleural effusions. Annu Rev Med. 1990;41:7–13.
2. Light RW. Parapneumonic effusions and empyema. Proc Am Thorac Soc. 2006;3(1):75–80.
3. Wang NS. Anatomy and physiology of the pleural space. Clin Chest Med. 1985;6(1):3–16.
4. Bryant RE, Salmon CJ. Pleural empyema. Clin Infect Dis. 1996;22(5):747–62; quiz 63-4.
5. Sellares J, Lopez-Giraldo A, Lucena C, Cilloniz C, Amaro R, Polverino E, et al. Influence of previous use of inhaled corticoids on the development of pleural effusion in community-acquired pneumonia. Am J Respir Crit Care Med. 2013;187(11):1241–8.
6. Heffner JE, Klein JS, Hampson C. Diagnostic utility and clinical application of imaging for pleural space infections. Chest. 2010;137(2):467–79.
7. Svigals PZ, Chopra A, Ravenel JG, Nietert PJ, Huggins JT. The accuracy of pleural ultrasonography in diagnosing complicated parapneumonic pleural effusions. Thorax. 2017;72(1):94–5.
8. Colice GL, Curtis A, Deslauriers J, Heffner J, Light R, Littenberg B, et al. Medical and surgical treatment of parapneumonic effusions: an evidence-based guideline. Chest. 2000;118(4):1158–71.
9. Shen KR, Bribriesco A, Crabtree T, Denlinger C, Eby J, Eiken P, et al. The American Association for Thoracic Surgery consensus guidelines for the management of empyema. J Thorac Cardiovasc Surg. 2017;153(6):e129–e46.
10. Rahman NM, Maskell NA, West A, Teoh R, Arnold A, Mackinlay C, et al. Intrapleural use of tissue plasminogen activator and DNase in pleural infection. N Engl J Med. 2011;365(6):518–26.
11. Wozniak CJ, Paull DE, Moezzi JE, Scott RP, Anstadt MP, York VV, et al. Choice of first intervention is related to outcomes in the management of empyema. Ann Thorac Surg. 2009;87(5):1525–30; discussion 30-1.
12. Potaris K, Mihos P, Gakidis I, Chatziantoniou C. Video-thoracoscopic and open surgical management of thoracic empyema. Surg Infect (Larchmt). 2007;8(5):511–7.
13. Cassina PC, Hauser M, Hillejan L, Greschuchna D, Stamatis G. Video-assisted thoracoscopy in the treatment of pleural empyema: stage-based management and outcome. J Thorac Cardiovasc Surg. 1999;117(2):234–8.
14. Mandal AK, Thadepalli H, Mandal AK, Chettipally U. Outcome of primary empyema thoracis: therapeutic and microbiologic aspects. Ann Thorac Surg. 1998;66(5):1782–6.
15. Majid A, Kheir F, Folch A, Fernandez-Bussy S, Chatterji S, Maskey A, et al. Concurrent intrapleural instillation of tissue plasminogen activator and dnase for pleural infection: a single-center experience. Ann Am Thorac Soc. 2016;13(9):1512–8.
16. Maskell NA, Davies CW, Nunn AJ, Hedley EL, Gleeson FV, Miller R, et al. U.K. Controlled trial of intrapleural streptokinase for pleural infection. N Engl J Med. 2005;352(9):865–74.
17. Tokuda Y, Matsushima D, Stein GH, Miyagi S. Intrapleural fibrinolytic agents for empyema and complicated parapneumonic effusions: a meta-analysis. Chest. 2006;129(3):783–90.

A 45-Year-Old Woman With Respiratory Failure and Septic Shock

38

Xavier E. Fonseca Fuentes, MD, Gaja F. Shaughnessy, MD, and Tobias Peikert, MD

Case Presentation

A 45-year-old woman with a history of multiple myeloma (MM), which was treated with autologous peripheral blood stem cell transplant complicated by delayed engraftment, was admitted to the hospital for hypoxemic respiratory failure and septic shock secondary to a central line–associated bloodstream infection due to methicillin-resistant *Staphylococcus aureus*. In addition, she had a history of recurrent symptomatic malignant pleural effusion due to MM that required an indwelling pleural catheter, which was eventually removed after pleurodesis 6 weeks before admission. The patient was initially admitted to the intensive care unit (ICU) because she briefly required therapy with vasopressors. Broad-spectrum antibiotic coverage was provided, the central line was removed, and the patient was transferred to a general care unit within 24 hours.

While in the hospital, she had persistent hypoxemia that required pulmonary consultation and evaluation on hospital day 7. On physical examination, she appeared chronically ill and had conversational dyspnea while receiving oxygen (4 L/min) through a nasal cannula. On

cardiovascular examination, she had tachycardia with no murmurs; she had bilateral crackles on pulmonary auscultation. Her abdomen was not tender or distended. On the anterior aspect of her right lower extremity she had erythematous to violaceous papules that coalesced into a large plaque. This lesion had been biopsied during this hospitalization, and results were pending. Relevant results from laboratory testing were leukopenia (without neutropenia), anemia, and a normal platelet count; mildly abnormal electrolyte results; and normal results on liver function tests. Computed tomography (CT) of the chest showed bilateral, predominantly peripheral, dense consolidations with additional patchy ground-glass opacities and intralobar septal thickening (Figure 38.1). The pleura was thickened, but there was no evidence of pleural effusion. Findings were unremarkable from bronchoscopy with bronchoalveolar lavage (BAL), and results from evaluation for an infectious process were negative. A CT-guided pleural biopsy was considered because of concern for a recurrence of MM, but the skin punch biopsy results, which were available on the same day as the procedure, were positive for MM, so a pleural biopsy was not attempted.

Figure 38.1   CT of the Chest

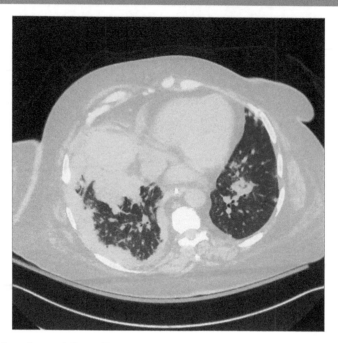

Axial view shows bilateral ground-glass infiltrates with areas of consolidation and right pleural thickening.

Questions

Multiple Choice (choose the best answer)

38.1. What would be the best initial test to confirm diagnosis?
a. Follow-up bronchoscopy with BAL
b. Open lung biopsy
c. CT-guided lung biopsy
d. Observation only
e. Ultrasound-guided diagnostic thoracentesis

38.2. If pleural effusion persists and if malignancy is still a strong consideration even without evidence from initial cytology, what would be the best next step?
a. Subsequent thoracentesis with cytology
b. Bone marrow biopsy
c. Biopsy of a lytic lesion
d. Video-assisted thoracic surgery
e. Evaluation of cell blocks from the initial thoracentesis

38.3. What test should be included in the initial evaluation of MM involvement in the pleural space?
a. Adenosine deaminase
b. Pleural fluid culture
c. Flow cytometry
d. Pleural fluid triglycerides
e. N-terminal pro-brain natriuretic peptide (NT-proBNP)

38.4. Which of the following would be the most useful for confirmation of the diagnosis?
a. Video-assisted thoracic surgery
b. Blind pleural biopsy
c. Pleural fluid protein electrophoresis
d. Positron emission tomography–CT
e. Pleural fluid cultures

38.5. Which statement describes the prognosis for a patient with MM and pleural involvement compared to the prognosis for a patient with MM and no pleural involvement?
a. The response to chemotherapy is better
b. The prognosis is poorer
c. Survival is longer
d. The response to radiotherapy is good
e. The prognosis is the same

Case Follow-up and Outcome

A trial of daratumumab and systemic corticosteroids was administered, but the patient showed no evidence of clinical improvement. Her overall condition deteriorated, and she was transferred back to the ICU for mechanical ventilation. While she was in the ICU, multifactorial acute kidney injury developed and she received renal replacement therapy. However, her condition did not improve and, after a care conference, the patient's family decided to begin comfort measures. Autopsy showed that MM had involved the right pleura.

Discussion

MM is a neoplastic plasma cell disorder characterized by clonal proliferation of malignant plasma cells in the bone marrow (1). The infiltration of bone marrow by plasma cells can lead to osteolytic lesions, osteopenia, and pathologic fractures but also can affect other organs.

Up to 46% of patients with MM have chest involvement (2). MM often affects bone structures or lung parenchyma and pleura, or it may occur as a solitary intramedullary or extramedullary lesion of neoplastic monoclonal plasma cells. In addition, various manifestations from treatment of MM can occur. Adverse effects of MM treatment include radiation pneumonitis, engraftment syndrome, and complications of stem cell transplant (diffuse alveolar hemorrhage, opportunistic infections, organizing pneumonia, acute lung injury, and graft-vs-host disease).

Pleural effusion occurs in approximately 6% of patients with MM (1). The cause can be multifactorial and affect other organs besides the lungs. Pleural effusion can occur with decompensated heart failure from amyloidosis, fluid overload from renal failure or hypoalbuminemia, infections and parapneumonic effusions, pulmonary embolism, lung infarct, and neoplasms.

Less than 1% of patients with MM have myelomatous involvement of the pleura (3). The mechanism for myelomatous pleural effusion is unclear, but several hypotheses have been proposed, including extension of the disease to the pleura from adjacent skeletal or lung parenchymal tumors, implantation of plasma cells on the pleura, and lymphatic obstruction from mediastinal lymph node infiltration (4). The time of onset varies and is usually associated with dyspnea and bone and chest pain. The effusion can be unilateral or bilateral, and its appearance can be serous, serohemorrhagic, or hemorrhagic. The pleural fluid is usually exudative with a predominance of lymphocytes. Diagnostic methods include detection of monoclonal proteins on serum and pleural fluid electrophoresis, identification of atypical plasma cells on pleural fluid cytology, histologic confirmation with pleural biopsy, and (most recently) flow cytometry and pleural fluid cytogenetics (5). However, flow cytometry and cytogenetic analysis of pleural fluid are considered only supplemental studies.

Treatment is not well defined but includes chemotherapy for MM, systemic corticosteroids, and drainage of recurrent pleural effusion with repeated therapeutic thoracentesis, chest thoracostomy tubes or an indwelling tunneled pleural catheter, and pleurodesis. The prognosis is poor despite aggressive treatment, and median survival is 4 months after diagnosis (6). The course is frequently aggressive, and the disease can be resistant to treatment and have a high chance of relapse.

Summary

Pleural involvement in MM is a rare condition that is frequently associated with a poor prognosis. The diagnostic strategy includes pleural fluid cytology and electrophoresis or histologic confirmation with pleural biopsy. Management involves treatment of MM and relief of respiratory symptoms with drainage of pleural fluid or pleurodesis.

Answers

38.1. Answer e.

In the right clinical context, the next step should be diagnostic thoracentesis to obtain pleural fluid for analysis. Current guidelines recommend the use of ultrasonographic imaging to perform this procedure. Ultrasonographic guidance increases the success rate of thoracentesis and reduces the risk of procedure-related complications, including pneumothorax. Because the early diagnosis of a malignant pleural effusion can affect clinical outcomes, open lung biopsy would not be the best initial test. Follow-up bronchoscopy, CT-guided lung biopsy, and observation alone would not be the best initial tests to confirm the diagnosis. Additional information is available in the medical literature (7).

38.2. Answer e.

The best next step would be to evaluate cell blocks from the initial thoracentesis (prepared through centrifugation and extraction of the cellular portion), which is a simple and cost-effective technique that increases the diagnostic yield. The sensitivity of pleural cytology for malignant pleural effusion is approximately 60%, and subsequent thoracentesis with cytologic analysis has a low diagnostic yield and is not recommended. Bone marrow biopsy, biopsy of a lytic lesion, and video-assisted thoracic surgery would not be the best next steps. Additional information is available in the medical literature (8,9).

38.3. Answer c.

Pleural effusion in MM can be related to pleural processes directly or to consequences of the involvement of other organs. In addition to pleural fluid cytology, flow cytometry can be considered an ancillary test. High levels of adenosine deaminase support the diagnosis of tuberculosis and can occur in other hematologic diseases. Myelomatous involvement of the pleura is rare and can be challenging to diagnose, so culturing pleural fluid and measuring levels of triglycerides would not be appropriate in the initial evaluation. The measurement of NT-proBNP is most useful for the investigation of cardiac disease. Additional information is available in the medical literature (10,11).

38.4. Answer a.

Video-assisted thoracic surgery is widely used not only for the diagnosis but also for the treatment of malignant pleural effusions. The diagnostic sensitivity is about 95%. Similarly, medical thoracoscopy can be useful in certain instances. The other answer choices would not be as useful. Additional information is available in the medical literature (8,12).

38.5. Answer b.

The prognosis is poor, and the reported median survival time is less than 4 months. Even with aggressive chemotherapy and radiotherapy, the response to treatment is poor. Additional information is available in the medical literature (6,13).

References

1. Palumbo A, Anderson K. Multiple myeloma. N Engl J Med. 2011 Mar 17;364(11):1046–60.

2. Kintzer JS Jr, Rosenow EC 3rd, Kyle RA. Thoracic and pulmonary abnormalities in multiple myeloma: a review of 958 cases. Arch Intern Med. 1978 May;138(5):727–30.

3. Alexandrakis MG, Passam FH, Kyriakou DS, Bouros D. Pleural effusions in hematologic malignancies. Chest. 2004 Apr;125(4):1546–55.

4. Al-Farsi K, Al-Haddabi I, Al-Riyami N, Al-Sukaiti R, Al-Kindi S. Myelomatous pleural effusion: case report and review of the literature. Sultan Qaboos Univ Med J. 2011 May;11(2):259–64. Epub 2011 May 15.

5. Rodriguez JN, Pereira A, Martinez JC, Conde J, Pujol E. Pleural effusion in multiple myeloma. Chest. 1994 Feb;105(2):622–4.

6. Kamble R, Wilson CS, Fassas A, Desikan R, Siegel DS, Tricot G, et al. Malignant pleural effusion of multiple myeloma: prognostic factors and outcome. Leuk Lymphoma. 2005 Aug;46(8):1137–42.

7. Feller-Kopman DJ, Reddy CB, DeCamp MM, Diekemper RL, Gould MK, Henry T, et al. Management of malignant pleural effusions: an official ATS/STS/

STR Clinical Practice Guideline. Am J Respir Crit Care Med. 2018 Oct 1;198(7):839–49.

8. Hooper C, Lee YC, Maskell N; BTS Pleural Guideline Group. Investigation of a unilateral pleural effusion in adults: British Thoracic Society Pleural Disease Guideline 2010. Thorax. 2010 Aug;65 Suppl 2:ii4–17.

9. Chen H, Li P, Xie Y, Jin M. Cytology and clinical features of myelomatous pleural effusion: three case reports and a review of the literature. Diagn Cytopathol. 2018 Jul;46(7):604–9. Epub 2018 Feb 5.

10. Zhang LL, Li YY, Hu CP, Yang HP. Myelomatous pleural effusion as an initial sign of multiple myeloma: a case report and review of literature. J Thorac Dis. 2014 Jul;6(7):E152–9.

11. Palmer HE, Wilson CS, Bardales RH. Cytology and flow cytometry of malignant effusions of multiple myeloma. Diagn Cytopathol. 2000 Mar;22(3):147–51.

12. DePew ZS, Wigle D, Mullon JJ, Nichols FC, Deschamps C, Maldonado F. Feasibility and safety of outpatient medical thoracoscopy at a large tertiary medical center: a collaborative medical-surgical initiative. Chest. 2014 Aug;146(2):398–405.

13. Cho YU, Chi HS, Park CJ, Jang S, Seo EJ, Suh C. Myelomatous pleural effusion: a case series in a single institution and literature review. Korean J Lab Med. 2011 Oct;31(4):225–30. Epub 2011 Oct 3.

An 81-Year-Old Man With Chronic Dyspnea and Recurrent Pleural Effusion

39

Mark S. Norton, MD, James P. Utz, MD, and Ryan M. Kern, MD

Case Presentation

An 81-year-old man with a past medical history of chronic obstructive pulmonary disease and coronary artery disease presented with chronic dyspnea and recurrent pleural effusion (PLEF) on the right. In the previous 3 months, he had undergone unilateral, large-volume thoracentesis on 3 occasions.

On presentation, the patient had chronic dyspnea, which improved after large-volume thoracentesis. He had not had cough, wheeze, fevers, chills, night sweats, unintentional weight loss, chest pain, orthopnea, dry eyes or mouth, dysphagia, joint or muscle pain, skin rash, or Raynaud phenomenon. He was a current smoker with a history of 65 pack-years and occupational asbestos exposure from automobile brakes when he worked as a mechanic. Results of pleural fluid analysis from another medical facility showed an elevated total protein level but no abnormal results for levels of lactate dehydrogenase (LDH),

glucose, and triglycerides; pH; or Gram stain and cultures. Lymphocytes were the predominant cell type. Cytologic findings were normal from the 2 most recent thoracenteses. On examination, the patient's oxygen saturation was 96% while he was breathing room air. The right lung base was dull on percussion with decreased breath sounds, but otherwise the lung sounds were clear. He did not have a murmur, jugular vein distention, lymphadenopathy, hepatosplenomegaly, clubbing, cyanosis, or edema. Chest radiography showed a moderately sized PLEF, which had recurred, but no additional parenchymal abnormalities were present.

Another large-volume thoracentesis was performed; the free-flowing effusion yielded 1,380 mL of clear, light pink fluid. Analysis of the pleural fluid showed the following: total protein, 5.9 g/dL (serum, 6.7 g/dL); lactate dehydrogenase, 100 U/L; pH 7.42; glucose within the reference range; lymphocytes, 66%; triglycerides, 7 mg/dL; and negative findings with Gram stain and cultures.

Questions

Multiple Choice (choose the best answer)

39.1. If each of the following patients presented with a PLEF, for which patient would thoracentesis be *least* indicated?
   a. Patient with fever, productive cough, and new lobar consolidation on chest radiography
   b. Patient with unintentional weight loss, a smoking history, and an ipsilateral spiculated nodule on chest imaging
   c. Patient with a new large PLEF and new hypoxic respiratory failure of unclear origin
   d. Patient with fatigue, cough, night sweats, and positive results on interferon-γ release assay
   e. Patient with left ventricular ejection fraction of 19%, weight gain, orthopnea, and jugular venous distention

39.2. Which of the following best characterizes the most recent pleural fluid analysis for the patient in the Case Presentation above?
   a. Simple parapneumonic effusion
   b. Lymphocyte-predominant exudative effusion
   c. Malignant PLEF
   d. Transudative effusion
   e. Empyema

39.3. Which statement best reflects how pleural fluid cytology should be used and interpreted if malignancy is suspected as the cause of the recurrent PLEF for the patient in the Case Presentation above?
   a. Continue to perform cytologic analysis on samples from each subsequent thoracentesis until a diagnosis can be made

   b. Subsequent cytologic evaluation is indicated if mesothelioma is considered a strong possibility
   c. Pleural fluid cytologic analysis is rarely helpful, and it probably should not have been performed for this patient
   d. Pleural fluid cytology is indicated, but the diagnostic sensitivity decreases considerably with each thoracentesis that yields negative results
   e. Pleural fluid cytology cannot be used to make a diagnosis of malignancy; only a tissue biopsy can be diagnostic

39.4. To evaluate a recurrent exudative PLEF of unknown cause, which procedure should be performed next?
   a. Contrast-enhanced computed tomography (CT) of the chest
   b. Bronchoscopy with bronchoalveolar lavage and transbronchial biopsy
   c. Thoracic surgery consultation for consideration of video-assisted thoracoscopic surgery for pleural biopsy
   d. Medical thoracoscopy (ie, pleuroscopy) with pleural biopsy
   e. Another thoracentesis

39.5. Which statement correctly describes the acquisition of pleural tissue?
   a. CT-guided biopsy of an area of pleural nodularity has a higher diagnostic sensitivity than medical thoracoscopy (ie, pleuroscopy)
   b. Pleuroscopy should be considered only as a last resort because the associated complication rate is high
   c. Pleuroscopy can potentially be used for both diagnosis and definitive management of a recurrent exudative PLEF
   d. Pleural biopsy is generally not recommended for the evaluation of a recurrent exudative PLEF of unclear etiology
   e. Blind pleural biopsy is noninferior to pleural biopsy with pleuroscopy for focal malignant pleural disease

Case Follow-up and Outcome

The patient's exudative PLEF from an unknown cause was extensively evaluated. Laboratory testing results were negative for connective tissue disease cascade, serum protein studies, inflammatory markers, interferon-γ release assay, HIV, and hepatitis. CT of the chest showed a large, uncomplicated, right-sided PLEF with a localized area of anteromedial pleural thickening with nodularity and a 2-mm nodule in the right upper lobe with no mediastinal or hilar adenopathy (Figure 39.1). Because laboratory testing did not suggest a clear diagnosis and because a pleural abnormality was identified on CT of the chest, medical pleuroscopy was performed; that procedure showed patches of nodular pleural thickening (Figure 39.2). Biopsy results from the pleural lesions were positive for MALToma. Follow-up positron emission tomographic (PET)-CT showed linear avidity along the right anteromedial pleura without evidence of extrapleural disease activity (Figure 39.3). The patient was given a diagnosis of primary pleural extranodal MALToma and had a favorable response to rituximab therapy.

Discussion

A commonly encountered entity, PLEF has more than 50 recognized causes, each of which requires a different treatment strategy (1). Therefore, a systematic investigation is necessary to help narrow the wide differential diagnosis to aid in rapid diagnosis and management. Generally, when the cause is benign and clinically apparent, such as when a patient has an exacerbation of congestive heart failure, invasive sampling is unnecessary unless the patient has atypical features or does not respond to conventional treatment (2). When the cause of a recurrent PLEF is unclear, diagnostic thoracentesis with pleural fluid analysis should be performed to classify the effusion as a transudate or an exudate according to the Light criteria (Box 39.1) (1). After classifying the fluid, further fluid analysis can help to narrow the differential diagnosis. For example, evaluation might include determining the number and type of white blood cells present, testing for triglycerides and glucose, and evaluating for infection with Gram stain, culture, and pH. For the patient described in the Case Presentation, pleural fluid analysis showed that the ratio of pleural total protein to

Figure 39.1   CT of the Chest

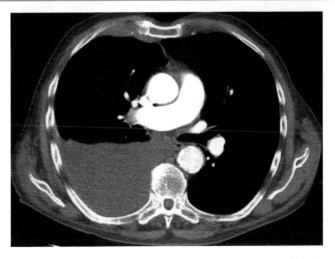

Axial view shows a large, uncomplicated, right-sided PLEF, an area of anteromedial pleural thickening with nodularity, and a 2-mm nodule in the right upper lobe without mediastinal or hilar adenopathy.

Figure 39.2   Medical Pleuroscopy

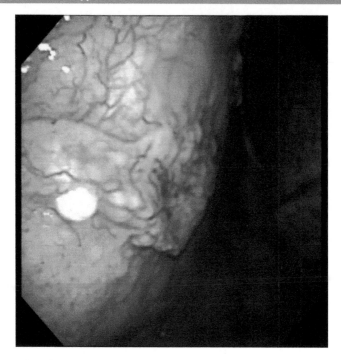

Photograph shows patches of nodular pleural thickening.

Figure 39.3   PET-CT of the Chest

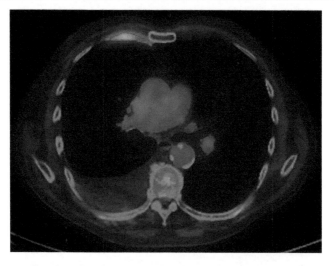

Axial view shows linear avidity along the right anteromedial pleura without evidence of extrapleural disease.

Box 39.1

Light Criteria

Pleural fluid is an exudate if 1 or more of the
   following criteria are met:
   The ratio of pleural total protein to serum total
      protein >0.5
   The ratio of pleural LDH to serum LDH >0.6
   The concentration of pleural LDH is more
      than two-thirds of the upper limit of the
      reference range for serum LDH

Data from Light RW. Clinical practice: pleural effusion.
N Engl J Med. 2002 Jun 20;346(25):1971-7.

serum total protein was 0.88, which meets the
criteria for an exudate. Furthermore, the patient
had lymphocytosis with 66% lymphocytes. Thus,
this collection of fluid was best described as a
lymphocyte-predominant exudative effusion.

Lymphocyte-predominant PLEF (where >50%
of cells are lymphocytes) is most commonly associated with malignancy (particularly lymphoma
if the percentage of lymphocytes is markedly
high) and tuberculosis worldwide (2). Other considerations include rheumatoid effusion, sarcoidosis, and chylothorax; however, a long-standing
PLEF usually accumulates lymphocytes, which
can be seen when effusions are due to chronic
heart failure, especially when patients have been
receiving loop diuretic therapy (1, 2). The wide
differential diagnosis underscores the importance of a thorough history and physical examination in addition to serologic investigations to
gain an understanding of the underlying cause of
the recurrent lymphocyte-predominant PLEF.

If malignancy is a consideration, pleural fluid
cytology should be performed because it can lead
to a definitive diagnosis for approximately 60%
of patients with malignant PLEF (2). However,
the diagnostic yield from the collection of cytologic samples on different occasions diminishes
with each negative result. The majority of positive results (65%) are obtained on the initial sampling; 27%, on the second sampling; and 5%, on
the third sampling (3). After the third sampling,

the diagnostic yield does not increase, so if 2 or
3 cytologic investigations have provided negative results, additional cytologic samples are not
recommended (2). Additionally, the sensitivity
of pleural fluid cytology depends on the underlying malignancy. For example, the diagnostic
sensitivity in adenocarcinoma is 78%; in mesothelioma, 32% (4).

If the cause of the recurrent exudative PLEF is
still unclear after pleural fluid analysis, CT of the
chest should be performed to further distinguish
between malignant and benign pleural disease.
For higher diagnostic sensitivity, CT should be
performed with a contrast medium before pleural
fluid drainage; that sequence allows for optimal
visualization of the pleura. The specificity for
focal or diffuse pleural abnormalities ranges from
88% to 100% for malignancy, and localization can
further guide more invasive diagnostic sampling
if necessary (5). Magnetic resonance imaging
(MRI) can also be used to help distinguish between benign disease and malignant disease, but
the diagnostic accuracy is not necessarily superior to that of CT (6). Furthermore, MRI is less accessible, more technically challenging, and more
costly. PET-CT is poor for differentiating malignant disease from benign disease because it has a
high rate of false-positive uptake owing to nonspecific pleural inflammation, which is seen with
both conditions (7). Bronchoscopy is not useful
in the evaluation of a recurrent exudative PLEF of
unclear etiology because it does not generally increase the diagnostic yield (2).

After advanced cross-sectional imaging with
dedicated CT of the chest has been performed,
tissue biopsy is the next step in the evaluation of
a recurrent exudative PLEF of unclear etiology.
Before advanced procedures with imaging guidance were widely available, blind biopsy of the
pleura was generally pursued, but the diagnostic
sensitivity of this procedure is only 47% (the sensitivity of blind biopsy of tuberculous pleuritis is
nearly 80%) (2). Needle biopsy of a pleural abnormality under CT guidance has much higher
sensitivity (87%) and a low complication rate
and is generally well tolerated. However, pleural
biopsy under direct visualization with medical

pleuroscopy has the highest diagnostic sensitivity of the 3 modalities (92%) (2,8). Pleuroscopy has the advantage of providing an opportunity for definitive management of the pleural space with procedures such as talc poudrage or placement of an indwelling pleural catheter, which can be performed at the end of the procedure. Furthermore, pleuroscopy is safe; the complication rate is 1.8% (8).

For the patient described in the Case Presentation, the methodical evaluation of the lymphocyte-predominant exudative PLEF of unclear etiology resulted in a swift diagnosis and effective treatment of primary pleural MALToma, a rare disease (9). This evaluation underscores the importance of approaching PLEF of unclear etiology with an evidence-based, systematic approach.

Summary

Recurrent exudative PLEF of unclear etiology is a commonly encountered entity with a wide differential diagnosis. Expedient evaluation and diagnosis are necessary to facilitate treatment, so a concise and systematic approach to evaluation is essential. Pleural fluid analysis is the first step because a lymphocyte-predominant exudate is most commonly associated with malignancy or tuberculosis; however, other causes must also be considered. Cytology is helpful and has a diagnostic sensitivity of 60%, but the sensitivity decreases considerably with each subsequent sampling, so cytology after the second or third sample is generally not useful. Advanced cross-sectional imaging with CT of the chest, preferably with a contrast agent, is needed if a diagnosis is not made after initial evaluation and analysis of the pleural fluid. This will help in differentiating between benign and malignant pleural disease and in providing guidance for tissue acquisition. Medical pleuroscopy is a safe and effective procedure for pleural biopsy, and it offers the unique opportunity for definitive management of the pleural space during the procedure with talc poudrage or placement of an indwelling pleural catheter if indicated.

Answers

39.1. Answer e.

Generally, when the cause is benign and clinically apparent, such as when a patient has an exacerbation of congestive heart failure, invasive sampling is unnecessary unless the patient has atypical features or does not respond to conventional treatment. Additional information is available in the medical literature (2).

39.2. Answer b.

Pleural fluid is exudative if 1 or more conditions are met for the Light criteria. For this patient, the ratio of pleural total protein to serum total protein was 0.88. A ratio greater than 0.5 confirms that the pleural fluid is an exudate. The differential leukocyte count from the pleural fluid showed a lymphocyte predominance of 66%. Lymphocyte-predominant PLEFs are defined as having more than 50% lymphocytes. Therefore, the patient had a lymphocyte-predominant exudative effusion. Additional information is available in the medical literature (1,2).

39.3. Answer d.

If patients have a malignant PLEF, pleural fluid cytology can lead to a definitive diagnosis for approximately 60% of patients. However, the diagnostic yield from the collection of cytologic samples on different occasions diminishes with each negative result. The majority of positive results (65%) are obtained on the initial sampling; 27%, on the second sampling; and 5%, on the third sampling. After the third sampling, the diagnostic yield does not increase. Additional information is available in the medical literature (3).

39.4. Answer a.

If the cause of the recurrent exudative PLEF is still unclear after pleural fluid analysis, CT of the chest should be performed to further distinguish between malignant and benign pleural disease. The specificity for focal or diffuse pleural abnormalities ranges from 88% to 100% for malignancy, and localization can further guide more invasive diagnostic sampling if necessary. Additional information is available in the medical literature (5).

39.5. Answer c.

Pleural biopsy under direct visualization with pleuroscopy has the highest diagnostic sensitivity (92%) of the 3 modalities (blind pleural biopsy, CT-guided biopsy, and medical pleuroscopy). Pleuroscopy has the advantage of providing an opportunity for definitive management of the pleural space with procedures such as talc poudrage or placement of an indwelling pleural catheter, which can be performed at the end of the procedure. Additional information is available in the medical literature (8).

References

1. Feller-Kopman D, Light R. Pleural Disease. N Engl J Med. 2018;378(8):740–51.
2. Hooper C, Lee YC, Maskell N, Group BTSPG. Investigation of a unilateral pleural effusion in adults: British Thoracic Society Pleural Disease Guideline 2010. Thorax. 2010;65 Suppl 2:ii4–17.
3. Garcia LW, Ducatman BS, Wang HH. The value of multiple fluid specimens in the cytological diagnosis of malignancy. Mod Pathol. 1994;7(6):665–8.
4. Porcel JM, Esquerda A, Vives M, Bielsa S. Etiology of pleural effusions: analysis of more than 3,000 consecutive thoracenteses. Arch Bronconeumol. 2014;50(5):161–5.
5. Leung AN, Muller NL, Miller RR. CT in differential diagnosis of diffuse pleural disease. AJR Am J Roentgenol. 1990;154(3):487–92.
6. Knuuttila A, Kivisaari L, Kivisaari A, Palomaki M, Tervahartiala P, Mattson K. Evaluation of pleural disease using MR and CT: with special reference to malignant pleural mesothelioma. Acta Radiol. 2001;42(5):502–7.
7. Duysinx B, Nguyen D, Louis R, Cataldo D, Belhocine T, Bartsch P, et al. Evaluation of pleural disease with 18-fluorodeoxyglucose positron emission tomography imaging. Chest. 2004;125(2):489–93.
8. Rahman NM, Ali NJ, Brown G, Chapman SJ, Davies RJ, Downer NJ, et al. Local anaesthetic thoracoscopy: British Thoracic Society Pleural Disease Guideline 2010. Thorax. 2010;65 Suppl 2:ii54–60
9. Ahmad H, Pawade J, Falk S, Morgan JA, Balacumaraswami L. Primary pleural lymphomas. Thorax. 2003;58(10):908–9.

A 46-Year-Old Woman With Progressive Shortness of Breath

Taylor T. Teague, MD, and David E. Midthun, MD

Case Presentation

A 46-year-old woman presented with progressive shortness of breath for the past 5 days. Three weeks earlier, she had undergone a Whipple resection for early-stage pancreatic adenocarcinoma and had no postoperative complications. Her past medical history included well-controlled hypertension and depression. Her only medications were amlodipine 5 mg daily and citalopram 20 mg daily. She had not had fevers, chills, cough, sick contacts, or recent travel. Upon presentation she was afebrile, and her heart rate was 96 beats/min; blood pressure, 128/82 mm Hg; and respiratory rate, 22 breaths/min. Oxygen saturation was 96% while she breathed room air. On lung auscultation breath sounds were decreased at the right lung base with dullness on percussion. Laboratory test results were normal for a complete blood cell count, basic metabolic profile, and liver enzymes. Chest radiographs are shown in Figures 40.1 and 40.2.

Figure 40.1   Chest Radiograph From 7 Months Before Presentation

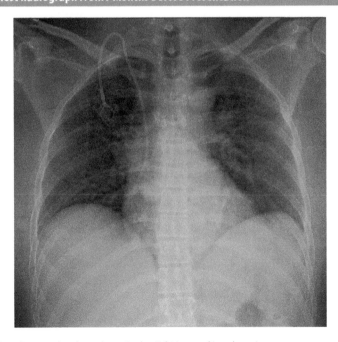

Anteroposterior view shows an implanted port in the right internal jugular vein.

Figure 40.2   Chest Radiograph Upon Presentation

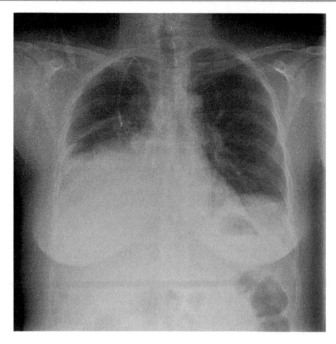

Anteroposterior view shows opacity on the right side and an implanted port in the right internal jugular vein.

Multiple Choice (choose the best answer)

40.1. For the patient described above, which of the following would be the best next step in the evaluation of the opacity on the right side of her chest?
  a. Ultrasound-guided thoracentesis
  b. Computed tomographic (CT) angiography of the chest
  c. CT of the abdomen and pelvis
  d. Transthoracic echocardiography
  e. Pulmonary function tests with bronchodilator challenge

40.2. Which of the following is most characteristic of chylothorax?
  a. Transudative effusion
  b. Pleural glucose concentration less than 40 mg/dL
  c. Pleural pH less than 7.2
  d. Pleural triglyceride concentration greater than 110 mg/dL
  e. Increased level of pleural fluid amylase

40.3. Which of the following is a risk factor for development of chylothorax?
  a. Pneumonectomy with lymph node dissection
  b. Acute pancreatitis
  c. Kidney failure
  d. Acute respiratory distress syndrome
  e. Pulmonary embolism

40.4. Which of the following is used in the treatment of chylothorax?
  a. Inhaled corticosteroids
  b. Long-acting muscarinic antagonist in combination with long-acting β-agonist inhaler
  c. Pneumonectomy
  d. Immunotherapy
  e. Low-fat, high-protein diet

40.5. Which of the following can result from a chronic, high-output chylothorax?
  a. Osteoporosis
  b. Fat-soluble vitamin deficiency
  c. Pancreatic insufficiency
  d. Liver failure
  e. Heart failure with decreased ejection failure

Case Follow-up and Outcome

The patient underwent bedside ultrasonography, which showed an anechoic fluid collection without septations. Bedside thoracentesis results are shown in Table 40.1. The pleural fluid appeared milky, so chylothorax was suspected and was then confirmed because the concentration of pleural fluid triglycerides exceeded 110 mg/dL. A 14F locking-loop pigtail catheter was inserted to manage the dyspnea and to facilitate pleural drainage. Over the next 24 hours, the output was 1,700 mL, so it was managed as a high-output chylothorax (ie, >1 L daily). She was given nothing by mouth, and total parenteral nutrition (TPN) was begun along with octreotide 150 mcg subcutaneously 3 times daily. An interventional radiologist performed lymphangiography, which showed a retroperitoneal lymphatic leak at the L2-L3 level. Lymphatic embolization was unsuccessful. Over the next 2 days, pleural output ceased, the pigtail catheter was removed, and the patient was discharged home. The pleural effusion did not recur.

Table 40.1   Pleural Fluid Analysis Results

Component	Finding
Appearance	Milky
Lactate dehydrogenase, U/L	211
Protein, g/dL	3.3
pH	7.45
Glucose, mg/dL	98
Triglycerides, mg/dL	671
Creatinine, mg/dL	0.5
Total nucleated cells, cells/µL	1,948
Neutrophils, %	23
Lymphocytes, %	46
Macrophages, %	31

Discussion

The differential diagnosis for unilateral pleural effusion is broad, but a thorough history and physical examination often provide clues to the cause (1). For the patient described above, the differential diagnosis was narrow because the new unilateral pleural effusion occurred after recent complex abdominal surgery.

Chylothorax develops when the flow of chyle through the lymphatic system (specifically the thoracic duct and its tributaries) is disrupted and chyle subsequently accumulates within the pleural space. Overall, chylothorax is a relatively rare cause of pleural effusions (2).

In general, chylothorax is classified as either traumatic or nontraumatic depending on the cause. *Traumatic* chylothorax is usually related to surgery, specifically thoracic or head and neck surgery. The chylothorax in the patient described above was considered to be traumatic and related to extensive lymphadenectomy associated with the recent Whipple procedure. *Nontraumatic* chylothorax includes malignancy (most commonly lymphoma) and other underlying diseases (eg, sarcoidosis, tuberculosis, or lymphangioleiomyomatosis). In addition, chylothorax may be idiopathic (2-4).

If chylothorax is suspected, definitive testing with thoracentesis and pleural fluid analysis should be performed. Although the fluid in chylothorax is classically described as appearing milky white, it often appears to be serous, serosanguineous, or bloody instead (5). On pleural fluid analysis, most chylous effusions are exudative with a predominance of lymphocytes (5). A pleural fluid triglyceride concentration that exceeds 110 mg/dL is diagnostic if a patient has clinical features consistent with the diagnosis (ie, pleural fluid with the classic milky appearance and associated risk factors). A pleural fluid triglyceride level less than 50 mg/dL essentially excludes the diagnosis if the patient has a compatible clinical presentation (ie, no risk factors). If the diagnosis is in doubt (triglycerides >50 mg/dL to

<110 mg/dL), further studies can be performed, such as lipoprotein electrophoresis to detect chylomicrons (6). The presence of chylomicrons confirms a diagnosis of chylothorax.

Once chylothorax is diagnosed, management is tailored to the underlying cause and the output. Foremost for a large effusion, pleural drainage should be performed to assist symptom control. However, use of repeated large-volume thoracentesis and a tunneled pleural catheter requires caution because large-volume removal of chyle may lead to immunodeficiency, fat-soluble vitamin deficiency, and volume depletion with possible kidney failure. If chylous output is low (<1 L daily), appropriate conservative measures include modifying the diet (to a low-fat, high-protein diet without long-chain triglycerides), initiating TPN, and administering somatostatin analogues (eg, octreotide). If chylous output is high (>1 L daily), the patient may require more aggressive measures such as pleurodesis (chemical or surgical), thoracic duct ligation, or thoracic embolization.

Summary

The differential diagnosis for unilateral pleural effusion is broad, but the history and physical examination findings help to narrow it. Chylothorax is a rare cause of pleural effusion, and the fluid may not appear chylous, so a high degree of awareness is required, especially when patients have compatible risk factors (ie, underlying malignancy or recent surgery). Pleural fluid from chylothorax usually has a milky appearance, exudative characteristics, and a predominance of lymphocytes. The diagnosis can be made confidently if the pleural fluid triglyceride level exceeds 110 mg/dL in the appropriate clinical context. Treatment is multimodal and incorporates conservative measures such as the use of dietary modification, TPN, and somatostatin analogues. If conservative therapy is unsuccessful, more aggressive measures, such as pleurodesis or thoracic duct ligation or embolization, can be pursued.

Answers

40.1. Answer a.

The patient's chest radiographs show a new right-sided opacity. On chest radiography, pleural effusions are apparent in the presence of about 200 mL of pleural fluid. After a new unilateral pleural effusion is identified, further evaluation should be performed with ultrasound-guided thoracentesis. Ultrasonographic guidance assists with site identification for thoracentesis, increases the likelihood of successful pleural fluid aspiration, and reduces complications. CT angiography of the chest is not warranted at this time, but if dyspnea persists after thoracentesis, CT angiography could be considered for further evaluation for pulmonary embolism. Given the abnormalities on the chest radiograph, initial evaluation with ultrasound-guided thoracentesis is warranted rather than CT of the abdomen and pelvis. Transthoracic echocardiography could be considered if heart failure were a strong possibility, and pulmonary function tests with bronchodilator challenge could be considered if obstructive lung disease, such as asthma or chronic obstructive pulmonary disease, were a strong possibility. Additional information is available in the medical literature (1).

40.2. Answer d.

Pleural triglyceride concentration greater than 110 mg/dL is diagnostic of a chylous effusion in a patient with compatible risk factors. On pleural fluid analysis, most chylous effusions are exudative rather than transudative. Pleural glucose concentration less than 40 mg/dL and pleural pH less than 7.2 are characteristic of empyema rather than chylothorax. An elevated pleural fluid amylase level is not characteristic of chylothorax but may be present with acute pancreatitis, pancreatic pseudocyst, esophageal rupture, ruptured ectopic pregnancy, or pleural malignancy. Additional information is available in the literature (1,5).

40.3. Answer a.

Depending on its cause, chylothorax can be classified as traumatic, nontraumatic, or idiopathic. *Traumatic* chylothorax is usually related to surgery, specifically thoracic or head and neck surgery. *Nontraumatic* chylothorax includes malignancy (most commonly lymphoma) and other underlying diseases (eg, sarcoidosis, tuberculosis, or lymphangioleiomyomatosis). The other conditions (acute pancreatitis, kidney failure, acute respiratory distress syndrome, and pulmonary embolism) can result in pleural effusion, but they are not considered risk factors for chylous effusion. Additional information is available in the medical literature (2,4).

40.4. Answer e.

Several treatment options are available for chylothorax. Conservative treatment measures include modifying the patient's diet (to a low-fat, high-protein diet without long-chain triglycerides), initiating TPN, and administering somatostatin analogues (eg, octreotide). Other more aggressive treatment measures include pleurodesis (chemical or surgical), thoracic duct ligation, and thoracic duct embolization. No evidence suggests that treatment of chylothorax should be based on inhaled corticosteroids, a long-acting muscarinic antagonist in combination with a long-acting β-agonist inhaler, pneumonectomy, or immunotherapy. Additional information is available in the medical literature (2,3).

40.5. Answer b.

Prolonged, large-volume removal of chyle may lead to immunodeficiency, fat-soluble vitamin deficiency, and volume depletion with possible kidney failure. However, no findings have suggested that prolonged drainage of pleural fluid results in osteoporosis, pancreatic insufficiency, liver failure, or heart failure with reduced ejection failure. Additional information is available in the medical literature (3).

References

1. Hooper C, Lee YC, Maskell N; BTS Pleural Guideline Group. Investigation of a unilateral pleural effusion in adults: British Thoracic Society Pleural Disease Guideline 2010. Thorax. 2010 Aug;65 Suppl 2:ii4–17.

2. McGrath EE, Blades Z, Anderson PB. Chylothorax: aetiology, diagnosis and therapeutic options. Respir Med. 2010 Jan;104(1):1–8.

3. Valentine VG, Raffin TA. The management of chylothorax. Chest. 1992 Aug;102(2):586–91.

4. Doerr CH, Allen MS, Nichols FC 3rd, Ryu JH. Etiology of chylothorax in 203 patients. Mayo Clin Proc. 2005 Jul;80(7):867–70.

5. Maldonado F, Hawkins FJ, Daniels CE, Doerr CH, Decker PA, Ryu JH. Pleural fluid characteristics of chylothorax. Mayo Clin Proc. 2009 Feb;84(2):129–33.

6. Hillerdal G. Chylothorax and pseudochylothorax. Eur Respir J. 1997 May;10(5):1157–62.

A 25-Year-Old Man With Sudden Onset of Severe Dyspnea

Bryan T. Kelly, MD, and John J. Mullon, MD

Case Presentation

A 25-year-old man with a history of chronic hypersensitivity pneumonitis and eosinophilic pneumonia, who was being evaluated for lung transplant, presented to the emergency department (ED) for a sudden onset of severe dyspnea. His medications included daily low-dose prednisone and azathioprine for immunosuppression. He had no recent sick contacts, cough, or fevers. In the ED, he required oxygen for hypoxemia, and he had hypotension, tachycardia, and tachypnea. On examination breath sounds were absent over the left lung field, and coarse sounds were present over the right side. Radiography of the chest (CXR) with a portable unit showed a large left-sided pneumothorax with a tension component (Figure 41.1).

Emergent needle thoracostomy provided symptomatic relief, and the patient's hemodynamic status improved. Subsequent CXR showed partial reexpansion of the lung. After the patient's condition stabilized, a 14F pigtail catheter was placed and attached to a water seal chest

| Figure 41.1 | CXR With a Portable Unit |

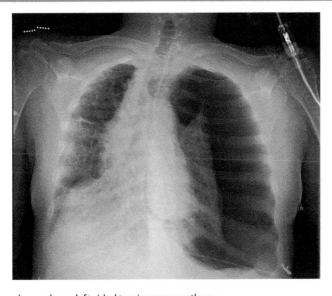

Anteroposterior view shows a large, left-sided tension pneumothorax.

drain with suction applied; a continuous air leak was present. Follow-up CXR showed adequate placement of the chest tube, but the size of the pneumothorax had increased, again with a mediastinal shift to the right. In the operating room the patient underwent urgent placement of an 18F chest tube, which was attached to a water seal chest drain with suction applied. On subsequent CXR, a tiny residual pneumothorax was present. Over the next few days, the 14F pigtail catheter became nonfunctional and the air leak from the 18F chest tube became intermittent; however, serial imaging showed that the left pneumothorax was larger, so a 28F surgical chest tube was placed and the nonfunctioning pigtail catheter was removed.

Questions

Multiple Choice (choose the best answer)

41.1. Which of the following is the safest location to perform emergent needle thoracostomy?
   a. Second intercostal space adjacent to the sternum
   b. Fifth intercostal space in the midclavicular line
   c. A site immediately adjacent to the xiphoid process
   d. Eighth intercostal space in the midaxillary line
   e. Second intercostal space in the midclavicular line

41.2. Which ultrasonographic finding could be used to rule out the presence of a pneumothorax?
   a. Lung pulse
   b. Identification of a lung point
   c. Barcode sign
   d. Identification of a pleural effusion
   e. Visualization of vertical artifacts arising from the chest wall

41.3. For which patient with a pneumothorax would simple aspiration of pleural air be most appropriate?
   a. A 23-year-old man with altered mental status after a motor vehicle accident
   b. A 63-year-old woman with chronic obstructive pulmonary disease (COPD) and a small pneumothorax with marked dyspnea

   c. A 24-year-old woman with cystic fibrosis and a large pneumothorax who is asymptomatic
   d. An 18-year-old man with a large pneumothorax and moderate shoulder pain but no dyspnea
   e. A 33-year-old asymptomatic woman with a small pneumothorax that was incidentally found on a preemployment physical examination

41.4. If each of the following patients had a pneumothorax that was treated with placement of a chest tube, for which patient would chemical pleurodesis with talc be contraindicated?
   a. A 23-year-old woman with cystic fibrosis awaiting lung transplant
   b. A 77-year-old man with COPD and a fully expanded lung while a water seal chest drain was in place
   c. A 54-year-old man whose lung was 70% reexpanded while a water seal chest drain was in place
   d. A 44-year-old female airline pilot with her first episode of primary spontaneous pneumothorax, which has resolved
   e. A 68-year-old man with lung cancer and malignant pleural effusion that has been completely evacuated with full lung expansion

41.5. What percentage of secondary spontaneous pneumothoraces with a prolonged air leak would be expected to resolve spontaneously within 2 weeks?
   a. 19%
   b. 39%
   c. 59%
   d. 79%
   e. 99%

Case Follow-up and Outcome

Despite the placement of a large-bore surgical chest tube, the patient had a persistent pneumothorax with a continuous air leak. After endobronchial valves were placed in the apical-posterior and anterior segments of the left upper lobe, the air leak decreased considerably and the lung reexpanded nearly completely (Figures 41.2 and 41.3). An intermittent air leak was treated successfully with a blood patch of 120 mL of venous blood instilled through the thoracostomy tube. A clamping trial was successful, so the thoracostomy tubes were removed, and the patient did not have further problems.

Discussion

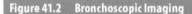

The lung is protected within the chest wall, from which it is separated by the pleura. The pleura has 2 components: the *visceral pleura*, which lines the lung, and the *parietal pleura*, which lines the

chest wall. The *pleural space* between the 2 layers is small and contains only a thin layer of fluid that provides lubrication as the pleural layers slide across each other during the respiratory cycle. A *pneumothorax* occurs when the pleural space is compromised with the introduction of air, which reduces lung expansion. Depending on factors such as the extent of the injury and the health of the underlying parenchyma, the presentation of a patient with a pneumothorax may range from asymptomatic to life-threatening.

The diagnosis of pneumothorax requires radiologic confirmation. Computed tomography (CT) is the gold standard, although its drawbacks include radiation exposure, cost, and time to diagnosis. Other diagnostic imaging includes CXR and ultrasonography. In a meta-analysis that compared ultrasonography and CXR, both had excellent specificity (>98%), but the sensitivity of ultrasonography (90.9%) was far higher than the sensitivity of CXR (50.2%) (1). However, CXR was performed with patients in the supine position, so the diagnostic accuracy of CXR may have been underestimated; when patients are in the upright position, CXR shows air within the pleural space at the apex of the lung.

Figure 41.2   Bronchoscopic Imaging

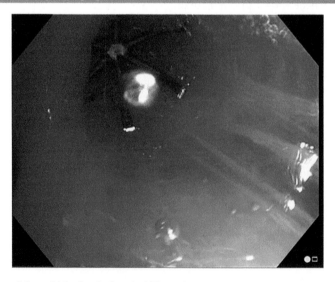

This view shows an endobronchial valve deployed within an airway.

Figure 41.3   CXR With a Portable Unit After Placement of 2 Endobronchial Valves

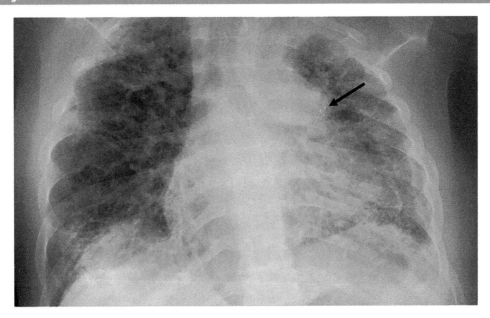

Anteroposterior view shows valves (arrow) and nearly complete reexpansion of the lung.

The use of ultrasonography for the diagnosis of pneumothorax requires experience but can be learned fairly easily. Sonographic findings that assist with the diagnosis or exclusion of pneumothorax include lung sliding, B lines, a lung pulse, and a lung point (2).

Pneumothoraces may be classified as *spontaneous* (occurring in the absence of an external cause), *iatrogenic* (due to a medical complication), or *traumatic* (from blunt force or penetrating injury to the chest wall). Spontaneous pneumothorax can be classified further as *primary* (occurring in the absence of underlying lung disease) or *secondary* (associated with a pulmonary abnormality). In addition to the cause of a pneumothorax, the degree of symptoms (particularly dyspnea) and the size are helpful in determining the appropriate management strategy.

Primary Spontaneous Pneumothorax

Primary spontaneous pneumothorax (PSP) occurs in patients without lung disease, but possible risk factors include male sex, tobacco use, tall stature, low body weight, and a positive family history of pneumothorax (3). Additionally, although some patients have PSP without recognized lung disease, most patients have apical blebs or bullae (or both) that are evident on further evaluation with CT or surgical thoracoscopy (3).

Given the lack of underlying lung disease in PSP, the clinical presentation tends to be more benign and pneumothorax is typically better tolerated than in patients with secondary spontaneous pneumothorax (SSP). Therefore, management decisions are made primarily according to symptoms in combination with pneumothorax size.

For many patients with PSP, an appropriate approach is conservative management, which includes supplemental oxygen and observation in the ED with close ambulatory follow-up; however, guidelines for treatment of PSP vary among professional societies (4-6). Guidelines from the American College of Chest Physicians (ACCP) published in 2001 suggest 1) observation if the pneumothorax is small (<3 cm at the apex) and the patient is clinically stable and 2) drainage with chest tube if the pneumothorax is large (≥3 cm at the apex) or if the patient is symptomatic (4). The British Thoracic Society (BTS) guidelines published in 2010 also recommend observation for pneumothoraces that are small (<2 cm at the hilum) if patients are not breathless; if a patient is breathless or has a large pneuomothorax (≥2 cm at the hilum), drainage with needle aspiration of up to 2.5 L of air is recommended, and a chest tube should be placed if clinical signs continue or the pneumothorax remains large (6). The European Respiratory Society suggests drainage with needle aspiration of the PSP (of any size) only if patients are symptomatic (5). When a chest tube is placed, the ACCP guidelines suggest placement of a Heimlich valve or the use of a water seal; the ACCP guidelines state that suction may be applied immediately, but the recommendation of the BTS guidelines is that suction should not be used routinely.

After PSP is treated successfully, about 30% of patients have a recurrence (7). Consensus recommendations vary on an opportune time for prevention of recurrence: Some advocate treatment after the first episode, while others recommend treatment only after a second event. Options for preventing recurrence include video-assisted thoracoscopic surgery for resection of identified blebs in combination with pleural abrasion, pleurectomy, or chemical pleurodesis (typically with talc) (7).

Secondary Spontaneous Pneumothorax

When an SSP occurs, lung function is already compromised, so SSPs are more difficult than PSPs for patients to tolerate. With this in mind, almost all SSPs require intervention; if conservative management is appropriate, close observation should occur within a hospital.

According to the ACCP guidelines, appropriate candidates for conservative management are those with a stable condition and small pneumothoraces (<3 cm at the apex), although

placement of a chest tube is still reasonable depending on the severity of the symptoms. The BTS guidelines recommend conservative management with close observation only for patients without breathlessness and with a small pneumothorax (<1 cm at the hilum).

For all other patients, pneumothorax drainage is recommended. For patients in stable condition with a large pneumothorax, the ACCP recommends placement of a medium-bore chest tube (16F-22F), although a small-bore chest tube (≤14F) may be considered. A large-bore chest tube (24F-28F) is recommended for patients in unstable condition with a large pneumothorax. The BTS guidelines suggest placement of a small-bore chest tube if patients have a large SSP or have breathlessness. In patients with a PSP measuring 1 to 2 cm at the hilum who do not have breathlessness, the BTS guidelines recommend first treating with needle aspiration to remove up to 2.5 L of air. After aspiration, continued observation is appropriate if CXR shows that the pneumothorax has decreased to less than 1 cm at the hilum; a chest tube should be placed if the pneumothorax remains larger than 1 cm.

After successful treatment of SSP, the majority of patients should undergo a definitive procedure to prevent recurrence (4). Historically pleurodesis has not been offered to certain patients with SSP because of concerns related to future transplant potential and disqualification from future transplant consideration. However, although surgical pleurodesis and chemical pleurodesis are associated with increased blood loss and early postoperative morbidity (including kidney and primary graft dysfunction after transplant), pleurodesis itself is not a contraindication to lung transplant, and intervention is unlikely to affect future acceptance for transplant (8).

Tension Pneumothorax

While most pneumothoraces may be observed or treated somewhat urgently, a tension pneumothorax is a medical emergency that must be treated as such. The pathophysiologic mechanism of a *tension pneumothorax* is that a rupture in the pleura allows air to enter during inspiration but not escape with expiration, so the intrapleural pressure steadily increases. Ultimately venous return to the heart is impaired, decreasing cardiac output and leading to shock (6).

Given the emergent nature of the disease, tension pneumothorax is primarily a clinical diagnosis, and treatment should not wait for confirmation from CXR, although the increased use of ultrasonography in certain practice settings may allow for prompt evaluation. Many situations may lead to a tension pneumothorax, but some of the most frequent include mechanical or noninvasive ventilation, trauma, cardiopulmonary resuscitation, SSPs, malfunctioning chest tubes, and hyperbaric oxygen therapy (6).

Treatment should include immediate drainage of air to decrease the intrapleural pressure and restore cardiac output. This may be accomplished by insertion of a chest tube or by placement of a flexible cannula in either the second intercostal space in the midclavicular line or the fifth intercostal space in the midaxillary line (either location is relatively safe from serious complications). If a flexible cannula becomes kinked as the lung reexpands, a tension pneumothorax may recur, so a chest tube should be placed immediately if this method is used for initial stabilization.

Iatrogenic Pneumothorax

An *iatrogenic pneumothorax* is a pneumothorax that occurs as a complication of a medical procedure; certain procedures carry more risk than others. In general, most iatrogenic pneumothoraces are well tolerated and will resolve spontaneously with observation; however, those that require intervention because of size or symptoms may be treated with needle aspiration nearly 90% of the time (6). An exception is iatrogenic pneumothoraces that occur in an intensive care unit (ICU) setting because they may be caused by or coexist with positive pressure from mechanical ventilation, which may lead to a tension pneumothorax. Therefore,

iatrogenic pneumothoraces that occur in an ICU setting almost certainly require placement of a chest tube (6).

Prolonged Air Leak

While most pneumothoraces that require chest tube drainage resolve quickly, the resolution of others is more prolonged. The term *prolonged air leak* (PAL) or *persistent air leak* is used to describe an air leak that has been present for more than approximately 5 days. For PAL, additional treatment strategies may be considered to facilitate resolution and hospital discharge; however, 100% of PSPs and 79% of SSPs resolve within 14 days with chest tube drainage alone (9).

An ambulatory drainage device such as a Heimlich valve is an option to facilitate hospital discharge if patients have adequate symptom control after chest tube placement, if their condition is stable with a water seal, and if they are amenable to close follow-up. These devices contain a 1-way valve that allows air to escape the thoracic cavity to the external environment while preventing external air entry. Functionally these devices serve the same purpose as maintaining a chest tube with a water seal, so the main reason for their use is to facilitate early hospital discharge rather than resolution of the PAL.

Surgical intervention is an option for patients if management with an ambulatory drainage device is not appropriate, if a PAL does not resolve, or if earlier definitive management is desired. This approach allows for identification and correction of the source of the air leak, and it provides the opportunity to prevent future recurrence through the removal of blebs or bullae and to perform mechanical pleurodesis.

When surgical management is not an option, chemical pleurodesis is an alternative with a high success rate for closing a PAL and preventing future recurrence of pneumothorax. Unlike surgical intervention, which may be performed when the lung has not reexpanded or when suction has been required for management, chemical pleurodesis should be performed only when the lung has reexpanded because treatment requires contact between the visceral and parietal pleurae.

Autologous blood patch is another option when surgical management is not the chosen strategy and the patient has contraindications to chemical pleurodesis. This strategy involves instillation of a patient's blood through the chest tube with the goal of resolving the air leak. The exact mechanism of action is unknown, but it is thought that the technique works through 1) coagulated blood directly sealing the air leak and 2) the blood products inducing inflammation that leads eventually to pleurodesis (10). Although the amount of blood required has not been agreed upon, the typical amount is about 100 mL of venous blood. The overall success rate for autologous blood patch is more than 90% (11), and less than 10% of patients have complications, which may include empyema, pain, and chest tube occlusion (12).

Another approach to PAL treatment is bronchoscopic intervention, of which the most common is the use of endobronchial valves (13). These devices, which may be situated in the lobar, segmental, and subsegmental bronchi, contain a 1-way valve that allows air and fluid to move past the valve into the proximal airway without allowing additional air to continue passing through the alveolopleural fistula. To determine the proper location for the valve, the airway is sequentially occluded and the air leak is observed to isolate the source by identifying the segments that, when occluded, reduce or eliminate the air leak. The valves may eventually be removed through subsequent bronchoscopy.

Summary

Pneumothorax is a common pulmonary disease that may occur spontaneously, iatrogenically, or traumatically. Although multiple guidelines exist to guide appropriate interventions, there is no overall consensus about when conservative treatment is appropriate, when intervention is necessary, or which intervention should be performed initially. However, the most widely accepted indication for therapy is the presence of clinically significant symptoms. If an alveolopleural fistula leads to prolonged air leaks, healing usually occurs within 2 weeks, but additional interventions may be pursued to treat an unresolved leak or to reduce morbidity.

Answers

41.1. Answer e.

The chest cavity houses several vital structures, and the introduction of a needle for thoracostomy increases the risk of complications. In the supine position, air in the pleural space tends to accumulate anteriorly. In the upright position, air tends to accumulate at the apex. On the basis of these facts and the locations of anatomical structures, the American College of Surgeons recommends that emergent needle thoracostomy be performed in the second intercostal space in the midclavicular line. Another acceptable location would be the fifth intercostal space but in the midaxillary line rather than the midclavicular line. Additional information is available in the medical literature (14).

41.2. Answer a.

Several ultrasonographic findings are useful for ruling out a pneumothorax. They include visualization of lung sliding, B-lines, and a lung pulse. A *lung pulse* is vertical movement of the pleural line in synchrony with the cardiac rhythm as cardiac motion is conducted through the lung to the pleural surface. *Lung sliding* is horizontal movement of the pleural line that indicates contact between the visceral and parietal pleurae. *B-lines* are vertical artifacts that arise from the pleural line as a result of the transmission of the ultrasound wave through lung tissue, which contains both air and fluid (which may be physiologic or pathologic). B-lines should not be confused with *E-lines*, which are artifactual vertical lines that do not arise from the pleural line; instead, they arise from the chest wall in patients with subcutaneous emphysema, which frequently accompanies pneumothorax. A *lung point* is an ultrasonographic

location where the transition of previously mentioned normal ultrasonographic findings disappear, indicating the presence of a pneumothorax with 100% specificity. Specifically, the lung point is where the lung and parietal pleura remain in contact. Additional information is available in the medical literature (2).

41.3. Answer d.

Simple aspiration of pleural air would be most appropriate for a patient deemed to be of lower risk. The 18-year-old man with a large pneumothorax and moderate shoulder pain but no dyspnea has a primary spontaneous pneumothorax and may symptomatically benefit from aspiration. He probably would not require chest tube insertion and may be observed for recurrence of pneumothorax after aspiration. The 33-year-old woman has a small pneumothorax and is asymptomatic; therefore, according to guidelines from the ACCP, BTS, and European Respiratory Society, no intervention is recommended and she may be observed. The other patients all warrant intervention. The patient with a pneumothorax after a motor vehicle accident has a traumatic pneumothorax; he would benefit from chest tube insertion and close monitoring as further investigation and management proceeds. The other 2 patients (the woman with COPD and the woman with cystic fibrosis) have secondary spontaneous pneumothoraces that are less likely to resolve quickly, so both patients would benefit from chest tube insertion for treatment and stabilization. Additional information is available in the medical literature (4-6).

41.4. Answer c.

When chemical pleurodesis is performed to prevent recurrence of a pneumothorax, the lung and chest wall must be in apposition to allow for chemical sclerosing of the pleural surfaces together. For the 54-year-old man with only 70% lung reexpansion, the likelihood of success would be low, so chemical pleurodesis should be avoided unless further lung reexpansion occurs first. Lung transplant candidates have historically been offered management aimed toward minimizing interventions on their thoracic cavity to avoid affecting their candidacy for transplant. However, such management has not been a critical factor in transplant consideration. Although interventions such as pleurodesis may increase complications such as bleeding, the Pulmonary Transplantation Council of the International Society for Heart and Lung Transplantation endorses appropriate pneumothorax prevention. For patients with a primary spontaneous pneumothorax, the general recommendation is to pursue pleurodesis after a recurrent episode rather than after an initial event; however, if a patient has a preference or a high-risk occupation, pleurodesis may be offered with the initial pneumothorax. A malignant pleural effusion may alter the efficacy of talc pleurodesis, particularly in high-output effusions, but it is not an absolute contraindication. Additional information is available in the medical literature (4,8,15).

41.5. Answer d.

If given sufficient time, the majority of secondary spontaneous pneumothoraces with a prolonged air leak will resolve spontaneously with supportive care. At 2 weeks, the pneumothorax would be expected to have resolved in 79% of patients. Additional information is available in the medical literature (9).

References

1. Alrajhi K, Woo MY, Vaillancourt C. Test characteristics of ultrasonography for the detection of pneumothorax: a systematic review and meta-analysis. Chest. 2012 Mar;141(3):703–8.
2. Volpicelli G. Sonographic diagnosis of pneumothorax. Intensive Care Med. 2011 Feb;37(2):224–32.
3. Hallifax RJ, Goldacre R, Landray MJ, Rahman NM, Goldacre MJ. Trends in the incidence and recurrence of inpatient-treated spontaneous pneumothorax, 1968-2016. JAMA. 2018 Oct 9;320(14):1471–80.
4. Baumann MH, Strange C, Heffner JE, Light R, Kirby TJ, Klein J, et al; AACP Pneumothorax Consensus Group. Management of spontaneous pneumothorax: an American College of Chest Physicians Delphi consensus statement. Chest. 2001 Feb;119(2):590–602.
5. Tschopp JM, Bintcliffe O, Astoul P, Canalis E, Driesen P, Janssen J, et al. ERS task force statement: diagnosis and treatment of primary spontaneous pneumothorax. Eur Respir J. 2015 Aug;46(2):321–35.
6. MacDuff A, Arnold A, Harvey J; BTS Pleural Disease Guideline Group. Management of spontaneous pneumothorax: British Thoracic Society Pleural Disease Guideline 2010. Thorax. 2010 Aug;65 Suppl 2:ii18–31.
7. Hallifax R, Janssen JP. Pneumothorax-time for new guidelines? Semin Respir Crit Care Med. 2019 Jun;40(3):314–22.
8. Weill D, Benden C, Corris PA, Dark JH, Davis RD, Keshavjee S, et al. A consensus document for the selection of lung transplant candidates: 2014: an update from the Pulmonary Transplantation Council of the International Society for Heart and Lung Transplantation. J Heart Lung Transplant. 2015 Jan;34(1):1–15.
9. Chee CB, Abisheganaden J, Yeo JK, Lee P, Huan PY, Poh SC, et al. Persistent air-leak in spontaneous pneumothorax: clinical course and outcome. Respir Med. 1998 May;92(5):757–61.
10. Ibrahim IM, Elaziz MEA, El-Hag-Aly MA. Early autologous blood-patch pleurodesis versus conservative management for treatment of secondary spontaneous pneumothorax. Thorac Cardiovasc Surg. 2019 Apr;67(3):222–6.
11. Chambers A, Routledge T, Bille A, Scarci M. Is blood pleurodesis effective for determining the cessation of persistent air leak? Interact Cardiovasc Thorac Surg. 2010 Oct;11(4):468–72.
12. Manley K, Coonar A, Wells F, Scarci M. Blood patch for persistent air leak: a review of the current literature. Curr Opin Pulm Med. 2012 Jul;18(4):333–8.
13. Mukhtar O, Khalid M, Shrestha B, Alhafdh O, Pata R, Bakhiet M, et al. Endobronchial valves for persistent air leak all-cause mortality and financial impact: US trend from 2012-2016. J Community Hosp Intern Med Perspect. 2019 Nov 1;9(5):397–402.
14. American College of Surgeons. Advanced trauma life support program for doctors (ATLS). 6th ed. Chicago (IL): American College of Surgeons; c1997. 444 p.
15. Rodriguez-Panadero F, Antony VB. Pleurodesis: state of the art. Eur Respir J. 1997 Jul;10(7):1648–54.

A 71-Year-Old Woman With Cough, Night Sweats, and Fevers

Hasan A. Albitar, MD, and Alice Gallo de Moraes, MD

Case Presentation

A 71-year-old woman with a previous medical history of hypertension and gastroesophageal reflux disease presented with a 1-month history of episodic, severe dry cough associated with fevers, night sweats, and decreased appetite. She did not think that she had lost weight or had hemoptysis or any relevant environmental or infectious exposures. On physical examination she had an elevated heart rate (118 beats/min), an elevated temperature (38 °C), and decreased breath sounds at the right lung base. Radiography of the chest showed moderate pleural effusion on the right with associated atelectasis in the middle and lower lobes of the right lung and increased prominence of the right hilum.

Questions

Multiple Choice (choose the best answer)

42.1. For the patient described above, what is the most appropriate next step?
   a. Perform diagnostic thoracentesis
   b. Measure the serum level of N-terminal pro-brain natriuretic peptide (NT-proBNP) and perform echocardiography
   c. Proceed with video-assisted thoracoscopic surgery (VATS) and pleural biopsy
   d. Administer systemic empirical antibiotic therapy without performing thoracentesis
   e. Perform positron emission tomographic (PET)–computed tomography (CT)

42.2. The patient described above underwent diagnostic thoracentesis, and the pleural fluid analysis results are shown in Table 42.Q2.

Table 42.Q2

Component	Finding
Volume, mL	500
Appearance of fluid	Slightly cloudy; straw colored
Total nucleated cell count, cells/µL	4,500
Lymphocytes, %	97
Lactate dehydrogenase (LDH), U/L	
Pleural fluid	732
Serum	190
Total protein, g/dL	
Pleural fluid	5.1
Serum	7.5
Pleural fluid pH	7.29
Cytology	Negative for malignancy

What is the most likely diagnosis?
   a. Connective tissue disease, such as rheumatoid arthritis or systemic lupus erythematosus (SLE)
   b. Acute pulmonary embolism (PE)
   c. Tuberculous pleural effusion (TPE)
   d. Heart failure with a transudate due to increased microvascular pressure
   e. Kidney or liver disease with a transudate due to decreased plasma oncotic pressure

42.3. Which of the following tests has the highest yield for supporting a diagnosis of pleural tuberculosis?
   a. Pleural fluid staining for acid-fast bacilli (AFB)
   b. Bacterial culture from pleural fluid sample
   c. Culture from induced sputum sample
   d. Pleural biopsy for bacterial culture in combination with histopathologic analysis
   e. Interferon-gamma release assay on pleural fluid

42.4. If *Mycobacterium tuberculosis* grew in a culture from pleural fluid, what would be the most appropriate initial treatment?
   a. Daily rifampin, isoniazid, pyrazinamide, and ethambutol
   b. Daily isoniazid and rifampin
   c. Intermittent therapy with rifampin, isoniazid, pyrazinamide, and ethambutol twice weekly
   d. Daily rifampin, ethambutol, pyrazinamide, and levofloxacin
   e. Daily isoniazid monotherapy

42.5. When patients begin daily therapy with rifampin, isoniazid, pyrazinamide, and ethambutol, which of the following is the *least* common adverse effect?
   a. Hyperuricemia
   b. Optic neuropathy
   c. Red or orange discoloration of body fluids
   d. Peripheral neuropathy
   e. Lung fibrosis

Case Follow-up and Outcome

The patient underwent diagnostic thoracentesis, and 500 mL of slightly cloudy, straw-colored fluid was collected. Results of pleural fluid analysis are summarized in Table 42.Q2. Given those results and the patient's symptoms of night sweats, fevers, and decreased appetite, the pleural effusion was thought to be due to *M tuberculosis*. When smears from the pleural fluid were stained for AFB, the results were negative. However, the mycobacterial culture grew *M tuberculosis*. The patient began receiving daily therapy with rifampin, isoniazid, pyrazinamide, and ethambutol for TPE.

Discussion

The second most common form of extrapulmonary tuberculosis (after lymphatic involvement) is TPE. Most commonly, it results from a delayed hypersensitivity reaction to mycobacteria or mycobacterial antigens in the pleural space (1).

Patients with TPE typically present with acute febrile illness with nonproductive cough and pleuritic chest pain. Night sweats and anorexia can also occur. Tuberculosis should be considered if patients present with such symptoms even if the patients live where the disease is not endemic and do not have risk factors for tuberculosis. TPE is usually unilateral and usually occurs on the right side (2).

A diagnosis of TPE can be definitively established when *M tuberculosis* is identified in the pleural fluid or in a pleural biopsy, and the diagnostic yield is higher with bacterial culture in combination with histopathologic analysis of biopsied pleural tissue. Several approaches can be used for pleural biopsy. *Percutaneous pleural biopsy* can be performed as closed pleural biopsy or under CT guidance. Closed pleural biopsy can be performed blindly or under ultrasonographic guidance. *Thoracoscopic pleural biopsy* can be performed as VATS or as medical thoracoscopy (also known as pleuroscopy). The sensitivities of these techniques are generally comparable. For example, Kirsch et al (3) reported the sensitivity of closed pleural biopsy as 87%, and Christopher et al (4) reported the sensitivity of thoracoscopic pleural biopsy as 100%. Closed pleural biopsy is generally preferred in geographic regions where TPE is common and in countries that lack the financial resources and infrastructure needed to perform thoracoscopic pleural biopsy.

Summary

TPE is an exudative effusion with a predominance of lymphocytes. When TPE is suspected, pleural fluid must be obtained and evaluated. The results of laboratory testing are usually characterized by elevated LDH concentration, low pH, and elevated protein concentration (almost invariably >3 g/dL). Pleural fluid glucose is usually 60 to 100 mg/dL (5). In addition, the pleural fluid adenosine deaminase (ADA) level can be checked when a diagnosis of TPE is suspected. The test has a high negative predictive value; an ADA level less than 40 IU/L virtually excludes a diagnosis of tuberculosis in patients with lymphocytic pleural effusions (6). Moreover, when the clinical suspicion for TPE is high, a presumptive diagnosis can be made without pathologic confirmation when the pleural effusion has a predominance of lymphocytes and an ADA level greater than 40 IU/L (7). In general, treatment of TPE is the same as standard treatment of active pulmonary tuberculosis (8). Finally, if the above evaluation does not yield a definitive diagnosis, pleural biopsy should be considered.

Answers

42.1. Answer a.

Performing diagnostic thoracentesis would be the most appropriate next step given this patient's presentation. Thoracentesis is helpful for differentiating between transudative and exudative pleural effusions and would be crucial for reaching the final diagnosis for this patient.

NT-proBNP is a sensitive marker for both systolic and diastolic heart failure. It has been effective for discriminating between transudates associated with congestive heart failure and transudates or exudates associated with other causes. However, this patient did not have a history of heart failure, and the presence of fevers and night sweats makes heart failure less likely cause of the patient's pleural effusion.

VATS can be used for the diagnosis and treatment of benign or malignant pleural diseases, but diagnostic thoracentesis can be used to establish the cause of the pleural effusion in this patient, and it carries a lower risk of complications than VATS. Therefore, the use of VATS and pleural biopsy before diagnostic thoracentesis would not be appropriate.

Parapneumonic effusions are pleural effusions that form in the pleural space adjacent to an area with pneumonia, and parapneumonic effusion would be in the differential diagnosis for this patient. However, in general, a parapneumonic effusion should be sampled to tailor antimicrobial treatment according to culture results and antimicrobial susceptibility and to guide the physician on whether insertion of a chest tube is indicated, so beginning empirical antibiotic therapy without performing thoracentesis would not be an appropriate next step.

The uptake of fluorodeoxyglucose F 18 (FDG) has been shown to be greater in malignant pleural effusions. However, the value of PET-CT in distinguishing benign disease from malignant disease is limited by false-positive results when patients have pleural inflammation (eg, pleural infection). Additional information is available in the medical literature (9,10).

42.2. Answer c.

The pleural fluid analysis findings are representative of an exudative pleural effusion. Tuberculosis is the most likely diagnosis; TPE is typically a lymphocyte-rich, exudative pleural effusion with low pH and elevated pleural fluid protein. This diagnosis is supported by a predominance of lymphocytes in the pleural fluid in addition to the patient's history of night sweats, fevers, and decreased appetite. Connective tissue diseases, such as rheumatoid arthritis and SLE, can cause exudative pleural effusions with a low pleural fluid pH; however, an autoimmune disease would be less likely given this patient's presentation. Acute PE can cause exudative pleural effusion; however, the patient has had symptoms for more than a month, so PE is less likely. Increased microvascular pressure can occur in heart failure, and decreased plasma oncotic pressure can occur in kidney and liver disease, but the pleural effusions in those diseases are typically transudative, not exudative. Additional information is available in the medical literature (11).

42.3. Answer d.

Pleural biopsy for bacterial culture in combination with histopathologic analysis provides the highest diagnostic yield (up to 93%) for supporting a diagnosis of pleural tuberculosis. The diagnostic yield is low for analysis of pleural fluid with staining for AFB (12%) and with culturing for bacteria (2%). The diagnostic yield of cultures from induced sputum varies from 20% to 52%, and the interferon-gamma release assay has variable diagnostic accuracy.

Nucleic acid amplification (NAA) assay is approved by the US Food and Drug Administration for use with sputum; however, some laboratories use NAA assays with pleural fluid (for which the assay is not approved). One meta-analysis reported a pooled sensitivity of 46.4% with NAA assays. Additional information is available in the medical literature (12,13).

42.4. Answer a.

In general, treatment of TPE is the same as treatment of active pulmonary tuberculosis, and it typically consists of an intensive phase and a continuation phase. During the intensive phase, isoniazid, rifampin, pyrazinamide, and ethambutol are given for 2 months. Ethambutol may be discontinued if the results of drug susceptibility studies reveal susceptibility to isoniazid, rifampin, and pyrazinamide before completion of the intensive phase. After the intensive phase, isoniazid and rifampin should be administered for at least an additional 4 months. Daily therapy is preferred over intermittent therapy, especially during the intensive phase, to reduce the risk of relapse and drug resistance.

Fluoroquinolones, particularly levofloxacin and moxifloxacin, are typically used as second-line agents in the treatment of tuberculosis. They are generally used when patients have contraindications or adverse effects to first-line agents or when the infection is drug resistant to those agents, and so they are inappropriate for initial treatment. Monotherapy with isoniazid for 9 months is used for treatment of latent tuberculosis, so that would be inappropriate in this situation. Additional information is available in the medical literature (14-16).

42.5. Answer e.

Lung fibrosis is not associated with any of the 4 antituberculous medications mentioned in the question. Hyperuricemia is an adverse effect of pyrazinamide. Optic neuropathy can occur with ethambutol. Rifampin causes red or orange discoloration of body fluids, and the use of isoniazid can be complicated by peripheral neuropathy. Additional information is available in the medical literature (14).

References

1. Leibowitz S, Kennedy L, Lessof MH. The tuberculin reaction in the pleural cavity and its suppression by antilymphocyte serum. Br J Exp Pathol. 1973 Apr;54(2):152–62.

2. Valdes L, Alvarez D, San Jose E, Penela P, Valle JM, Garcia-Pazos JM, et al. Tuberculous pleurisy: a study of 254 patients. Arch Intern Med. 1998 Oct 12;158(18):2017–21.

3. Kirsch CM, Kroe DM, Azzi RL, Jensen WA, Kagawa FT, Wehner JH. The optimal number of pleural biopsy specimens for a diagnosis of tuberculous pleurisy. Chest. 1997 Sep;112(3):702–6.

4. Christopher DJ, Dinakaran S, Gupta R, James P, Isaac B, Thangakunam B. Thoracoscopic pleural biopsy improves yield of Xpert MTB/RIF for diagnosis of pleural tuberculosis. Respirology. 2018 Jul;23(7):71–7.

5. Berger HW, Mejia E. Tuberculous pleurisy. Chest. 1973 Jan;63(1):88–92.

6. Jimenez Castro D, Diaz Nuevo G, Perez-Rodriguez E, Light RW. Diagnostic value of adenosine deaminase in nontuberculous lymphocytic pleural effusions. Eur Respir J. 2003 Feb;21(2):220–4.

7. Sahn SA, Huggins JT, San Jose ME, Alvarez-Dobano JM, Valdes L. Can tuberculous pleural effusions be diagnosed by pleural fluid analysis alone? Int J Tuberc Lung Dis. 2013 Jun;17(6):787–93.

8. Zhai K, Lu Y, Shi HZ. Tuberculous pleural effusion. J Thorac Dis. 2016 Jul;8(7):E486–94.

9. Zhou Q, Ye ZJ, Su Y, Zhang JC, Shi HZ. Diagnostic value of N-terminal pro-brain natriuretic peptide for pleural effusion due to heart failure: a meta-analysis. Heart. 2010 Aug;96(15):1207–11.

10. Duysinx B, Nguyen D, Louis R, Cataldo D, Belhocine T, Bartsch P, et al. Evaluation of pleural disease with 18-fluorodeoxyglucose positron emission tomography imaging. Chest. 2004 Feb;125(2):489–93.

11. Feller-Kopman D, Light R. Pleural disease. N Engl J Med. 2018 Feb 22;378(8):740–51.

12. Conde MB, Loivos AC, Rezende VM, Soares SL, Mello FC, Reingold AL, et al. Yield of sputum induction in the diagnosis of pleural tuberculosis. Am J Respir Crit Care Med. 2003 Mar 1;167(5):723–5.

13. Denkinger CM, Schumacher SG, Boehme CC, Dendukuri N, Pai M, Steingart KR. Xpert MTB/RIF assay for the diagnosis of extrapulmonary tuberculosis: a systematic review and meta-analysis. Eur Respir J. 2014 Aug;44(2):435–46.

14. Nahid P, Dorman SE, Alipanah N, Barry PM, Brozek JL, Cattamanchi A, et al. Official American Thoracic Society/Centers for Disease Control and Prevention/Infectious Diseases Society of America Clinical Practice Guidelines: treatment of drug-susceptible tuberculosis. Clin Infect Dis. 2016 Oct 1;63(7):e147–95.

15. Maitre T, Petitjean G, Chauffour A, Bernard C, El Helali N, Jarlier V, et al. Are moxifloxacin and levofloxacin equally effective to treat XDR tuberculosis? J Antimicrob Chemother. 2017 Aug 1;72(8):2326–33.

16. Yew WW, Chan CK, Chau CH, Tam CM, Leung CC, Wong PC, et al. Outcomes of patients with multidrug-resistant pulmonary tuberculosis treated with ofloxacin/levofloxacin-containing regimens. Chest. 2000 Mar;117(3):744–51.

A 57-Year-Old Woman With Progressively Decreasing Oxygen Saturation After Liver Transplant

Govind Panda, MD, and Bhavesh M. Patel, MD

Case Presentation

A 57-year-old woman with cirrhosis due to non-alcoholic steatohepatitis with associated esophageal varices, ascites, hepatorenal syndrome, and hepatic hydrothorax was admitted for elective deceased-donor orthotopic liver transplant. On preoperative evaluation she had a large pleural effusion on the right side (Figure 43.1). She was breathing room air comfortably (oxygen saturation as measured by pulse oximetry [Spo_2] >90%) and was asymptomatic from a respiratory standpoint.

Figure 43.1   Preoperative Radiograph of the Chest

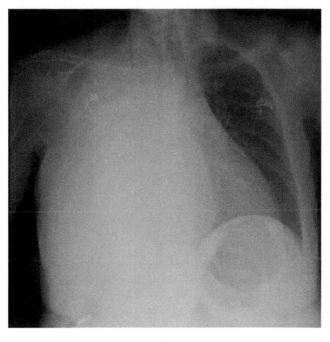

Anteroposterior view shows a large right-sided pleural effusion preoperatively.

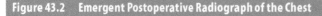

Figure 43.2   Emergent Postoperative Radiograph of the Chest

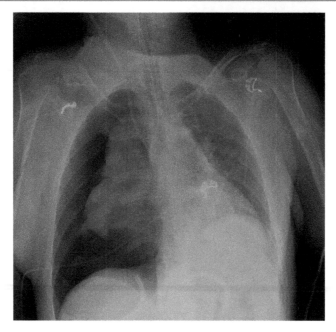

Anteroposterior view shows a large right-sided tension pneumothorax.

The transplant surgery team decided to forego preoperative thoracentesis and planned for intraoperative thoracentesis. The liver transplant was uncomplicated and successful, requiring a minimal quantity of blood products. At the conclusion of the procedure, 3 L of pleural effusion was evacuated with a drain placed through the right side of the diaphragm with subsequent removal and primary repair. When the patient arrived in the intensive care unit (ICU) postoperatively, she had an endotracheal tube in place. The Spo_2 immediately began to progressively decrease to about 75%, and the ventilator alarms for elevated peak pressure were triggered. Her blood pressure began to decrease. Immediate ultrasonography of the lungs showed a lack of lung sliding; an emergent radiograph of the chest is shown in Figure 43.2.

Questions

Multiple Choice (choose the best answer)

43.1. Which ultrasonographic sign is most diagnostic for pneumothorax?
   a. Absence of lung pulse
   b. Presence of lung sliding
   c. Absence of lung sliding
   d. Absence of B-lines
   e. Presence of lung point sign

43.2. Which of the following best describes lung ultrasonography in comparison with chest radiography as an imaging tool for the diagnosis of pneumothorax?
   a. Ultrasonography is less sensitive
   b. Ultrasonography is less specific
   c. Ultrasonography is more sensitive
   d. Ultrasonography and radiography are equal in sensitivity and specificity
   e. Neither imaging tool is sensitive or specific for pneumothorax

43.3. If a patient has a tension pneumothorax and is hemodynamically unstable, what would be the first step in emergent treatment?
   a. Chest tube placement in the triangle of safety of the affected hemithorax
   b. Chest tube placement in the second intercostal space at the midclavicular line of the affected hemithorax
   c. Rapid needle decompression in the fourth or fifth rib space slightly anterior to the midaxillary line or the second intercostal space at the midclavicular line of the affected hemithorax
   d. Administration of an intravenous fluid bolus and vasopressor
   e. Oxygen therapy for Spo$_2$ greater than 90%

43.4. Which of the following statements correctly describes chest tube placement for pneumothorax?
   a. Small-bore chest tubes are effective for treatment of pneumothorax
   b. Only large-bore chest tubes are effective in decompression of pneumothorax
   c. Large-bore chest tubes cause less pain at insertion than small-bore chest tubes
   d. Small-bore chest tubes result in more complications than large-bore tubes for treatment of pneumothorax
   e. Chest tubes are contraindicated for the treatment of pneumothorax

43.5. According to the Advanced Trauma Life Support guidelines, what needle length is recommended for needle decompression of tension pneumothorax?
   a. 5 cm for a small adult patient; 8 cm for a large adult patient
   b. 4 cm
   c. 3 cm
   d. 2 cm
   e. 1 cm

Case Follow-up and Outcome

Needle decompression was attempted in the right second intercostal space at the midclavicular line, but the catheter became kinked in the subcutaneous tissue and did not enter the pleural space. Needle decompression, with subsequent placement of a small-bore pigtail chest tube in the fifth intercostal space slightly anterior to the midaxillary line, provided immediate pleural decompression accompanied by the release of a large gush of air and improvement in the patient's Spo₂ and hemodynamic status. Chest radiography was used to confirm that placement of the chest tube was appropriate (Figure 43.3). Later that day, when the patient had hemodynamic and respiratory stability, she was extubated. The chest tube was placed on continuous suction. An air leak that persisted for several days was thought to be due to possible lung injury from

intraoperative thoracentesis. After approximately 1 week the air leak gradually resolved, the chest tube was removed, and the patient was discharged. Follow-up chest radiography showed complete resolution of the pneumothorax.

Discussion

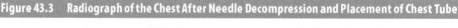

Pneumothorax can be diagnosed rapidly at the bedside with lung ultrasonography and is included in many diagnostic protocols for the evaluation of critically ill patients who have respiratory or hemodynamic compromise (eg, Extended Focused Assessment With Sonography in Trauma [eFAST], Rapid Ultrasound in Shock [RUSH], and Bedside Lung Ultrasound in Emergency [BLUE]). Diagnosis relies on the absence of several easily evaluated lung

Figure 43.3   Radiograph of the Chest After Needle Decompression and Placement of Chest Tube

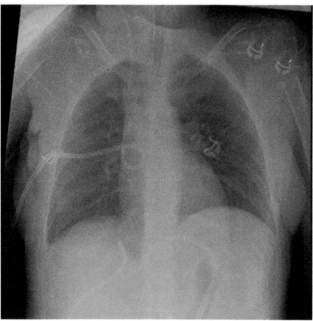

Anteroposterior view provides confirmation of proper placement of the right-sided chest tube with complete resolution of the pneumothorax.

findings: lung sliding, B-lines, and lung pulse. However, the most convincing finding is the presence of *lung point*, which is the location where the area with lung sliding meets the adjacent area without lung sliding. The lung point defines the anatomical boundaries of the pneumothorax (1). Both lung ultrasonography and chest radiography have good specificity for the diagnosis of pneumothorax; however, lung ultrasonography has much greater sensitivity than chest radiography (0.87 vs 0.46) as shown in several meta-analyses (2,3). Major guidelines advocate the use of lung ultrasonography in the diagnosis of pneumothorax (1,4).

Tension pneumothorax develops when a 1-way-valve air leak in the lung or chest wall is present and air under pressure becomes trapped in the pleural space. The trapped air causes complete collapse of the affected lung, a mediastinal shift, and decreased venous return and cardiac output, resulting in obstructive shock (5).

Treatment of tension pneumothorax includes emergent needle decompression of the affected pleural space. The traditional site suggested for needle decompression is the second intercostal space at the midclavicular line. However, postmortem computed tomographic (CT) studies have shown that this anterior approach may be prone to catheter kinking and increased rates of failed penetration of the pleural cavity (6). Furthermore, accurate identification of the midclavicular line is challenging, and clinicians often incorrectly identify a point medial to the midclavicular line with the landmark technique and put vital mediastinal structures at risk (7). The fourth or fifth intercostal space at the anterior axillary line has been suggested as a better location for needle decompression because CT studies have shown that the chest wall is approximately 1.3 cm thinner at this location (8). Either the anterior axillary line or a location slightly anterior to the midaxillary line can be used. This lateral approach can also facilitate the first step in subsequent chest tube placement if a Seldinger over-the-wire technique is used to place the chest tube. Tactical Combat Casualty Care guidelines recognize the lateral approach as an acceptable site for needle decompression (9). A large-bore catheter at least 5 cm (2 inches) long should be used to ensure pleural space entry, and longer needles up to 8 cm may be needed for patients with a larger body habitus according to recent Advanced Trauma Life Support guidelines (5). Larger catheters enter the pleural cavity more consistently, but they may increase the risk of adverse events such as penetration of the liver or lung.

Large-bore chest tubes have been used traditionally in the treatment of pneumothorax, but small-bore chest tubes have increased in popularity because they are less invasive. Small-bore chest tubes, which may be as effective as large-bore chest tubes, are less painful during insertion for the treatment of simple pneumothorax (10). Guidelines for the treatment of pneumothorax advocate the use of a chest tube of a size that is appropriate for the clinical stability of the patient (11). Other considerations are the clinician's clinical judgment and familiarity with chest tubes.

Summary

Tension pneumothorax is a life-threatening diagnosis that can be made accurately at the bedside with lung ultrasonography. Treatment consists of emergent needle decompression of the pleural space in the second intercostal space at the midclavicular line or in the fifth intercostal space at the anterior axillary line with a long, large-bore needle and immediate placement of a chest tube.

Answers

43.1. Answer e.

The lung point sign is a specific finding for the diagnosis of pneumothorax. The absence of lung sliding may be suggestive but is not specific for pneumothorax. Additional information is available in the medical literature (12).

43.2. Answer c.

In multiple studies and a meta-analysis, lung ultrasonography has been shown to be more sensitive than chest radiography for the diagnosis of pneumothorax. However, the accuracy of the diagnosis depends on the skill of the practitioner. Additional information is available in the medical literature (13).

43.3. Answer c.

Rapid needle decompression is recommended as the first step in emergent treatment of tension pneumothorax. A chest tube should be placed after needle decompression. Additional information is available in the medical literature (5).

43.4. Answer a.

Chest tube size depends on the size of the patient and the indication for placement. A small-bore catheter is sufficient for most patients who have primary spontaneous pneumothorax. One meta-analysis showed that the success rate was similar between small-bore pigtail catheters and large-bore catheters for primary and secondary spontaneous pneumothoraces, but the complication rate was lower with small-bore chest tubes. Additional information is available in the medical literature (14).

43.5. Answer a.

The size of the needle depends on the body habitus of the patient. Depending on the body habitus of the adult patient, a 5- to 8-cm needle should be used. A 5-cm over-the-needle catheter will reach the pleural space more than 50% of the time, whereas an 8-cm over-the-needle catheter will reach the pleural space more than 90% of the time. Additional information is available in the medical literature (5).

References

1. Volpicelli G, Elbarbary M, Blaivas M, Lichtenstein DA, Mathis G, Kirkpatrick AW, et al; International Liaison Committee on Lung Ultrasound (ILC-LUS) for International Consensus Conference on Lung Ultrasound (ICC-LUS). International evidence-based recommendations for point-of-care lung ultrasound. Intensive Care Med. 2012 Apr;38(4):577–91.

2. Ebrahimi A, Yousefifard M, Mohammad Kazemi H, Rasouli HR, Asady H, Moghadas Jafari A, et al. Diagnostic accuracy of chest ultrasonography versus chest radiography for identification of pneumothorax: a systematic review and meta-analysis. Tanaffos. 2014; 13(4):29–40.

3. Alrajab S, Youssef AM, Akkus NI, Caldito G. Pleural ultrasonography versus chest radiography for the diagnosis of pneumothorax: review of the literature and meta-analysis. Crit Care. 2013 Sep 23;17(5):R208.

4. Mowery NT, Gunter OL, Collier BR, Diaz JJ Jr, Haut E, Hildreth A, et al. Practice management guidelines for management of hemothorax and occult pneumothorax. J Trauma. 2011 Feb;70(2):510–8.

5. American College of Surgeons. (ATLS) Advanced Trauma Life Support: student course manual. 10th edition. Chicago (IL): American College of Surgeons; c2018. 420 p.

6. Harcke HT, Mabry RL, Mazuchowski EL. Needle thoracentesis decompression: observations from post-mortem computed tomography and autopsy. J Spec Oper Med. 2013 Winter;13(4):53–8.

7. Ferrie EP, Collum N, McGovern S. The right place in the right space? Awareness of site for needle thoracocentesis. Emerg Med J. 2005 Nov;22(11):788–9.

8. Inaba K, Ives C, McClure K, Branco BC, Eckstein M, Shatz D, et al. Radiologic evaluation of alternative sites for needle decompression of tension pneumothorax. Arch Surg. 2012 Sep;147(9):813–8.

9. Anonymous A. TCCC Updates: Tactical Combat Casualty Care guidelines for medical personnel: 3 June 2015. J Spec Oper Med. 2015 Fall;15(3):129–47.

10. Kulvatunyou N, Erickson L, Vijayasekaran A, Gries L, Joseph B, Friese RF, et al. Randomized clinical trial of pigtail catheter versus chest tube in injured patients with uncomplicated traumatic pneumothorax. Br J Surg. 2014 Jan;101(2):17–22.

11. Baumann MH, Strange C, Heffner JE, Light R, Kirby TJ, Klein J, et al; AACP Pneumothorax Consensus Group. Management of spontaneous pneumothorax: an American College of Chest Physicians Delphi consensus statement. Chest. 2001 Feb;119(2):590–602.

12. Lichtenstein D, Meziere G, Biderman P, Gepner A. The "lung point": an ultrasound sign specific to pneumothorax. Intensive Care Med. 2000 Oct;26(10): 1434–40.

13. Ding W, Shen Y, Yang J, He X, Zhang M. Diagnosis of pneumothorax by radiography and ultrasonography: a meta-analysis. Chest. 2011 Oct;140(4): 859–866. Epub 2011 May 5.

14. Chang SH, Kang YN, Chiu HY, Chiu YH. A Systematic Review and Meta-Analysis Comparing Pigtail Catheter and Chest Tube as the Initial Treatment for Pneumothorax. Chest. 2018 May;153(5):1201–1212. Epub 2018 Feb 13.

Interventional Pulmonology

A 79-Year-Old Woman With Shortness of Breath, Fatigue, Near Syncope, and Chest Tightness

44

Amanda J. McCambridge, MD, Samuel F. Ekstein, and Kaiser G. Lim, MD

Case Presentation

A 79-year-old woman presented to the emergency department (ED) with a 2-week history of progressive shortness of breath at rest and during activity in addition to fatigue, near syncope, and intermittent chest tightness. Her past medical history included bilateral intraocular B-cell lymphoma with orbital recurrence and subsequent central nervous system metastases, for which she was receiving pomalidomide after her use of rituximab was discontinued because of rituximab-induced demand ischemia. Her history also included coronary artery disease, myocardial infarction and stent placement several years earlier, ischemic cardiomyopathy (ejection fraction, 30%-35%), hypertension, and hyperlipidemia. In the ED she was afebrile without vital sign abnormalities. She had not had cough, recent sick contacts, fevers, or lower extremity swelling. Radiography of the chest showed a large right-sided pleural effusion and associated atelectasis. She was admitted to the medical unit.

Right-sided thoracentesis yielded fluid (600 mL) that was exudative according to lactate dehydrogenase criteria but did not show evidence of malignancy or infection. The patient had progressive shortness of breath. Five days later computed tomography (CT) of the chest showed reaccumulation of the right-sided pleural effusion and collapse of the right upper lobe (RUL) with intralobar hypoattenuation, which suggested intrapulmonary abscess (Figure 44.1). Bronchoscopy showed torsion and distortion of the bronchus intermedius and right lower lobe (RLL), causing extrinsic compression at the takeoff of the RUL, which was the source of mucopurulent secretions (Figure 44.2). Subsequent high-resolution CT showed torsion of the upper, middle, and lower lobes; the upper lobe had collapsed and was located in the right lower medial aspect of the chest, and the RLL was occupying much of the superior aspect of the chest. A ventilation-perfusion (V̇/Q) scan showed a marked decrease in perfusion and ventilation of the right lung compared to the left, which was consistent with right lung torsion.

Figure 44.1   Thoracic Imaging of Pulmonary Torsion

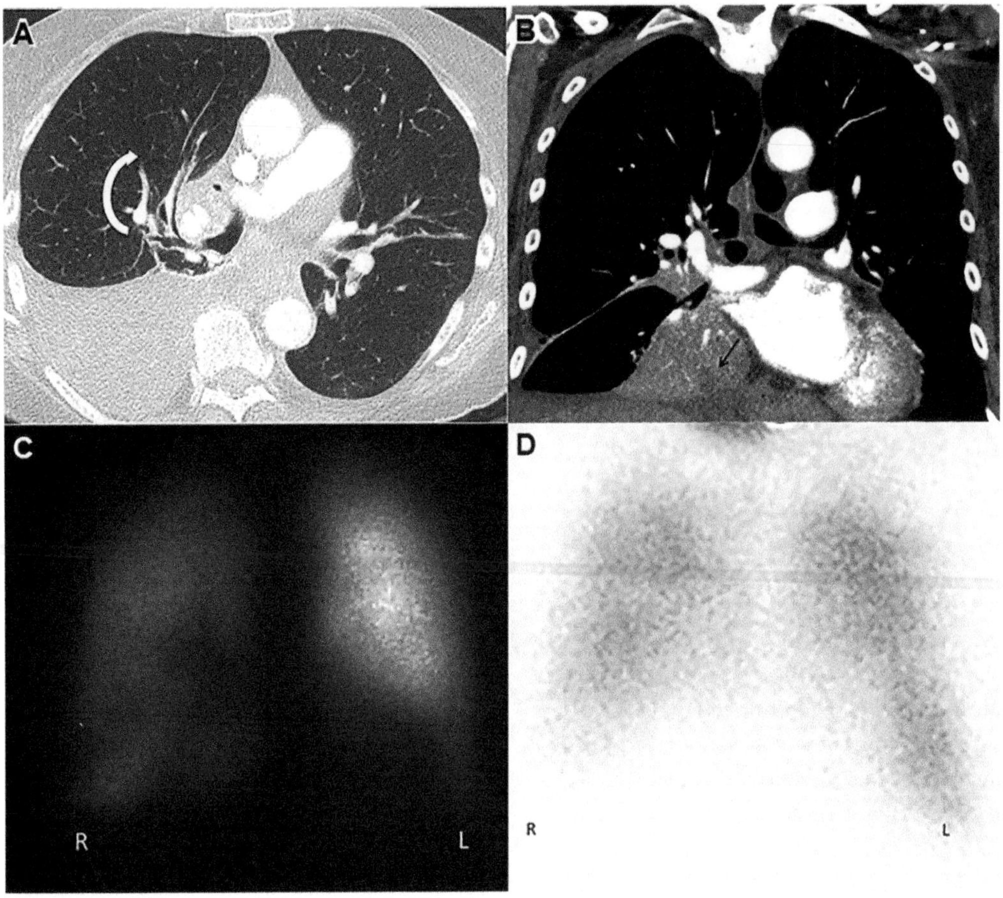

A, Axial CT of the chest shows clockwise swirling (curved arrow) around the right hilum with distortion of the bronchovascular bundle. Moderate right pleural effusion is present. B, Coronal CT image shows inferomedial rotation of the collapsed RUL with internal hypoattenuation because of a juxtadiaphragmatic abscess (arrow). C, Coronal view from anterior technetium Tc 99m macroaggregated albumin perfusion imaging shows markedly decreased lung perfusion on the right compared to the left. D, Coronal view from a corresponding xenon Xe 133 V̇/Q scan shows hypoventilation of the right lung. L indicates left; R, right.

(From Ekstein SF, McCambridge A, Edell ES, Koo CW, Blackmon SH. Case of spontaneous whole-lung torsion with literature review. J Thorac Dis. 2018 Sep;10[9]:E690-3; used with permission).

Figure 44.2   Bronchoscopy Findings in Pulmonary Torsion

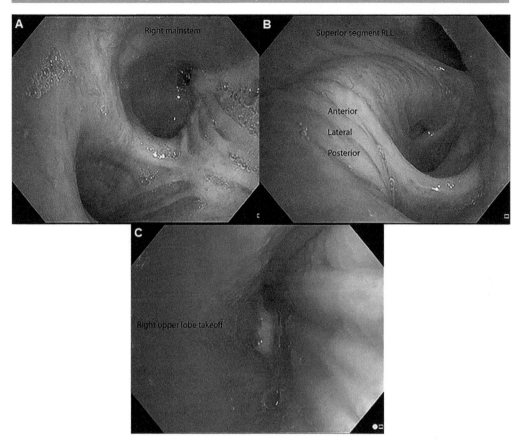

A, The main carina has purulent material draining from the right mainstem bronchus. B, The anatomy of the RLL is distorted because of the clockwise torsion. C, The takeoff of the RUL appears extrinsically compressed and has purulent secretions.

(From Ekstein SF, McCambridge A, Edell ES, Koo CW, Blackmon SH. Case of spontaneous whole-lung torsion with literature review. J Thorac Dis. 2018 Sep;10[9]:E690-3; used with permission).

Questions

Multiple Choice (choose the best answer)

44.1. What is considered the best noninvasive test for diagnosis of pulmonary torsion?
a. Bronchoscopy
b. Positron emission tomography (PET)-CT
c. High-resolution CT angiography of the chest
d. V̇/Q scan
e. Magnetic resonance imaging (MRI) of the chest

44.2. A 54-year-old man was involved in a head-on automobile collision. He had never smoked, and his past medical history was notable for hypertension. On presentation in the ED he was in respiratory distress. Breath sounds were present bilaterally, and oxygen saturation was 87% while he breathed room air, but it increased to 90% with supplemental oxygen (5 L/min). His blood pressure was 98/62 mm Hg. Noncontrast CT of the chest showed distorted anatomy with torsion of the right middle lobe (RML). What would be the best next step in management?
a. CT angiography
b. V̇/Q scan
c. Empirical full-dose anticoagulation
d. Intubation and emergent thoracic surgery
e. Bronchoscopy

44.3. A 4-year-old girl had sudden-onset respiratory distress. Her past medical history was unremarkable. Spontaneous torsion of the RUL was identified. The absence of which of the following structures most likely allowed the pulmonary torsion to occur?
a. Inferior pulmonary ligament
b. Left ligament
c. Visceral pleura
d. Central diaphragmatic tendon
e. Superior pulmonary ligament

44.4. A 72-year-old man presented to the ED with a 4-hour history of shortness of breath. He had a smoking history of 66 pack-years. He said that 5 years ago he was told that he had a "spot" on his lung that should be monitored, but he never made a follow-up appointment. His oxygen saturation as measured by pulse oximetry was 90% while he breathed supplemental oxygen (3 L/min); otherwise, his vital signs were within normal limits. Breath sounds were equal bilaterally. CT angiography of the chest showed collapse of the RUL and associated torsion of the RML. The radiologist identified a possible abnormality near the origin of the bronchus intermedius but suggested further investigation because the torsion obscured full visualization. What would be the next step in evaluation of the cause of the RUL collapse?
a. PET-CT
b. Bronchoscopy
c. V̇/Q scan
d. Thoracotomy
e. Ultrasonograpy of the chest

44.5. Which of the following is *not* usually considered a complication of pulmonary torsion?
a. Vascular thromboembolic disease
b. Hemorrhagic infarction
c. Intrapulmonary abscess formation
d. Delayed-onset reactive airway disease
e. Sepsis

Case Follow-up and Outcome

After consultation with the thoracic surgery service, video-assisted lobectomy of the RUL was performed. The RUL had extensive abscess formation, the inferior pulmonary ligament was intact, and the hilum was rotated 90° (Figures 44.3 and 44.4). The remaining lung was sutured into place. The patient did not have complications and was discharged home.

Figure 44.3   Intraoperative Photographs

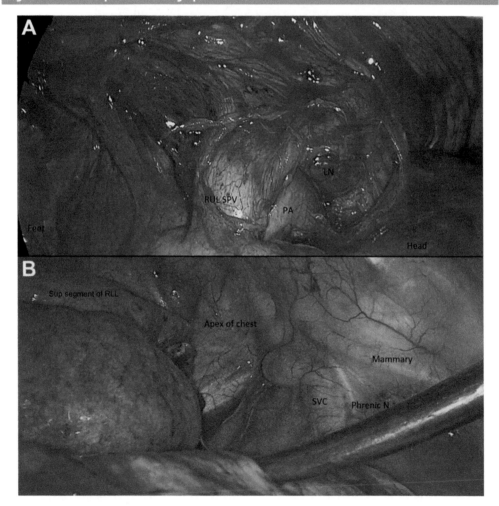

A, The anatomy is shown after the pleura was dissected from the hilum and the RUL was untwisted. The RUL superior pulmonary vein (SPV) is displaced caudally, and the azygous vein is displaced cranially. B, The entire lung is rotated 180° clockwise, as seen by the position of the RLL in the apex of the chest. LN indicates lymph node; N, nerve; PA, pulmonary artery; Sup, superior; SVC, superior vena cava.

(From Ekstein SF, McCambridge A, Edell ES, Koo CW, Blackmon SH. Case of spontaneous whole-lung torsion with literature review. J Thorac Dis. 2018 Sep;10[9]:E690-3; used with permission.)

Figure 44.4   Gross Specimen of RUL After Resection

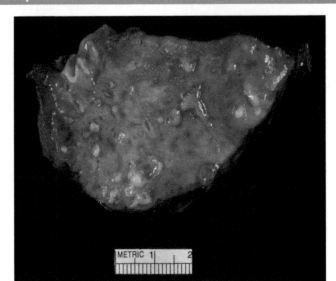

The RUL had extensive abscess formation.

(From Ekstein SF, McCambridge A, Edell ES, Koo CW, Blackmon SH. Case of spontaneous whole-lung torsion with literature review. J Thorac Dis. 2018 Sep;10[9]:E690-3; used with permission.)

Discussion

Pulmonary torsion, an extremely rare event, occurs when a lobe or the whole lung rotates around a bronchovascular pedicle and results in airway obstruction and vascular compromise (1-3). This torsion usually occurs as a complication of surgery or chest trauma and is most commonly associated with torsion of the RML after lobectomy of the RUL (4). Spontaneous torsion is even more uncommon, and only 10 cases have been published (1-3,5-9). Diagnosis is typically based on contrast CT of the chest and bronchoscopy (6). CT of the chest with a contrast agent allows identification of the relationships among the trachea, bronchi, and pulmonary arteries and often shows the twisted path of the affected vessels. Bronchoscopy can be used to identify bronchial torsion and endobronchial lesions if they are present. Definitive diagnosis is made through thoracoscopic exploration (6).

Pulmonary torsion can be life threatening; the reported mortality rate is 22%. Complications typically begin with occlusion of the pulmonary vein, preventing venous return and promoting thrombosis formation. Bronchial occlusion leads to the development of postobstructive pneumonia and abscess formation. With compromise of the pulmonary artery, early-onset hemorrhagic infarction and necrosis are expected, with rapid progression to respiratory failure and shock (5,6). Prompt intervention with thoracic surgery is recommended for definitive management (5,6).

In patients who have spontaneous pulmonary torsion, the inferior pulmonary ligament is frequently absent congenitally. This ligament is a reflection of the mediastinal parietal pleura extending from the hilum to the dome of the diaphragm and from the mediastinum to the medial surface of the lower lobe. The ligament holds the lower lobes of the lung in position.

Surprisingly, the condition of the patient described above remained stable even though she had whole-lung torsion, RUL collapse with abscess formation, and vascular compromise. She did not require oxygen supplementation or cardiovascular support. Another unexpected result was that her inferior pulmonary ligament remained intact.

Summary

Pulmonary torsion is a rare but potentially life-threatening condition. It usually occurs after intrathoracic surgery or chest trauma, but it can occur spontaneously. Diagnosis is made with the use of contrast CT of the chest or bronchoscopy, and urgent or emergent definitive management with thoracic surgery is usually required.

Answers

44.1. Answer c.

Although pulmonary torsion is quite rare, the medical literature suggests that CT angiography is the most reliable noninvasive test for diagnosis. Use of CT angiography allows for evaluation of the pulmonary vasculature with an intravenous contrast agent and usually for identification of abrupt discontinuation of flow at the site of torsion. A V̇/Q scan can also be used, but it is used more often for surgical planning than for diagnosis of torsion. Bronchoscopy is a reasonable procedure for confirming a suspected torsion and for evaluating an endobronchial lesion as a possible cause of the torsed lung, but it is more invasive than CT angiography and would not be the best first test. PET-CT and MRI of the chest have not traditionally been used in the diagnosis of pulmonary torsion. Additional information is available in the medical literature (6).

44.2. Answer d.

Emergent thoracic surgery is considered the treatment of choice for pulmonary torsion. Torsion usually compromises the blood supply to the lung, and as the duration of torsion increases, the rate of complications increases. These complications include infarction, thromboembolic disease, infection, sepsis, and death. Although CT angiography or a V̇/Q scan may be performed during evaluation of pulmonary torsion, imaging would not preclude the need for emergent surgery, especially if shock is developing. Many patients with pulmonary torsion receive full-dose anticoagulation because of the increased risk of thromboembolic disease. However, because shock was developing in the patient described in this question, he would most likely need urgent surgery, so therapeutic anticoagulation

should be delayed. Bronchoscopy may be performed intraoperatively, but the procedure should not delay definitive management. Additional information is available in the medical literature (5,6).

44.3. Answer a.

Spontaneous pulmonary torsion is often associated with congenital absence of the inferior pulmonary ligament. This is a triangular sheet of parietal and visceral pleura that extends from the hilum to the dome of the hemidiaphragm and connects the medial surface of the lower lobe to the mediastinum. There is no superior pulmonary ligament. The left ligament is anatomically bound by the esophagus and, posteriorly, by the descending aorta, but it does not directly attach to the lower lobe of the lung. The central diaphragmatic tendon is located just anterior to the midline of the diaphragm. During inspiration this tendon is drawn inferiorly with diaphragmatic contraction. This expands the chest cavity and leads to a negative intrathoracic pressure, allowing air to flow into the lungs. Absence of this tendon would not be associated with the development of spontaneous pulmonary torsion. Additional information is available in the medical literature (1,2).

44.4. Answer b.

Bronchoscopy would be the best next step in evaluation. The patient's hemodynamic status is stable, and CT angiographic findings suggest that an endobronchial abnormality may be present. Therefore, evaluation with bronchoscopy may be useful for identifying the cause of the torsion and biopsying the abnormality to evaluate for cancer. The patient will probably still need to undergo thoracic surgical intervention, and in clinical practice bronchoscopy may be performed at surgery. Relieving the endobronchial obstruction may help to prevent recurrence. PET-CT may also be performed later in his care because he may have lung cancer. PET-CT would be useful for identification of metabolic activity and metastatic disease but not for current management. A V̇/Q scan is occasionally used in surgical planning for pulmonary torsion, but it would not be the best next step for this patient. Ultrasonography of the chest would not be diagnostically useful if a patient had pulmonary torsion. Additional information is available in the medical literature (3,5).

44.5. Answer d.

Pulmonary torsion carries serious and potentially life-threatening complications, including the development of venous thromboembolic disease, postobstructive pneumonia and abscess formation, septic shock, hemorrhagic pulmonary infarction, and death. However, delayed-onset reactive airway disease related to pulmonary torsion has not been reported. Additional information is available in the medical literature (5,6).

References

1. Shorr RM, Rodriguez A. Spontaneous pulmonary torsion. Chest. 1987 Jun;91(6):927–8.
2. Ternes T, Trump M, de Christenson MR, Howell G, Stewart J. Spontaneous middle-lobe torsion. Radiol Case Rep. 2015 Dec 7;8(1):812.
3. Bell MT, Kelmenson DA, Vargas D, Meguid RA. Spontaneous pulmonary torsion secondary to left upper lobe malignancy. J Thorac Oncol. 2015 Nov;10(11): 1653–4.
4. Sung HK, Kim HK, Choi YH. Re-thoracoscopic surgery for middle lobe torsion after right upper lobectomy. Eur J Cardiothorac Surg. 2012 Sep;42(3):582–3.
5. Chrysou K, Gioutsos K, Filips A, Schmid R, Schmid RA, Kocher GJ. Spontaneous right whole-lung torsion secondary to bronchial carcinoma: a case report. J Cardiothorac Surg. 2016 Jul 14;11(1):107.
6. Irie M, Okumura N, Nakano J, Fujiwara A, Noguchi M, Kayawake H, et al. Spontaneous whole-lung torsion after massive pleural effusion and atelectasis. Ann Thorac Surg. 2014 Jan;97(1):329–32.
7. Kanayama M, Osaki T, Nishizawa N, Nakagawa M, So T, Kodate M. Idiopathic spontaneous pulmonary torsion of the lingula: a case report. Int J Surg Case Rep. 2017;37: 205–7.
8. Kita Y, Go T, Nii K, Matsuura N, Yokomise H. Spontaneous torsion of the right upper lung lobe: a case report. Surg Case Rep. 2017 Dec;3(1):37.
9. Raynaud C, Lenoir S, Caliandro R, Raffenne L, Validire P, Gossot D. Spontaneous middle lobe torsion secondary to pleural effusion. Chest. 2009 Jul;136(1): 281–3.

A 49-Year-Old Woman With Coital Hemoptysis[a]

Laura Piccolo Serafim, Ryan D. Clay, MD, and James P. Utz, MD

Case Presentation

A 49-year-old woman presented with a history of 4 recent episodes of dyspnea, chest discomfort, and hemoptysis related to intercourse. She reported coughing up a small amount of bright red blood on 3 of the 4 occasions (on the fourth, she tasted blood in the back of her throat), and she had not made any changes of practice during intercourse, such as breath-holding or autoasphyxiation. Additionally, she reported having dyspnea and discomfort between the shoulder blades after walking 10 blocks and occasional episodes of diaphoresis. Her past medical history included hypertension, type 2 diabetes, and obesity (body mass index, 35.4; calculated as weight in kilograms divided by height in meters squared). She said that she did not use tobacco or recreational drugs and that she rarely drank alcohol and had not traveled recently. Her current medications were low-dose aspirin, lisinopril, metformin, and insulin.

After the second episode of hemoptysis she sought care at an emergency department, where computed tomography (CT) of the chest showed a bilateral diffuse pattern of ground-glass opacities, a small pulmonary cyst, and no endobronchial lesions (Figure 45.1). Laboratory testing was pertinent for anemia (hemoglobin, 11.8 g/dL), leukocytosis (16.6×10^9/L), increased level of C-reactive protein (2.7 mg/L), and negative results on testing for lupus anticoagulant. She was treated with azithromycin as an outpatient, and CT of the chest 12 days later showed total resolution of the ground-glass opacities that had been present previously (Figure 45.2).

On physical examination the patient's heart rate was 124 beats/min, and she had a holosystolic murmur. Results were negative for antineutrophil cytoplasmic autoantibody and antinuclear antibody, and results were normal for pulmonary function testing. Findings on transthoracic echocardiography at rest included a normal ejection fraction, concentric left ventricular hypertrophy, a moderately dilated inferior vena cava with reduced inspiratory collapse, and no evidence of pulmonary hypertension or valvular disease. Stress echocardiography showed evidence of myocardial ischemia with exertional wall motion abnormalities and a decrease in left ventricular ejection fraction from 60% to 50% without electrocardiographic changes. The test was terminated at 4.9 metabolic equivalent tasks because the patient had presyncope.

The patient was admitted to the cardiology service because of concern for severe multivessel coronary artery disease. Catheterization of the left side of her heart showed evidence of mild coronary artery disease. Subsequent magnetic resonance imaging (MRI) of the heart showed a normal ejection fraction with evidence of concentric ventricular hypertrophy (wall thickness, 13-15 mm) and diffuse delayed subendocardial enhancement. On catheterization of the right side of the heart, pulmonary capillary wedge pressure was greatly increased at rest; with exercise, the pulmonary mean artery and

---

[a] Case presented in poster form at the CHEST Annual Meeting, Toronto, Canada, October 31, 2017.

Figure 45.1   CT of the Chest After the Second Episode of Hemoptysis

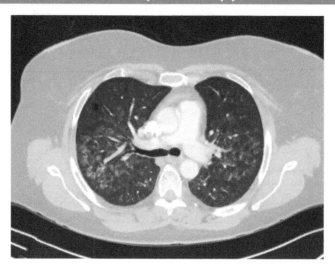

This image shows diffuse ground-glass opacities bilaterally.

(From Clay RD, Utz JP. Coital hemoptysis due to cardiac AL amyloidosis. Mayo Clin Proc. 2018 Jun;93[6]:811-12; used with permission of Mayo Foundation for Medical Education and Research.)

Figure 45.2   CT of the Chest After 12 Days of Treatment

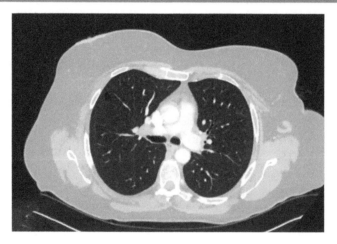

In this image, the ground-glass opacities have resolved.

(From Clay RD, Utz JP. Coital hemoptysis due to cardiac AL amyloidosis. Mayo Clin Proc. 2018 Jun;93[6]:811-12; used with permission of Mayo Foundation for Medical Education and Research.)

Table 45.1	Findings From Catheterization of the Right Side of the Heart	
Pressure	At rest, mm Hg	With exercise (80 W), mm Hg
Pulmonary capillary wedge	20	42
Right atrial	13	27
Atrial	118/56	181/80
Pulmonary artery	38/16	64/33
Mean pulmonary artery	27	50

pulmonary capillary wedge pressures increased further (Table 45.1).

Serum protein electrophoresis with immunofixation showed a small peak for monoclonal lambda protein. Assessment of kappa and lambda light chains showed an abnormally low ratio of kappa to lambda. On 24-hour urine protein electrophoresis, the urine protein level was increased and an M-protein spike was present in the beta fraction. Congo red staining of a biopsy sample from the right ventricle showed amyloid deposition with interstitial deposits and a moderate pericellular pattern.

Questions

Multiple Choice (choose the best answer)

45.1. In the differential diagnosis for hemoptysis, which of the following is most frequently associated with coital hemoptysis?
a. Neoplasia
b. Dieulafoy lesion
c. Bronchiectasis
d. Tuberculosis
e. Heart failure

45.2. Which of the following correctly describes the diagnosis of this patient's condition?
a. Low-voltage QRS complexes on the electrocardiogram (ECG) in addition to ventricular hypertrophy on echocardiography are sufficient for the diagnosis
b. Myocardial biopsy is always required for the diagnosis
c. The absence of a thickened ventricular wall on echocardiography excludes the diagnosis
d. A classic finding in patients who have this condition is subendocardial late gadolinium enhancement on MRI of the heart
e. Cardiac uptake on bone scintigraphy is highly specific for the diagnosis, so

assessment for monoclonal proteins would be redundant

45.3. Which of the following is useful for determining the prognosis for patients with this condition?
a. Urine microscopy
b. Serum ferritin
c. Troponin and N-terminal pro–brain natriuretic peptide (NT-proBNP) levels
d. Fibrinogen and D-dimer tests
e. Erythrocyte sedimentation rate

45.4. Which drug class has the strongest indication for treatment of heart failure associated with this condition?
a. β-Blockers
b. Angiotensin-converting enzyme (ACE) inhibitors
c. Digitalis
d. Loop diuretics
e. Nondihydropyridine calcium channel blockers

45.5. Which test would be important for identifying the underlying cause of amyloid deposition and for guiding treatment?
a. Cardiac MRI
b. Bone marrow biopsy
c. Endomyocardial tissue polymerase chain reaction
d. Fat pad aspirate with Congo red staining
e. Electroneuromyography

Case Follow-up and Outcome

A diagnosis of cardiac amyloidosis was made. Mass spectrometry showed a peptide profile consistent with deposition of AL amyloid (lambda type). The sinus tachycardia and holosystolic murmur were attributed to severe anemia.

The patient began therapy with a loop diuretic and a low dose of a calcium channel blocker to decrease ventricular preload, stiffness, and afterload. A bone survey showed spotty lucencies throughout the calvarium, pelvis, and proximal portions of the humeri. On bone marrow biopsy, the finding of 15% lambda light chain–restricted plasma cells was consistent with multiple myeloma. Chemotherapy was initiated with cyclophosphamide, bortezomib, and dexamethasone, and autologous stem cell transplant was planned.

Discussion

Hemoptysis has a broad differential diagnosis that includes structural and infectious pulmonary abnormalities, vasculitis, cardiovascular causes, neoplasm, trauma, iatrogenic causes, and foreign bodies. Hemoptysis that occurs exclusively during or after coitus is rare and is usually associated with a cardiovascular cause (1). During sexual activity, increased cardiovascular demand is accompanied by increases in heart rate, right ventricular systolic and diastolic pressures, and pulmonary artery pressures (2). Hemoptysis may develop if increased pulmonary venous and capillary pressures lead to capillary rupture (2). In patients with heart failure and pulmonary hypertension, these alterations are more prominent during sexual activity than during other forms of exercise (2). Also, in patients with ischemic heart disease, left ventricular function might be transiently impaired during intercourse and lead to pulmonary venous congestion and hemoptysis (1).

Amyloidosis is characterized by the extracellular deposition of beta-amyloid fibril in tissues,

either locally or systemically, and it is classified according to the type of fibrillin deposited. Cardiac involvement is most commonly seen in transthyretin amyloidosis and immunoglobulin light chain amyloidosis (also called AL amyloidosis) (3). It is characterized by restrictive cardiomyopathy, and its presence portends a poor prognosis for patients who have systemic amyloidosis (4,5). Patients present with fatigue and weakness, impaired exercise tolerance, heart failure, and arrhythmia (4).

When patients have cardiac amyloidosis, typical findings include low-voltage QRS complexes on ECG and left ventricular hypertrophy on echocardiography (6). Other findings may include increased wall thickness in both ventricles, normal or small left ventricular cavity size with preserved ejection fraction, and biatrial enlargement, but the absence of increased ventricular wall thickness does not exclude cardiac amyloidosis (6). The classic finding on cardiac MRI is a pattern of global transmural or subendocardial late gadolinium enhancement (6).

Definitive diagnosis requires cardiac biopsy; however, if typical cardiac features are identified with noninvasive testing, a noncardiac tissue sample with positive staining for amyloid fibril is sufficient to assume the diagnosis of amyloid cardiomyopathy (5,6). Immunohistochemical analysis is needed for assessment of the origin of the amyloid fibrils and for treatment guidance (5). If AL amyloidosis is diagnosed, the underlying plasma cell dyscrasia should be assessed with additional testing that includes bone marrow biopsy, serum and urine protein electrophoresis with immunofixation, and serum free light chain assay (6).

Treatment of cardiac amyloidosis comprises diuretics and salt restriction, but overdiuresis should be prevented because of the risk of hypotension and azotemia due to preload dependence (4,6). The use of β-blockers and ACE inhibitors is contraindicated because in patients with cardiac amyloidosis, cardiac output is dependent on heart rate (the stroke volume is fixed), and, if the patient has an underlying autonomic neuropathy, neurohormonal blockade can result in severe hypotension (6). The underlying plasma cell dyscrasia must also be treated.

Summary

Coital hemoptysis is rare, but when it is present, a cardiac cause should be assumed until proved otherwise. Cardiac amyloidosis has a nonspecific presentation and should be part of the differential diagnosis when a patient has heart failure with preserved ejection fraction. Cardiac amyloidosis is frequently present in patients who have systemic AL amyloidosis. Management involves treating the heart failure with diuretics and identifying and treating the underlying cause of the amyloid deposition.

Answers

45.1. Answer e.

Postcoital hemoptysis is an uncommon presentation infrequently described in the literature. The cause is usually cardiac (eg, heart failure, mitral valve disease, or coronary artery disease) because of the increased demands on the cardiovascular system with sexual activity, particularly the increased sympathetic activation and increased ventricular and pulmonary vascular pressures. Cases resulting from pulmonary hypertension and lymphangioleiomyomatosis have also been reported. Although lung neoplasia, bronchiectasis, and tuberculosis are all known causes of hemoptysis, they are not typically associated with a postcoital presentation. Dieulafoy lesions are abnormally large submucosal arteries of the gastrointestinal tract and are not part of the differential diagnosis of hemoptysis. Additional information is available in the medical literature (1,2,7).

45.2. Answer d.

Cardiac MRI, although insufficient for the diagnosis of cardiac amyloidosis, may show the highly characteristic appearance of subendocardial late gadolinium enhancement, and with disease progression a transmural myocardial enhancement pattern may be identified. When echocardiographic findings are inconclusive, cardiac MRI may be diagnostically useful.

Although ECG and echocardiographic findings may suggest the possibility, they are insufficient for the diagnosis. Myocardial biopsy is not required for the diagnosis when findings for the presence and type of cardiac amyloidosis are highly indicative (eg, an amyloid-positive noncardiac tissue sample and typical cardiac features, the presence of grade 2 or 3 myocardial radiotracer uptake on bone scintigraphy without the finding of

monoclonal proteins, or cardiac MRI findings in patients with diagnosed AL amyloidosis). Some patients with cardiac amyloidosis (especially AL cardiomyopathy) may present with minimal or no ventricular wall thickening on echocardiography; this finding is considered to be due to the direct toxicity of immunoglobulin light chains, predominant vascular involvement, or primarily endocardial involvement.

Cardiac uptake on bone scintigraphy is a valuable diagnostic tool for transthyretin amyloidosis if there is grade 2 or 3 cardiac uptake or a heart to contralateral chest ratio greater than 1.5. However, this modality can also be positive in AL amyloidosis, so it should be interpreted only in the context of negative findings from a monoclonal protein screen.

Additional information is available in the medical literature (5,6,8-10).

45.3. Answer c.

Multiple prognostic models have been developed for patients with AL amyloidosis. However, models incorporating NT-proBNP (the Mayo 2004, Mayo 2004 with European modification, and Mayo 2012 staging systems) or BNP (the Boston University biomarker scoring system) and cardiac troponin are the ones easily applied in clinical practice. Urine microscopy, serum ferritin, fibrinogen, D-dimer, and erythrocyte sedimentation rate are not useful for determining prognosis for patients with AL amyloidosis. Additional information is available in the medical literature (11-13).

45.4. Answer d.

Management of edema with loop diuretics is the established therapy for heart failure in patients with cardiac amyloidosis, although diuretics should be used cautiously so they do not further impair systemic perfusion with preload reduction in patients who have a fixed stroke volume. No definitive data support the use of ACE inhibitors and angiotensin receptor blockers for these patients. Patients with cardiac amyloidosis may not tolerate β-blockers because of heart rate dependence to maintain cardiac output. The same is true for nondihydropyridine calcium channel blockers because they also bind amyloid fibrils, potentially leading to heart block. Even though digoxin might be used in selected circumstances, its use in patients with cardiac amyloidosis is linked to potential binding to amyloid fibrils and toxicity. Additional information is available in the medical literature (6,8).

45.5. Answer b.

Bone marrow biopsy is important for the assessment of patients with AL amyloidosis because it provides information about the underlying plasma cell dyscrasias and guidance for the therapeutic approach. Cardiac MRI findings may be suggestive of cardiac amyloidosis, but they do not help in differentiating the type of fibrils or the cause of their accumulation. Endomyocardial tissue polymerase chain reaction is important in the evaluation of cardiac viral infections, but it is not usually useful for investigating the cause of amyloidosis. Fat pad aspiration biopsy is an important part of the diagnostic workup, but Congo red staining by itself does not provide information related to the type of fibril. Electroneuromyography is part of the evaluation of peripheral neuropathy frequently encountered with systemic amyloidosis but does not provide specific information about the cause. Additional information is available in the medical literature (9,14,15).

References

1. Fuks L, Shitrit D, Amital A, Fox BD, Kramer MR. Postcoital hemoptysis: our experience and review of the literature. Respir Med. 2009 Dec;103(12):1828–31.
2. Shafter AM, Elkoustaf RA. Post-coital hemoptysis due to silent coronary artery disease. J Clin Case Rep, 2017;7(6):972.
3. Ruberg FL, Berk JL. Transthyretin (TTR) cardiac amyloidosis. Circulation. 2012 Sep 4;126(10):1286–300.
4. Czeyda-Pommersheim F, Hwang M, Chen SS, Strollo D, Fuhrman C, Bhalla S. Amyloidosis: modern cross-sectional imaging. Radiographics. 2015 Sep-Oct;35(5):1381–92.
5. Izumiya Y, Takashio S, Oda S, Yamashita Y, Tsujita K. Recent advances in diagnosis and treatment of cardiac amyloidosis. J Cardiol. 2018 Feb;71(2):135–43.
6. Bejar D, Colombo PC, Latif F, Yuzefpolskaya M. Infiltrative cardiomyopathies. Clin Med Insights Cardiol. 2015 Jul 8;9(Suppl 2):29–38.
7. Kesieme EB, Okonkwo BC, Okokhere PO, Prisadov G, Aigbe E, Affusim C. Postcoital haemoptysis: a case report and a review of the literature. Case Rep Med. 2013;2013:189326. Epub 2013 May 8.
8. Kittleson MM, Maurer MS, Ambardekar AV, Bullock-Palmer RP, Chang PP, Eisen HJ, et al; American Heart Association Heart Failure and Transplantation Committee of the Council on Clinical Cardiology. Cardiac amyloidosis: evolving diagnosis and management: a scientific statement from the American Heart Association. Circulation. 2020 Jul 7;142(1):e7–e22.
Epub 2020 Jun 1. Erratum in: Circulation. 2021 Jul 6;144(1):e10. Erratum in: Circulation. 2021 Jul 6;144(1):e11.
9. Grogan M, Dispenzieri A, Gertz MA. Light-chain cardiac amyloidosis: strategies to promote early diagnosis and cardiac response. Heart. 2017 Jul;103(14):1065–72. Epub 2017 Apr 29.
10. Maceira AM, Joshi J, Prasad SK, Moon JC, Perugini E, Harding I, et al. Cardiovascular magnetic resonance in cardiac amyloidosis. Circulation. 2005 Jan 18;111(2):186–93. Epub 2005 Jan 3.
11. Dispenzieri A, Gertz MA, Kyle RA, Lacy MQ, Burritt MF, Therneau TM, et al. Serum cardiac troponins and N-terminal pro-brain natriuretic peptide: a staging system for primary systemic amyloidosis. J Clin Oncol. 2004 Sep 15;22(18):3751–7.
12. Lilleness B, Ruberg FL, Mussinelli R, Doros G, Sanchorawala V. Development and validation of a survival staging system incorporating BNP in patients with light chain amyloidosis. Blood. 2019 Jan 17;133(3):215–23. Epub 2018 Oct 17.
13. Kumar S, Dispenzieri A, Lacy MQ, Hayman SR, Buadi FK, Colby C, et al. Revised prognostic staging system for light chain amyloidosis incorporating cardiac biomarkers and serum free light chain measurements. J Clin Oncol. 2012 Mar 20;30(9):989–95. Epub 2012 Feb 13.
14. Palladini G, Merlini G. What is new in diagnosis and management of light chain amyloidosis? Blood. 2016 Jul 14;128(2):159–68. Epub 2016 Apr 6.
15. Palladini G, Milani P, Merlini G. Management of AL amyloidosis in 2020. Blood. 2020 Dec 3;136(23):2620–7.

Transplantation

A 60-Year-Old Man With Fever, Cough, and Fatigue 2 Months After Bilateral Lung Transplant

Matthew J. Cecchini, MD, PhD, and Anja C. Roden, MD

Case Presentation

A 60-year-old man was admitted to the hospital with low-grade fever, cough, increased sputum production, and fatigue. His history included bilateral lung transplant for idiopathic pulmonary fibrosis 2 months before presentation. Computed tomography (CT) showed increased left-sided pleural effusion, consolidation in the lingula, and nodular areas of infiltrate in the left upper and lower lung lobes.

His tacrolimus levels were above the therapeutic target. At 1 month after transplant, no evidence of rejection was apparent on transbronchial lung biopsy (TBLB). At admission, TBLB showed perivascular chronic inflammation with a predominance of lymphocytes (Figure 46.1) and evidence of acute lung injury, including intra-alveolar fibrin and organizing fibrinous pneumonia (Figures 46.2 and 46.3).

Figure 46.1   High-Power Photomicrograph Showing Perivascular Chronic Inflammation With Scattered Eosinophils

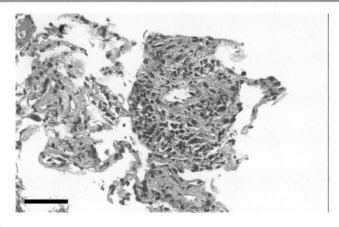

Hematoxylin-eosin; scale bar = 60 μm.

Figure 46.2   Photomicrograph Showing Abundant Organizing Intra-alveolar Fibrin

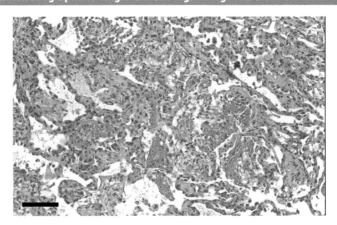

Hematoxylin-eosin; scale bar = 100 μm.

Figure 46.3   High-Power Photomicrograph Showing Intra-alveolar Fibrin and Type 2 Pneumocyte Hyperplasia

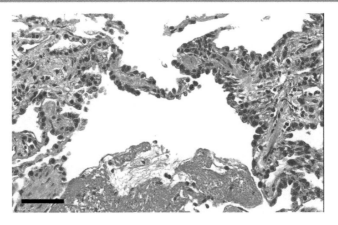

Hematoxylin-eosin; scale bar = 60 μm.

Multiple Choice (choose the best answer)

46.1. According to the TBLB findings described above in the Case Presentation, what is the International Society for Heart and Lung Transplantation (ISHLT) grade of acute cellular rejection?
a. A0
b. A1
c. A2
d. A3
e. A4

46.2. According to the ISHLT, what is the minimum number of allograft TBLB pieces containing well-expanded alveolated lung parenchyma that is required for assessment of acute rejection?
a. No minimum
b. 2
c. 3
d. 5
e. 20

46.3. Staining for which of the following should be used to assess for antibody-mediated rejection (AMR)?
a. C4d
b. CD68
c. Fibrin
d. Immunoglobulin (Ig)A
e. IgG

46.4. What is the ISHLT grade of an allograft biopsy that shows multiple small vessels surrounded by more than 3 concentric rings of mononuclear inflammatory cells without extension into the adjacent interalveolar septa?
a. A0
b. A1
c. A2
d. A3
e. A4

46.5. What is the typical management for patients with grade A2 rejection?
a. Follow-up biopsy
b. Increased immunosuppression
c. Decreased immunosuppression
d. Plasmapheresis
e. No change in management

Case Follow-up and Outcome

Owing to the high-grade rejection (A4), the patient was treated with methylprednisolone. His immunosuppressive therapy was changed from tacrolimus, azathioprine, and prednisone to tacrolimus, mycophenolate mofetil, and prednisone. At 2 weeks and at 1.5 months, follow-up TBLB showed evidence of A1 rejection; at 4 months, TBLB findings indicated grade A0 for rejection.

Discussion

Allograft rejection is a major complication of lung transplant and can cause graft dysfunction and failure (1). A relatively common event, allograft rejection occurs in 29% of patients in the first year after transplant (2). Allograft rejection is classified as cell-mediated rejection or AMR; however, cell-mediated rejection is more common in the lung. Cell-mediated rejection can occur over a broad time frame from days to years after transplant. Although AMR can occur from weeks to more than a year after transplant, the majority of cases have been reported to occur within the first year (3).

The clinical signs and symptoms of patients with allograft rejection are variable; some patients are asymptomatic, and others may have dyspnea, fever, and leukocytosis. Consequently, infectious causes are often ranked high on the differential diagnosis list. Tissue diagnosis is the gold standard for establishing a diagnosis of allograft rejection. TBLB and occasionally cryobiopsies have been used for assessment of allograft rejection (4). ISHLT requires at least 5 pieces of well-expanded alveolated lung parenchyma for adequate assessment of acute cellular rejection (5). This requirement is usually accomplished only if the bronchoscopist samples more than 5 pieces of lung parenchyma.

In acute cellular rejection, a characteristic mononuclear inflammatory cell infiltrate involves both the vasculature and the small airways. The vascular component is graded with the A score; the small airways component is graded with the B score. Vascular rejection is scored from A0 (no rejection) to A4 (high-grade rejection). *A1* rejection is characterized by vessels that are surrounded by a thin ring of mononuclear cells (2-3 layers thick). In grade *A2*, more than 3 layers of mononuclear cells are present. In grade *A3*, the inflammatory cell infiltrate extends into the adjacent interalveolar septa. Grade *A4*, characterized by perivascular mononuclear cell infiltrates, often shows morphologic evidence of an acute lung injury such as organizing pneumonia, fibrinous pneumonia, or diffuse alveolar damage (or any combination of these 3). Eosinophils are usually present with grades A3 and A4 (which are also considered high-grade rejection). Small-airways rejection is graded from B0 to B2R. *B1R* is defined as a chronic inflammatory infiltrate (predominantly lymphocytes) in the submucosa of bronchioles; *B2R* is characterized as marked inflammation that also involves the mucosa and is accompanied by mucosal changes such as erosion, ulceration, or squamous metaplasia.

Generally patients with rejection of grade A2 or higher are treated with increased immunosuppression; however, some patients with grade A1 rejection, depending on the clinical features, may also be treated with increased immunosuppression (6).

Morphologic mimics of rejection include infection, aspiration, drug toxicity, harvest (reperfusion) injury, posttransplant lymphoproliferative disease, and recurrent primary disease. Therefore, when an infectious cause is possible, stains for fungi, acid-fast bacteria, and viruses should be used.

No specific histologic features have been identified for AMR in lung allografts. However, AMR is an important cause of graft dysfunction and failure in some patients. AMR is thought to be due to preformed or de novo recipient antibodies that recognize donor-specific antigens.

While C4d deposition, evaluated with either immunohistochemistry or immunofluorescence, might suggest AMR, this finding is not specific or sensitive. Therefore, the diagnosis of AMR requires a combination of donor-specific antigen testing, the finding of C4d deposition, histologic findings that suggest AMR (including neutrophilic capillaritis, neutrophilic margination, high-grade rejection [A3 or A4], and acute lung injury), and clinical signs of graft dysfunction (7-9). Treatment of patients with AMR may include plasmapheresis and, in some patients, rituximab or intravenous immunoglobulin.

Summary

Acute cellular rejection is a common and important cause of graft dysfunction and failure after lung transplant. It is graded histologically according to the degree of inflammation surrounding the vessels and small airways. Patients with high-grade A4 rejection also have features of acute lung injury. Even mild rejection is often treated with increased immunosuppression. Infectious causes and other mimics of rejection should always be considered.

Answers

46.1. Answer e.

The biopsy showed perivascular mononuclear cell infiltrates with morphologic evidence of acute lung injury, including
intra-alveolar fibrin and organizing fibrinous
pneumonia. Morphologic evidence of acute
lung injury in combination with perivascular
inflammation is diagnostic of high-grade rejection (grade 4). Additional information is
available in the medical literature (1).

46.2. Answer d.

As defined by the ISHLT, at least 5 pieces of
well-expanded alveolated lung parenchyma
are required for adequate assessment of acute
cellular rejection. Additional information is
available in the medical literature (5).

46.3. Answer a.

The finding of C4d deposition, with either
immunohistochemistry or immunofluorescence, can suggest AMR. However, this
finding is not specific or sensitive, and the
diagnosis of AMR requires a combination
of graft dysfunction, donor-specific antigen
testing, the finding of C4d deposition,
and histologic findings that suggest AMR.
Additional information is available in the
medical literature (7-9).

46.4. Answer c.

A2 is the grade of an allograft biopsy that
shows multiple small vessels with more
than 3 layers of mononuclear cells without
extension into the adjacent interalveolar
septa. Additional information is available
in the medical literature (1).

46.5. Answer b.

Patients with rejection of grade A2 or
higher are typically treated with increased
immunosuppression. Additional information is available in the medical literature (6).

References

1. Roden AC, Aisner DL, Allen TC, Aubry MC, Barrios RJ, Beasley MB, et al. Diagnosis of acute cellular rejection and antibody-mediated rejection on lung transplant biopsies: a perspective from members of the Pulmonary Pathology Society. Arch Pathol Lab Med. 2017 Mar;141(3):437–44.

2. Yusen RD, Edwards LB, Kucheryavaya AY, Benden C, Dipchand AI, Goldfarb SB, et al. The Registry of the International Society for Heart and Lung Transplantation: Thirty-second Official Adult Lung and Heart-Lung Transplantation Report--2015; focus theme: early graft failure. J Heart Lung Transplant. 2015 Oct;34(10):1264–77.

3. Witt CA, Gaut JP, Yusen RD, Byers DE, Iuppa JA, Bennett Bain K, et al. Acute antibody-mediated rejection after lung transplantation. J Heart Lung Transplant. 2013 Oct;32(10):1034–40.

4. Roden AC, Kern RM, Aubry MC, Jenkins SM, Yi ES, Scott JP, et al. Transbronchial cryobiopsies in the evaluation of lung allografts: do the benefits outweigh the risks? Arch Pathol Lab Med. 2016 Apr;140(4):303–11.

5. Stewart S, Fishbein MC, Snell GI, Berry GJ, Boehler A, Burke MM, et al. Revision of the 1996 working formulation for the standardization of nomenclature in the diagnosis of lung rejection. J Heart Lung Transplant. 2007 Dec;26(12):1229–42.

6. Martinu T, Pavlisko EN, Chen DF, Palmer SM. Acute allograft rejection: cellular and humoral processes. Clin Chest Med. 2011 Jun;32(2):295–310.

7. Wallace WD, Li N, Andersen CB, Arrossi AV, Askar M, Berry GJ, et al. Banff study of pathologic changes in lung allograft biopsy specimens with donor-specific antibodies. J Heart Lung Transplant. 2016 Jan;35(1):40–8.

8. Levine DJ, Glanville AR, Aboyoun C, Belperio J, Benden C, Berry GJ, et al. Antibody-mediated rejection of the lung: a consensus report of the International Society for Heart and Lung Transplantation. J Heart Lung Transplant. 2016 Apr;35(4):397–406.

9. Roux A, Levine DJ, Zeevi A, Hachem R, Halloran K, Halloran PF, et al. Banff Lung Report: current knowledge and future research perspectives for diagnosis and treatment of pulmonary antibody-mediated rejection (AMR). Am J Transplant. 2019 Jan;19(1):21–31.

Tara Tarmey, MB, BCh, BAO, Anja C. Roden, MD,
and Cassie C. Kennedy, MD

Case Presentation

A 59-year-old man presented with progressive shortness of breath and fatigue. He had undergone bilateral lung transplant 18 months earlier for idiopathic pulmonary fibrosis. His symptoms had been progressing slowly for the past year, and at presentation he had dyspnea on mild exertion (New York Heart Association class III). He had not had fevers, productive cough, recent travel or sick contacts, chest pain, or syncope. He had adhered to his therapy of immunosuppression medication and prophylactic antimicrobials. His past medical history also included chronic kidney disease (stage 3), coronary artery disease, hyperlipidemia, type 2 diabetes, and obstructive sleep apnea.

The posttransplant clinical course had been complicated with multiple episodes of acute rejection and recurrent infections, which included *Pseudomonas* infection, aspergillosis, and cytomegalovirus pneumonia. Consequently, balancing his immunosuppression regimen was a challenge, and his maintenance therapy was tacrolimus and prednisone alone. Other medications included routine prophylactic antimicrobials (posaconazole and sulfamethoxazole-trimethoprim), aspirin, rosuvastatin, metoprolol, furosemide, and insulin.

Physical examination findings included a regular heart rhythm without murmurs, gallops, or rubs and diminished breath sounds bilaterally. Other physical examination findings were unremarkable. Results of routine laboratory testing were similar to the patient's baseline results. Blood culture results were negative. The tacrolimus level was 7.7 ng/mL (target, 5-8 ng/mL). Chest radiography showed small bilateral pleural effusions and bibasilar opacities (Figure 47.1). High-resolution computed tomography (HRCT) showed patchy ground-glass opacities bilaterally, consolidative opacities in the left lower lobe, small pleural effusions bilaterally, and pleural thickening (Figure 47.2). Pulmonary function tests showed a sustained, progressive decrease in pulmonary function, with a forced expiratory volume in the first second of expiration (FEV_1) that decreased from 3.55 L at baseline to 1.63 L. Bronchoscopy with bronchoalveolar lavage (BAL) and transbronchial biopsy did not show evidence of acute rejection or infection.

Figure 47.1   Chest Radiograph

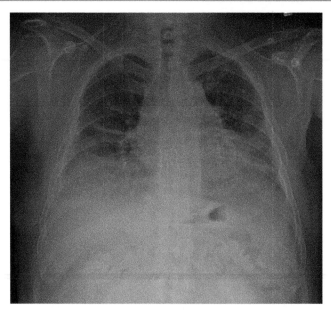

Anteroposterior view shows small bilateral pleural effusions, bibasilar opacities, and linear atelectasis in the right lower zone. A transcatheter aortic valve replacement is in situ.

Figure 47.2   HRCT of the Chest

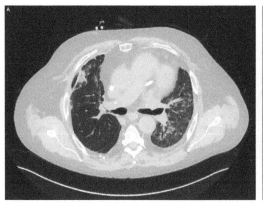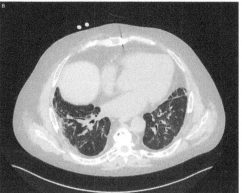

Axial imaging on lung windows through the upper (A) and lower (B) lobes shows bilateral ground-glass opacities and small pleural effusions. Two cardiac monitoring leads overlie the right anterior chest wall (B).

Questions

Multiple Choice (choose the best answer)

47.1. Which of the following statements correctly describes acute rejection after lung transplant?
  a. Negative findings on transbronchial biopsy exclude acute rejection
  b. The absence of ground-glass opacities on CT suggests an alternative diagnosis
  c. Asymptomatic patients with A1 rejection always require an increase in immunosuppression
  d. Humoral rejection is more common than acute rejection
  e. Acute rejection can be excluded if pulmonary function is stable according to results from spirometry

47.2. Which of the following is *not* an indication for extracorporeal photopheresis (ECP)?
  a. Cutaneous T-cell lymphoma
  b. Graft-vs-host disease
  c. Kaposi sarcoma
  d. Scleroderma
  e. Solid organ transplant

47.3. Which of the following is *not* a management consideration in chronic lung allograft dysfunction (CLAD)?
  a. Switching from cyclosporine to tacrolimus for long-term immunosuppression

  b. A trial of azithromycin
  c. Consideration of antireflux surgery for patients with confirmed gastroesophageal reflux disease
  d. Retransplant for end-stage CLAD that is refractory to all other therapies
  e. Sustained therapy with high doses of systemic corticosteroids

47.4. Which of the following is consistent with the restrictive phenotype of CLAD?
  a. A stable ratio of FEV_1 to forced vital capacity (FVC)
  b. A stable total lung capacity (TLC)
  c. Failure to achieve at least 80% of the predicted value of FEV_1 after transplant
  d. Increased level of donor-specific antibody
  e. Concomitant infection

47.5. Which of the following is *not* true about CLAD?
  a. Bronchiolitis obliterans (BO) is the characteristic histologic feature of grade C rejection
  b. Transbronchial biopsy is always sufficiently sensitive for the detection of BO
  c. Grade D rejection is characterized by fibrointimal thickening of arteries and veins
  d. At least 5 fragments of well-expanded alveolated lung are required for an adequate biopsy
  e. Recurrent acute rejection is a risk factor for CLAD

Case Follow-up and Outcome

After acute rejection and infection were excluded, a diagnosis of CLAD restrictive phenotype was made on the basis of the sustained decrease in FEV_1 and the persistent pulmonary infiltrates on imaging. The patient was discharged with oxygen for use at home, azithromycin was added to his medications, and a referral was arranged for pulmonary rehabilitation. His functional status and FEV_1 continued to decrease, so the decision was made to begin ECP therapy. After the patient had an initial mild improvement in symptoms, his condition continued to worsen during the next year, and he had multiple hospital admissions for recurrent infection and a progressive worsening in kidney function. After a family conference, the patient declined hemodialysis and was transitioned to palliative care.

Discussion

Compared to patients with transplants of other solid organs, patients with lung transplant have inferior long-term outcomes; the current median survival is 6 years (1). Survival is limited by both graft-related and non–graft-related factors. The causes of complications can be broadly divided into surgical, infectious, immunologic, and neoplastic. Infection is the leading cause of morbidity and mortality in the first 6 months after transplant; thereafter, allograft failure is the leading cause of death.

Late-onset or worsening dyspnea after transplant has a broad differential diagnosis. The main clinical considerations include acute rejection, CLAD, infection, aspiration, and airway complications such as bronchial stenosis, pulmonary embolism, posttransplant lymphoproliferative disorder, and recurrence of the primary disease.

Acute allograft rejection or dysfunction is a common complication, and more than one-third of patients have an episode of acute rejection in the first year after transplant (2). Acute cellular rejection is the most common subtype and is driven by T-lymphocyte recognition of foreign major histocompatibility complexes or human leukocyte antigens (HLAs). Humoral-mediated (or antibody-mediated) rejection is due to the binding of preformed or de novo antibodies that are directed against antigens expressed on the donor organ cells. The risk is greatest in the first few months after transplant and gradually decreases with time. Patients with a history of acute rejection have an increased risk for subsequent episodes of acute rejection. Other risk factors include HLA mismatch and different immunosuppression regimens; higher rates have been reported for cyclosporine-based regimens compared to tacrolimus-based regimens.

When patients are asymptomatic, the diagnosis is made from surveillance transbronchial biopsy. Symptoms are nonspecific and include dyspnea, cough, and fever. Results on spirometry may be normal or indicate airflow obstruction with a decrease in FEV_1 or restriction with a decrease in FVC and FEV_1. Findings on chest radiography, when present, are nonspecific and include perihilar opacities and pleural effusions. The main reason to perform chest radiography is to exclude an alternative diagnosis. HRCT is somewhat more sensitive, and findings include ground-glass opacities, interlobular septal thickening, and pleural effusions. The absence of ground-glass opacities on HRCT strongly suggests an alternative diagnosis. Bronchoscopy with BAL and transbronchial biopsy, including samples from multiple lobes and segments of the allograft, are required for confirmation of the diagnosis. Multiple samples are necessary because the distribution of abnormal tissue can be irregular, so that sampling bias is a possibility, and negative biopsy findings do not exclude acute rejection.

The International Society for Heart and Lung Transplantation (ISHLT) categorizes rejection according to the following grades: A, acute rejection; B, small airways rejection or lymphocytic bronchiolitis; C, chronic airways rejection; and D, chronic vascular rejection (3). The severity of acute rejection is graded from A0 (none) to A4 (severe). The decision to treat is based on clinical and histopathologic severity. Moderate (A3) or severe (A4) rejection is generally treated, but the approach varies for minimal (A1) or mild (A2) rejection and is often guided by other clinical considerations. The typical regimen for treating acute rejection includes high doses of parenteral glucocorticoids, and clinical improvement is expected within 24 to 48 hours. The patient's immunosuppressive regimen must then be reviewed to ensure that it is optimal and to prevent recurrent episodes of acute rejection, which is an established risk factor for CLAD (4).

According to the ISHLT, CLAD is defined as a substantial and persistent decrease ($\geq$20%) in the FEV_1 value from the baseline value (5). The baseline value is determined as the mean of the best 2 posttransplant FEV_1 measurements taken more than 3 weeks apart.

Potentially reversible triggers, such as infection or acute rejection, should be excluded first. A diagnosis of probable CLAD can be made if the FEV_1 remains impaired on subsequent testing at least 3 weeks after the initial decrease from baseline despite adequate treatment of any secondary causes. CLAD is confirmed if the abnormalities persist beyond 3 months.

Subtyping and staging of CLAD aid prognostication and tailored treatment planning. The most common manifestation of CLAD is an obstructive phenotype, previously termed *BO syndrome*, which is associated with 1) a decrease in the FEV_1 of 20% or more from baseline, 2) airflow limitation (FEV_1/FVC <0.7), and 3) the absence of persistent pulmonary opacities. Signs of air trapping, mosaic attenuation, and bronchiectasis can be seen on imaging. Up to 30% of patients have a restrictive pattern of CLAD, previously termed *restrictive allograft syndrome*, which is characterized by 1) a decrease of at least 20% in FEV_1, 2) a decrease in TLC of at least 10% from baseline, and 3) persistent radiologic pulmonary opacities. The restrictive phenotype is associated with inferior clinical outcomes (6). In some patients, the pattern may be mixed, and in others the pattern may be undefined; for example, a patient with an obstructive defect may have persistent pulmonary opacities without decreased TLC. The

Table 47.1	Staging of CLAD
Stage	FEV_1 compared to baseline, %
0	>80
1	>65–80
2	>50–65
3	>35–50
4	$\leq$35

underlying pathology of the obstructive phenotype is considered to be BO. The pathology of restrictive CLAD may include airway obliteration, parenchymal fibroelastosis (including intra-alveolar fibroelastosis with or without BO), fibrotic nonspecific interstitial pneumonia, fibrosis-induced subpleural or paraseptal emphysema, acute lung injury (eg, diffuse alveolar damage or acute fibrinous and organizing pneumonia), and acute rejection (5). CLAD is staged according to a comparison of the present FEV_1 with the baseline FEV_1 (Table 47.1).

The limited treatment options for CLAD include modifying the immunosuppressive regimen, beginning a trial of azithromycin, or treating gastroesophageal reflux disease. For selected patients who have advanced CLAD, retransplant may be the only option, but those patients tend to have higher postoperative mortality and decreased peak lung function when compared to patients after the first transplant (7). Other therapeutic options include total lymphoid radiotherapy or ECP; the best results occur when patients have the obstructive phenotype.

Summary

The differential diagnosis is broad when patients have late-onset dyspnea after lung transplant. After acute and reversible causes have been excluded, CLAD is an important consideration if the patient has a marked, sustained decrease in FEV_1. Early recognition and appropriate subtyping of CLAD aid in providing a prognosis and tailoring the therapy.

Answers

47.1. Answer b.

HRCT features of acute rejection are non-specific and include ground-glass opacities, interlobular septal thickening, and new or increasing pleural effusions. The absence of ground-glass opacities almost excludes acute rejection and should prompt consideration of an alternative differential diagnosis. Prompt improvement on imaging with 48 hours of intravenous corticosteroid therapy supports a diagnosis of acute rejection. In acute rejection the abnormal tissue is irregularly distributed, and therefore biopsy results can be negative. Acute rejection is more common than humoral rejection. Spirometry results are nonspecific and may be normal or indicate airflow obstruction (with a decrease in FEV_1) or restriction (with a decrease in FVC and FEV_1). Additional information is available in the medical literature (8).

47.2. Answer c.

ECP has been in clinical use for over 30 years after it received US Food and Drug Administration approval for the palliative treatment of the Sézary syndrome variant of cutaneous T-cell lymphoma in 1988. Additional indications that have been successfully introduced into clinical practice since then include graft-vs-host disease, scleroderma, and solid organ transplant. ECP is not indicated in the management of Kaposi sarcoma. Additional information is available in the medical literature (9).

47.3. Answer e.

Episodes of acute rejection, pneumonia, and cytomegalovirus infection have all been shown to predispose patients to CLAD, and therefore adequate immunosuppression and infection prophylaxis are essential preventive measures. In addition, every effort should be made to prevent or treat gastroesophageal reflux disease given its known association with chronic rejection. When CLAD is diagnosed, the patient's calcineurin inhibitor or nucleotide blocking agent (or both) can be changed to a different drug in the same class; if that does not help, substitution with sirolimus or everolimus can be considered. Approximately 35% of patients with obstructive CLAD have a response to macrolides and an improvement in FEV_1 of at least 10%. Therefore, a trial of azithromycin can be considered if CLAD is suspected. Select patients with end-stage CLAD that is refractory to all other therapies may be considered for retransplant, although survival rates are worse than with primary transplant. Sustained treatment with high doses of corticosteroid therapy has not been shown to improve outcomes but is associated with numerous and frequently severe adverse effects. Additional information is available in the medical literature (10-13).

47.4. Answer a.

Definite CLAD is defined as a decrease in FEV_1 of at least 20% from the reference FEV_1 that persists for more than 3 months despite treatment of secondary causes of allograft dysfunction such as infection, acute rejection, or airway stenosis. The restrictive pattern of CLAD is characterized by 1) a decrease of at least 20% in FEV_1, 2) a decrease in TLC of at least 10% from baseline, and 3) persistent radiologic pulmonary opacities. Unlike in kidney transplant, in lung transplant there is less evidence of the effect of anti-HLA mismatches on CLAD. However, in recent studies anti-HLA donor-specific antibodies were associated with poor outcome after lung transplant and were implicated with CLAD, although they are not a specific marker for the restrictive pattern. Additional information is available in the medical literature (6,14).

47.5. Answer b.

The ISHLT categorizes rejection according to the following grades: A, acute rejection; B, small airways rejection or lymphocytic bronchiolitis; C, chronic airways rejection; and D, chronic vascular rejection. Grade A is defined by the presence of perivascular mononuclear cell infiltrates with or without endotheliitis and is an important risk factor for the development of CLAD. Grade B applies only to small airways, such as the terminal or respiratory bronchioles, and is defined by inflammation of the small airways with a lymphocytic infiltrate. Grade C is characterized by narrowing of the small airways due to fibrosis. Grade D, which is not applicable to transbronchial biopsies since they lack vessels of sufficient size, is characterized by thickened pulmonary arteries and veins due to fibrointimal connective tissue. In symptomatic patients bronchoscopy with transbronchial biopsy is the gold standard for evaluation of acute rejection. However, the disease process is often diffuse and heterogeneously distributed, so sampling bias may produce a false-negative result. Standard practice is to obtain at least 5 samples of well-expanded alveolated lung tissue. Additional information is available in the medical literature (3,15,16).

References

1. Chambers DC, Yusen RD, Cherikh WS, Goldfarb SB, Kucheryavaya AY, Khusch K, et al; International Society for Heart and Lung Transplantation. The Registry of the International Society for Heart and Lung Transplantation: Thirty-fourth Adult Lung and Heart-Lung Transplantation Report-2017; focus theme: allograft ischemic time. J Heart Lung Transplant. 2017 Oct;36(10):1047–59.

2. Martinu T, Pavlisko EN, Chen DF, Palmer SM. Acute allograft rejection: cellular and humoral processes. Clin Chest Med. 2011 Jun;32(2):295–310.

3. Stewart S, Fishbein MC, Snell GI, Berry GJ, Boehler A, Burke MM, et al. Revision of the 1996 working formulation for the standardization of nomenclature in the diagnosis of lung rejection. J Heart Lung Transplant. 2007 Dec;26(12):1229–42.

4. Speich R, van der Bij W. Epidemiology and management of infections after lung transplantation. Clin Infect Dis. 2001 Jul 1;33 Suppl 1:S58–65.

5. Glanville AR, Verleden GM, Todd JL, Benden C, Calabrese F, Gottlieb J, et al. Chronic lung allograft dysfunction: definition and update of restrictive allograft syndrome: a consensus report from the Pulmonary Council of the ISHLT. J Heart Lung Transplant. 2019 May;38(5):483–92.

6. Verleden SE, Vos R, Vanaudenaerde BM, Verleden GM. Chronic lung allograft dysfunction phenotypes and treatment. J Thorac Dis. 2017 Aug;9(8):2650–9.

7. Halloran K, Aversa M, Tinckam K, Martinu T, Binnie M, Chaparro C, et al. Comprehensive outcomes after lung retransplantation: a single-center review. Clin Transplant. 2018 Jun;32(6):e13281.

8. Krishnam MS, Suh RD, Tomasian A, Goldin JG, Lai C, Brown K, et al. Postoperative complications of lung transplantation: radiologic findings along a time continuum. Radiographics. 2007 Jul-Aug;27(4):957–74.

9. Cho A, Jantschitsch C, Knobler R. Extracorporeal photopheresis: an overview. Front Med (Lausanne). 2018 Aug 27;5:236.

10. Kroshus TJ, Kshettry VR, Savik K, John R, Hertz MI, Bolman RM 3rd. Risk factors for the development of bronchiolitis obliterans syndrome after lung transplantation. J Thorac Cardiovasc Surg. 1997 Aug;114(2):195–202.

11. D'Ovidio F, Mura M, Tsang M, Waddell TK, Hutcheon MA, Singer LG, et al. Bile acid aspiration and the development of bronchiolitis obliterans after lung transplantation. J Thorac Cardiovasc Surg. 2005 May;129(5):1144–52.

12. Parada MT, Alba A, Sepulveda C. Everolimus in lung transplantation in Chile. Transplant Proc. 2010 Jan-Feb;42(1):328–30.

13. Meyer KC, Raghu G, Verleden GM, Corris PA, Aurora P, Wilson KC, et al; ISHLT/ATS/ERS BOS Task Force Committee; ISHLT/ATS/ERS BOS Task Force Committee. An international ISHLT/ATS/ERS clinical practice guideline: diagnosis and management of bronchiolitis obliterans syndrome. Eur Respir J. 2014 Dec;44(6):1479–503. Epub 2014 Oct 30.

14. Tissot A, Danger R, Claustre J, Magnan A, Brouard S. Early identification of chronic lung allograft dysfunction: the need of biomarkers. Front Immunol. 2019 Jul 17;10:1681.

15. Roden AC, Tazelaar HD. Pathology of lung rejection: cellular and humoral mediated. In: Raghu G, Carbone R, editors. Lung transplantation: evolving knowledge and new horizons. Cham, Switzerland: Springer; 2018. p. 209–230. (Online book.)

16. Greer M, Werlein C, Jonigk D. Surveillance for acute cellular rejection after lung transplantation. Ann Transl Med. 2020 Mar;8(6):410.

A 64-Year-Old Man With Back Spasms and Dyspnea 3 Weeks After Lung Transplant

Jessica Lau, MD

Case Presentation

A 64-year-old man presented with back spasms and dyspnea. His past medical history included end-stage idiopathic pulmonary fibrosis for which he had undergone left lung transplant 3 weeks earlier. Pathologic examination findings were consistent with usual interstitial pneumonia. The posttransplant course was complicated by atrial fibrillation with a rapid ventricular rate, which was treated with amiodarone. When surveillance bronchoscopy was performed 2 weeks after transplant, the anastomosis appeared healthy without evidence of stenosis, dehiscence, excessive formation of granulation tissue, fistula, infection, or malacia.

Radiography of the chest showed a persistent left-sided pleural effusion. Thoracentesis yielded 380 mL of viscous, serosanguinous fluid. The pleural fluid had a glucose level less than 2 mg/dL, pH 7.24, and increased levels of total nucleated cells, lactate dehydrogenase, and protein. A pigtail catheter was placed, and therapy was started with broad-spectrum antibiotics. The pleural fluid culture was positive for *Mycoplasma hominis*, and the antibiotic therapy was adjusted.

Computed tomography (CT) of the chest without an intravenous contrast agent showed a hydropneumothorax of the left side with many loculi. After a thoracic surgeon was consulted, the patient underwent video-assisted thoracoscopic surgery and decortication on the left side. His right arm swelled from a deep vein thrombosis related to a peripherally inserted central catheter. A heparin infusion was started, but a left-sided hemothorax developed and required another left thoracotomy and evacuation of the clot. Although chest tube output gradually decreased, a moderate to large left-sided pneumothorax developed. The pneumothorax resolved with placement of chest tubes and use of suction.

Questions

Multiple Choice (choose the best answer)

48.1. Which of the following is the most common airway complication after lung transplant?
   a. Exophytic granulation tissue
   b. Bronchial stenosis
   c. Anastomotic dehiscence
   d. Bronchomalacia
   e. Fistula formation

48.2. Which of the following is the gold standard for diagnosis of anastomotic dehiscence?
   a. Radiography of the chest
   b. CT of the chest
   c. Pulmonary function testing
   d. Video-assisted thoracoscopic surgery
   e. Bronchoscopy

48.3. Which of the following is *not* an established risk factor for airway complications after lung transplant?

   a. Infection with *Aspergillus fumigatus*
   b. Telescoping surgical technique
   c. Immunosuppressive therapy with sirolimus
   d. High body mass index
   e. Prolonged mechanical ventilation

48.4. Which of the following is an early airway complication of lung transplant?
   a. Bronchial stenosis at 2 months
   b. Bronchial stenosis at 4 months
   c. Anastomotic infection at 6 months
   d. Anastomotic infection at 8 months
   e. Anastomotic infection at 10 months

48.5. According to current data, when should surveillance bronchoscopy be performed after lung transplant?
   a. At 2 months
   b. At 4 months
   c. At 12 months
   d. At 18 months
   e. At 24 months

Case Follow-up and Outcome

The patient's hospitalization coincided with his routine 1-month follow-up, which included posttransplant bronchoscopy for inspection of the anastomosis, bronchoalveolar lavage with the immunocompromised host protocol, and transbronchial biopsies. Findings included necrosis of the donor bronchus immediately beyond the anastomosis and dehiscence of the anastomosis. A bifurcated silicone stent was placed in the distal portion of the left mainstem bronchus with bifurcations into the left upper lobe and left lower lobe bronchi. The posttransplant corticosteroid dosage was decreased to promote anastomotic healing. CT of the chest was used for surveillance of the graft because transbronchial biopsy was not performed.

Discussion

Airway complications are an important cause of morbidity and death among patients after lung transplant. In the absence of standardized definitions or a universal grading system, the reported incidence ranges up to 33%. Overall, though, the incidence of airway complications has decreased through the establishment of modified surgical techniques, medical advances, and improvements in graft preservation (1).

Airway complications, which can be classified as *early* (<3 months) or *late* (>3 months), include bronchial stenosis, exophytic granulation tissue, anastomotic necrosis and dehiscence, infection, tracheobronchomalacia, and fistula formation. The most common airway complication is bronchial stenosis. Bronchial stenosis and malacia tend to occur later, after the anastomosis has healed. Anastomotic necrosis and dehiscence commonly occurs earlier and is related to ischemia (1).

Only two-thirds of patients have symptoms related to anastomotic complications (2). Bronchoscopy is used for diagnosis, although

imaging of the chest with CT and radiography may be helpful. Management requires a multidisciplinary approach and ranges from conservative medical therapy to bronchoscopic or surgical intervention. Exophytic granulation tissue may result from an infection, which will heal after treatment with appropriate therapy (3). Management of bronchial stenosis includes balloon bronchoplasty, electrocautery or laser therapy, and self-expanding metallic or silicone stents. Surgical management includes reconstruction of the bronchial anastomosis (1,4).

Partial anastomotic dehiscence can be managed with surveillance and antibiotic therapy. Larger partial anastomotic dehiscence is managed with placement of a self-expanding metallic stent or a bifurcated silicone stent. Typically, the stent is removed 6 to 8 weeks after the anastomosis heals. Complete anastomotic dehiscence is usually repaired surgically (4).

Various surgical techniques for the anastomosis have been described as *telescoping* or *end to end*. Telescoping techniques are no longer favored because of the increased risk of airway complications, so anastomoses are now made end to end (5). Sirolimus is associated with impaired wound healing, which can lead to anastomotic complications. Other recognized risk factors include acute rejection and fungal and bacterial infections (6).

Summary

Lung transplant is an effective option in the treatment of end-stage lung disease, but pulmonary complications can arise after transplant and lead to serious morbidity and death. The present case highlights the importance of recognizing the more subtle complications of transplant such as airway complications. Pulmonary complications do not occur in isolation, though, so it is important to recognize that in the patient described above, the presence of empyema and the later development of a pneumothorax may have been signs of anastomotic complications.

Answers

48.1. Answer b.

Airway complications include bronchial stenosis, granulation tissue formation, anastomotic necrosis and dehiscence, focal infection, tracheobronchomalacia, and fistula formation. Of these complications, the most common is bronchial stenosis. Additional information is available in the medical literature (1).

48.2. Answer e.

Diagnosis of anastomotic dehiscence requires bronchoscopic visualization. CT of the chest may provide additional information related to, for example, bronchial wall defects or collections of air or fluid in the mediastinum or subcutaneous tissue. Additional information is available in the medical literature (3).

48.3. Answer d.

Risk factors for airway complications after lung transplant include primary graft dysfunction, acute rejection, infection or colonization with *A fumigatus*, telescoping surgical technique, immunosuppressive therapy with sirolimus, prolonged mechanical ventilation, and single-lung ventilation. High body mass index is not a risk factor. Additional information is available in the medical literature (5,6).

48.4. Answer a.

Early airway complications are those diagnosed within 3 months of transplant. Complications that occur after 3 months are considered *late* complications. Additional information is available in the medical literature (3).

48.5. Answer c.

Timing of surveillance bronchoscopy may vary, but according to the International Society for Heart and Lung Transplantation, the most common schedule is to perform bronchoscopy at 4 weeks, 3 months, 6 months, and 12 months after lung transplant. Additional information is available in the medical literature (7).

References

1. Santacruz JF, Mehta AC. Airway complications and management after lung transplantation: ischemia, dehiscence, and stenosis. Proc Am Thorac Soc. 2009 Jan 15;6(1):79–93.

2. Murthy SC, Blackstone EH, Gildea TR, Gonzalez-Stawinski GV, Feng J, Budev M, et al; Members of Cleveland Clinic's Pulmonary Transplant Team. Impact of anastomotic airway complications after lung transplantation. Ann Thorac Surg. 2007 Aug;84(2):401–9.

3. Cho EN, Haam SJ, Kim SY, Chang YS, Paik HC. Anastomotic airway complications after lung transplantation. Yonsei Med J. 2015 Sep;56(5):1372–8.

4. Ahmad S, Shlobin OA, Nathan SD. Pulmonary complications of lung transplantation. Chest. 2011 Feb;139(2):402–11.

5. Van De Wauwer C, Van Raemdonck D, Verleden GM, Dupont L, De Leyn P, Coosemans W, et al. Risk factors for airway complications within the first year after lung transplantation. Eur J Cardiothorac Surg. 2007 Apr;31(4):703–10.

6. Groetzner J, Kur F, Spelsberg F, Behr J, Frey L, Bittmann I, et al. Munich Lung Transplant Group. Airway anastomosis complications in de novo lung transplantation with sirolimus-based immunosuppression. J Heart Lung Transplant. 2004 May;23(5):632–8.

7. Martinu T, Koutsokera A, Benden C, Cantu E, Chambers D, Cypel M, et al; Bronchoalveolar Lavage Standardization Workgroup. International Society for Heart and Lung Transplantation consensus statement for the standardization of bronchoalveolar lavage in lung transplantation. J Heart Lung Transplant. 2020 Nov;39(11):1171–90. Epub 2020 Jul 15.

Vascular Diseases

A 57-Year-Old Man With a History of Recurrent Epistaxis and Arteriovenous Malformations

Vivek N. Iyer, MD, MPH, and Vaibhav Ahluwalia, MBBS

Case Presentation

A 57-year-old man presented with a long-standing history of epistaxis and a previous diagnosis of hereditary hemorrhagic telangiectasia (HHT). The patient reported having multiple episodes of severe epistaxis weekly for about 10 years. He had severe iron deficiency anemia that involved numerous hospitalizations over the preceding few years, and he had received 32 units of blood through transfusions in the past year. Previous treatments included embolization of the right and left sphenopalatine arteries and several nasal laser cauterization procedures, none of which controlled the epistaxis.

The patient's family history was notable for HHT in 2 of his brothers and his 2 children. His other medical comorbidities included hypertension, depression, insomnia, acute coronary syndrome (previously treated with dual antiplatelet therapy), and chronic biventricular heart failure (ejection fraction, 25%-30%). The dual antiplatelet therapy was terminated prematurely because the severity of the epistaxis increased markedly. After that therapy was discontinued, he had an out-of-hospital cardiac arrest and subsequently underwent implantation of a defibrillator.

On physical examination, the patient's resting room air oxyhemoglobin saturation was 93%. He had several classic features of HHT, including a few scattered telangiectasias on his palate and bilateral telangiectasias in his nose.

Computed tomography (CT) of the chest and abdomen showed multiple liver and pancreatic arteriovenous malformations (AVMs) and a large pulmonary AVM. A branch of the right upper lobe pulmonary artery had a large filling defect consistent with an acute pulmonary embolism. Echocardiography confirmed a high-output cardiac failure state (cardiac index, 4.8 L/min/m^2).

The following results from a complete blood cell count and other tests (with reference ranges) were consistent with iron deficiency anemia: hemoglobin, 9.7 g/dL (13-17 g/dL); hematocrit, 32.5% (41%-50%); serum iron, 14 µg/dL (60-170 µg/dL); and ferritin, 11 µg/L (12-300 µg/L).

Questions

Multiple Choice (choose the best answer)

49.1. Which of the following is *not* a cardinal feature of HHT?

a. Spontaneous and recurrent epistaxis
b. Mucocutaneous telangiectasias on the lips, tongue, and oral mucosal surfaces
c. Visceral AVMs involving the lungs, liver, brain, and intestinal tract
d. Coagulopathies
e. AVMs involving the spinal cord

49.2. How is HHT inherited?

a. Autosomal dominant inheritance with variable penetrance
b. Autosomal recessive inheritance with variable penetrance
c. X-linked recessive
d. Polygenic inheritance
e. Unknown

49.3. Which of the following is *not* part of the Curaçao criteria for diagnosis of HHT?

a. Epistaxis
b. Family history of HHT
c. Acute coronary syndrome
d. AVMs
e. Telangiectasias

49.4. Which medications are *not* helpful in the treatment of HHT-related bleeding?

a. Antiangiogenic agents (eg, bevacizumab)
b. Antifibrinolytic agents (eg, tranexamic acid)
c. Nasal lubricating and moistening agents
d. Aspirin and other nonsteroidal anti-inflammatory drugs (NSAIDs)
e. Pazopanib

49.5. Which of the following is *not* a complication of HHT?

a. Stroke
b. High-output cardiac failure
c. Anemia
d. Hypoxemia
e. Pancreatitis

Case Follow-up and Outcome

The diagnosis of HHT was confirmed according to the Curaçao criteria (1). These clinical criteria for the diagnosis of HHT include the following:

1. Recurrent, spontaneous nosebleeds (epistaxis)
2. Multiple mucocutaneous telangiectases on the skin of the hands, lips, or face or inside the nose or mouth (*telangiectases* are small vascular lesions that blanch under direct pressure)
3. AVMs or telangiectases in 1 or more visceral organs, including the lungs, brain, liver, intestines, stomach, and spinal cord
4. A family history of HHT (ie, a first-degree relative, such as brother, sister, parent, or child, with HHT according to the Curaçao criteria or genetic testing)

Patients who meet at least 3 of the 4 Curaçao criteria are considered to have *definite* HHT, whereas those meeting 2 of the 4 criteria are considered to have *possible* HHT.

A detailed discussion was undertaken with the patient to help him understand treatment options that would improve the epistaxis, severe iron deficiency anemia, and high-output cardiac failure. A protocol for bevacizumab was initiated at a dose of 5 mg/kg intravenously (IV) every 2 weeks for a total of 6 doses. After those 6 doses, maintenance doses were administered once monthly as needed for recurrent bleeding.

On a follow-up visit, the severity of the epistaxis had decreased by more than 90%. The hemoglobin level was normal, and, with initiation of the IV bevacizumab therapy, the patient no longer needed blood transfusions. He was then referred to an interventional radiologist for embolization of his left lower lobe pulmonary AVM (PAVM), which was successfully embolized on a subsequent visit without complications.

Discussion

HHT, also known as Osler-Weber-Rendu disease (2), is an autosomal dominant multisystem vascular disorder with variable penetrance characterized by the presence of telangiectasias on mucocutaneous surfaces and AVMs in visceral organs. The most common complications associated with HHT are spontaneous and recurrent epistaxis and gastrointestinal tract bleeding, which often result in severe iron deficiency anemia. The abnormal shunting of blood across PAVMs can result in hypoxemia and central nervous system (CNS) complications such as brain abscesses and embolic strokes. Primary brain AVMs occur frequently in patients with HHT and carry a risk of spontaneous rupture that can result in catastrophic CNS complications and considerable morbidity and mortality. However, embolic events occurring through undetected or untreated PAVMs are also a major cause of CNS complications among patients with HHT and can manifest as brain abscesses and CNS embolic events. Liver vascular malformations can cause various complications, including high-output cardiac failure, biliary ischemia, and hepatic failure.

The Second International Guidelines for the Diagnosis and Management of Hereditary Hemorrhagic Telangiectasia were recently published. They provide updated diagnostic and management guidelines on several HHT-related topics (3).

HHT-associated sequence variations occur in the *ENG* (HHT1), *ACVRL1* (HHT2), and *SMAD4* genes (1). Among the people who have definite HHT according to the Curaçao criteria, 80% to 90% carry a pathogenic HHT variation in 1 of these 3 genes, but about 10% to 15% of patients have negative test results even though their clinical findings are consistent with HHT. Family members of affected persons should undergo confirmatory genetic testing of the known mutation found in the index case. Appropriate screening tests can then be undertaken for those whose test results are positive for HHT.

Although HHT cannot be cured, the most important manifestations of HHT, including epistaxis, gastrointestinal tract bleeding, and high-output cardiac failure, are all treatable. With therapy, patients can lead normal lives.

Recurrent epistaxis, often the earliest presenting symptom of HHT, can start in early childhood and almost always appears before the age of 40 to 50 years. The severity of epistaxis, which can evolve over time, can range from minor bleeding to life-threatening blood loss resulting in severe anemia and a need for repeated blood transfusions. The *epistaxis severity score* is a valuable tool for tracking epistaxis severity and can help determine whether therapies are appropriate. Although the US Food and Drug Administration has not approved therapies for HHT, several treatment options have shown clinical promise. These include 1) drugs that block blood vessel growth (antiangiogenics), such as IV bevacizumab (4-6), pazopanib (7), and pomalidomide, and 2) drugs that slow the disintegration of clots, such as tranexamic acid (8).

At the time of diagnosis, all patients with HHT should undergo early and systematic screening for HHT-related AVMs at an HHT Center of Excellence. The initial screening tests often include magnetic resonance imaging of the brain, CT of the chest, echocardiography, a complete blood cell count, and iron studies. Not all AVMs require treatment (9). Treatment options for AVMs depend on the size and location of the AVMs and include embolization (for PAVMs), laser ablation (for nasal telangiectasias), and stereotactic radiosurgery (Gamma Knife) or neurosurgical resection for brain AVMs.

Patients with HHT do not have a shortened life expectancy, but their quality of life is affected because of the effects of epistaxis, chronic gastrointestinal tract bleeding, anemia, and symptomatic liver vascular malformations (10). Although HHT is the second most common inherited bleeding disorder in the US, it is often neglected in standardized testing and clinical teaching modules. The result has been low clinical awareness of this entity, which can cause prolonged diagnostic and therapeutic delays for affected patients.

Summary

HHT is an autosomal dominant vascular disorder characterized by epistaxis, mucocutaneous telangiectasias, and visceral AVMs. Spontaneous and recurrent epistaxis is a cardinal symptom of HHT, and its presence should alert the clinician to the possibility of HHT. Antiangiogenic therapies have been very effective for the management of HHT-related epistaxis and gastrointestinal tract bleeding. Patients and their family members with HHT should seek care at an accredited HHT Center of Excellence, where a comprehensive plan for screening diagnostic tests and discussions about therapeutic options can be undertaken without delay.

Answers

49.1. Answer d.

The cardinal manifestations of HHT include spontaneous and recurrent epistaxis; mucocutaneous telangiectasias involving areas such as the lips, tongue, fingertips, oral mucosa, and nose; and visceral AVMs typically involving the lungs, liver, brain, intestinal tract, and occasionally spinal cord. Although these telangiectasias and AVMs result in spontaneous rupture and associated bleeding, coagulopathy itself is not the cause of the bleeding in patients with HHT. Additional information is available in the medical literature (11).

49.2. Answer a.

HHT is an autosomal dominant multisystemic vascular disorder with variable penetrance. The disease is typically caused by genetic sequence variations in 1 of the following 3 genes: *ENG*, *ACVRL1*, and *SMAD4*. Epistaxis, the cardinal manifestation of HHT, typically occurs in early childhood but can be delayed up to the age of 40 or 50 years. Because the disease has a dominant inheritance pattern, in each generation of an affected family, typically at least 1 member has the disease. However, members of the same family and even siblings may have markedly different symptom profiles despite having the same genetic mutation. Additional information is available in the medical literature (1).

49.3. Answer c.

The Curaçao criteria for HHT are used for the diagnosis of HHT in a clinical setting. A clinical diagnosis of *definite* HHT is made if 3 or more of the criteria are met. If 2 of the 4 criteria are met, the diagnosis is *possible* HHT, and if fewer than 2 are met, HHT is *unlikely*. These criteria are the following: 1) recurrent, spontaneous nosebleeds (epistaxis) or recurrent bleeding from other sites, which may be mild to severe; 2) multiple telangiectases on the skin of the hands, lips, or face or inside the nose or mouth (telangiectases are small vascular lesions that blanch under direct pressure); 3) AVMs or telangiectases in 1 or more internal organs, including the lungs, brain, liver, intestines, stomach, and spinal cord; and 4) a family history of HHT (ie, first-degree relative such as brother, sister, parent, or child who meets these same criteria for definite HHT or has received a diagnosis after genetic testing). Although patients with HHT may have high-output cardiac failure due to diffuse liver vascular malformations, acute coronary syndromes are not a presenting or diagnostic feature of HHT. Additional information is available in the medical literature (11).

49.4. Answer d.

Aspirin and other NSAIDs typically worsen HHT-related epistaxis and gastrointestinal tract bleeding. The other treatments listed are effective for the management of HHT-related vascular complications, such as epistaxis (nasal lubricating solutions), and for gastrointestinal tract bleeding and epistaxis (tranexamic acid). Systemic antiangiogenic agents, such as bevacizumab, a vascular endothelial growth factor inhibitor, have been remarkably effective in the treatment of severe HHT-related bleeding and iron deficiency anemia. IV bevacizumab results in significantly increased hemoglobin levels, a marked decrease in the degree of epistaxis and gastrointestinal tract bleeding, and significantly improved quality of life. IV bevacizumab has also been helpful in patients with high-output cardiac failure from symptomatic liver vascular malformations. Pazopanib, a tyrosine kinase inhibitor, has also been shown to have significant beneficial effects in HHT-related bleeding. Additional information is available in the medical literature (12).

49.5. Answer e.

Common complications of HHT include anemia (from epistaxis and gastrointestinal tract bleeding), hypoxemia (from shunting through PAVMs), brain abscesses and stroke (from embolic events through PAVMs), and high-output cardiac failure (from liver AVMs creating a direct connection between the hepatic arteries and hepatic veins). Although pancreatic AVMs can be found on screening tests, pancreatitis is not a complication associated with HHT. Additional information is available in the medical literature (10).

References

1. Kritharis A, Al-Samkari H, Kuter DJ. Hereditary hemorrhagic telangiectasia: diagnosis and management from the hematologist's perspective. Haematologica. 2018;103(9):1433–43.
2. Kuhnel T, Wirsching K, Wohlgemuth W, Chavan A, Evert K, Vielsmeier V. Hereditary hemorrhagic telangiectasia. Otolaryngol Clin North Am. 2018; 51(1):237–54.
3. Faughnan ME, Mager JJ, Hetts SW, Palda VA, Lang-Robertson K, Buscarini E, et al. Second International Guidelines for the diagnosis and management of hereditary hemorrhagic telangiectasia. Ann Intern Med. 2020;173(12):989–1001.
4. Robert F, Desroches-Castan A, Bailly S, Dupuis-Girod S, Feige JJ. Future treatments for hereditary hemorrhagic telangiectasia. Orphanet J Rare Dis. 2020;15(1):4.
5. Al-Samkari H, Kasthuri RS, Parambil JG, Albitar HA, Almodallal YA, Vazquez C, et al. An international, multicenter study of intravenous bevacizumab for bleeding in hereditary hemorrhagic telangiectasia: the InHIBIT-Bleed study. Haematologica. 2021; 106(8):2161–9.
6. Iyer VN, Apala DR, Pannu BS, Kotecha A, Brinjikji W, Leise MD, et al. Intravenous bevacizumab for refractory hereditary hemorrhagic telangiectasia-related epistaxis and gastrointestinal bleeding. Mayo Clin Proc. 2018;93(2):155–66.
7. Faughnan ME, Gossage JR, Chakinala MM, Oh SP, Kasthuri R, Hughes CCW, et al. Pazopanib may reduce bleeding in hereditary hemorrhagic telangiectasia. Angiogenesis. 2019;22(1):145–55.
8. Geisthoff UW, Seyfert UT, Kubler M, Bieg B, Plinkert PK, Konig J. Treatment of epistaxis in hereditary hemorrhagic telangiectasia with tranexamic acid - a double-blind placebo-controlled cross-over phase IIIB study. Thromb Res. 2014;134(3):565–71.
9. Brinjikji W, Iyer VN, Wood CP, Lanzino G. Prevalence and characteristics of brain arteriovenous malformations in hereditary hemorrhagic telangiectasia: a systematic review and meta-analysis. J Neurosurg. 2017;127(2):302–10.
10. Thompson KP, Nelson J, Kim H, Pawlikowska L, Marchuk DA, Lawton MT, et al. Predictors of mortality in patients with hereditary hemorrhagic telangiectasia. Orphanet J Rare Dis. 2021;16(1):12.
11. Shovlin CL, Guttmacher AE, Buscarini E, Faughnan ME, Hyland RH, Westermann CJ, et al. Diagnostic criteria for hereditary hemorrhagic telangiectasia (Rendu-Osler-Weber syndrome). Am J Med Genet. 2000;91(1):66–7.
12. Hammill AM, Wusik K, Kasthuri RS. Hereditary hemorrhagic telangiectasia (HHT): a practical guide to management. Hematology Am Soc Hematol Educ Program. 2021;2021(1):469–77.

A 68-Year-Old Woman With Dyspnea and Pleuritic Chest Pain[a]

Phillip J. Gary, MD, and Yewande E. Odeyemi, MBBS

Case Presentation

A 68-year-old woman presented to the emergency department with shortness of breath on exertion, which began several days before. On the morning of presentation, she awoke with severe shortness of breath, sharp pleuritic chest pain, and light-headedness. She did not have associated leg swelling or leg discomfort. She described an increasingly sedentary lifestyle over the previous several months, which did not include travel or surgery. She did not take any hormonal supplementation. She did not have a personal history of venous thromboembolism or malignancy. Her medical history included hypertension with a baseline systolic blood pressure near 140 mm Hg and hyperlipidemia. Relevant family history included coronary artery disease and cancer in her father and no family history of venous thromboembolism. She was retired, she had never smoked, and she drank 2 or 3 alcoholic drinks per evening.

Her vital signs were as follows: sinus tachycardia (112 beats/min); blood pressure, 99/83 mm Hg; respiratory rate, 22 breaths/min; and oxygen saturation as measured by pulse oximetry, 93% while breathing room air. She appeared acutely ill and in moderate respiratory distress. On cardiac examination she had sinus tachycardia without murmurs or rubs. She did not have jugular venous distention, her lungs were clear on auscultation, and she did not have reproducible chest wall tenderness. Her abdomen was distended but not tender, and bowel sounds were normal. Her extremities appeared normal and symmetric without edema or tenderness, but her skin was mottled.

Laboratory test results included the following: white blood cell count, 19.9×10^9/L; hemoglobin, 15.0 g/dL; platelets, 336×10^9/L; creatinine, 0.75 mg/dL; total bilirubin, 0.4 mg/dL; alanine aminotransferase, 92 U/L; aspartate aminotransferase, 108 U/L; troponin T, 150 ng/L; N-terminal pro–brain natriuretic peptide (NT-proBNP), 144 pg/mL; lactate, 3.1 mmol/L; and D-dimer, 3,073 ng/mL. Electrocardiography showed sinus tachycardia (112 beats/min), right bundle-branch block, an $S_1Q_3T_3$ pattern, T-wave inversions in leads III and aVF, and ST-depression in leads V_4 through V_6. Results from chest radiography were unremarkable. Computed tomographic (CT) angiography of the chest showed bilateral segmental and subsegmental pulmonary embolism (PE) with an occlusive thrombus in the left main pulmonary artery, leftward deviation of the interventricular septum, a right ventricle (RV) to left ventricle ratio greater than 1.0, and reflux of contrast material into the inferior vena cava (IVC). Bedside ultrasonography showed a severely enlarged RV with decreased systolic function and RV free wall hypokinesis with apical sparing. These findings were confirmed with formal transthoracic echocardiography, which showed estimated cardiac index, 1.52 L/min/m^2; RV systolic pressure, 48 mm Hg; moderate to severe tricuspid valve regurgitation; and enlarged inferior vena cava with no inspiratory collapse.

---

[a] Virtual poster at the 7th Annual Pulmonary Embolism Symposium, October 15-16, 2021.

Questions

Multiple Choice (choose the best answer)

50.1. According to American Heart Association (AHA) guidelines, how should one classify this patient's PE?
   a. Subsegmental PE
   b. Low-risk PE
   c. Submassive PE without RV strain
   d. Submassive PE with RV strain
   e. Massive PE

50.2. In which clinical scenario is testing for inherited thrombophilia *not* warranted?
   a. PE develops in a 65-year-old patient who is undergoing active therapy for cancer
   b. PE and portal vein thrombosis develop in a 65-year-old patient
   c. PE develops in a 30-year-old patient whose mother had deep vein thrombosis (DVT) at age 40 years
   d. DVT develops in a 40-year-old patient who has had a recent transient ischemic attack
   e. Recurrent DVT occurs in a 40-year-old patient who has a history of warfarin-induced skin necrosis

50.3. Which patients should have an inferior vena cava (IVC) filter placed?

   a. Patients who have PE and a contraindication to anticoagulation or a prolonged interruption in anticoagulation
   b. Patients who present with PE and concomitant DVT
   c. Patients who have PE and a high risk for decompensation
   d. Patients who have PE and cancer
   e. All patients who have PE or DVT

50.4. If a patient has massive PE and no contraindication to thrombolysis, what dose of alteplase should be administered?
   a. 10 mg over 15 minutes
   b. 100 mg over 2 hours or 0.6 mg/kg over 15 minutes (maximum, 50 mg)
   c. Continuous infusion of 10 mg/h until the patient shows clinical improvement
   d. 75 mg over 1 hour
   e. 100 mg over 2 minutes

50.5. *Post-PE syndrome* is defined as persistent dyspnea, exercise limitation, and impaired quality of life that persist longer than how many months after therapeutic anticoagulation?
   a. 1
   b. 2
   c. 3
   d. 4
   e. 6

Case Follow-up and Outcome

The patient's description of vague abdominal pain prompted CT of the abdomen and pelvis with an intravenous contrast agent, which showed moderate-volume ascites. Ultrasonography of the abdomen showed nonocclusive portal vein thrombosis. Lower extremity venous ultrasonography showed acute DVT in the right common femoral vein. The patient's systolic blood pressure remained above 90 mm Hg, but this was a decrease of nearly 50 mm Hg from baseline, and the patient had evidence of hypoperfusion, including cool and mottled extremities, lactic acidosis, elevated transaminase values, and a decreased cardiac index (1.52 L/min/m^2). After she was treated with 50 mg intravenous alteplase, her hemodynamic status improved. Owing to the unclear cause of the newly discovered ascites, paracentesis was performed. Cytology of the ascitic fluid was consistent with metastatic adenocarcinoma, and immunohistochemical markers supported an ovarian primary origin. After the patient's treatment was transitioned to therapeutic enoxaparin, she underwent therapy for metastatic ovarian cancer.

Discussion

Risk stratification of patients presenting with acute PE is important because of the associated mortality of those with high-risk presentations who need more intensive monitoring and treatment. For patients with PE classified as *massive* (AHA) or *high-risk* (American College of Chest Physicians [ACCP] and European Society of Cardiology [ESC]), 30-day mortality is estimated to be 30% to 60% (1-3). For patients with PE classified as *submassive* (AHA) or *intermediate-risk* (ACCP and ESC), 30-day mortality may be as high as 14% (3,4).

For all patients presenting with massive or high-risk PE, intravenous tissue plasminogen activator (tPA) should be administered promptly unless the patient has a contraindication (5-7). After thrombolysis, parenteral anticoagulation should be resumed with a transition to long-term therapy, the duration of which depends on various factors that are beyond the scope of this discussion. If the patient has a contraindication to systemic thrombolysis or anticoagulation, consideration should be given to emergent management that uses a multidisciplinary approach with a catheter-directed or surgical approach to thromboembolectomy (depending on the availability and expertise at the institution). The degree of the patient's hemodynamic instability may also require vasopressor or inotropic support, pulmonary vasodilators, mechanical circulatory support, or extracorporeal membrane oxygenation. The use of endotracheal intubation requires caution because of the serious risk of hemodynamic collapse due to RV failure.

Current guidelines are not definitive for the management of submassive or intermediate-risk PE. Although many patients have a response to therapeutic anticoagulation alone, a subgroup has a higher risk for decompensation and death and, after consideration is given to the bleeding risk, will benefit from thrombolysis. Data are limited, though, for long-term outcomes of patients with post-PE syndrome, chronic thromboembolic pulmonary hypertension (CTEPH), or chronic thromboembolic disease (CTED) (8,9). Therefore, for each patient various clinical factors should be considered (eg, presence of tachycardia or profound bradycardia; oxygen requirements; levels of troponin, NT-proBNP, BNP, and lactate; and various echocardiographic and CT parameters) and the PE severity index (PESI) or simplified PESI should be calculated (10,11).

The acute condition of these patients presents challenges in decisions. However, the formation of multidisciplinary PE response teams has improved mortality and access to more advanced therapies without a change in major bleeding (12,13).

Summary

Patients presenting with acute PE require immediate risk stratification to determine the need for more intensive monitoring and consideration of additional therapies besides only anticoagulation. Thorough investigation can help stratify seemingly borderline cases, which, at some institutions, may be arbitrated by multidisciplinary teams. In most cases, testing for inherited thrombophilias is not warranted in the acute setting, and the use of IVC filters should be avoided unless the patient has a contraindication to anticoagulation. Many patients with symptomatic acute PE have persistent dyspnea and exercise limitations that often warrant further testing to rule out CTEPH or CTED.

Answers

50.1. Answer e.

AHA guidelines categorize PE according to various hemodynamic, biomarker, and imaging parameters. Patients have *massive PE* if their systolic blood pressure is less than 90 mm Hg for 15 minutes, if their systolic blood pressure is 40 mm Hg below baseline, if they require inotropic or vasopressor support, or if they have profound bradycardia or evidence of shock. *Subsegmental PE* is distinguished from *submassive PE* radiographically by the presence of a thrombus only in a subsegmental pulmonary artery branch. Subsegmental PE, described in the ACCP guidelines as *low-risk PE*, is typically diagnosed incidentally, and the patients often do not require anticoagulation. Patients who do not meet the above criteria are considered to have submassive PE with or without evidence of RV strain. RV strain is determined according to cardiac biomarkers (including troponin, NT-proBNP, and BNP levels), electrocardiography, echocardiography, and CT. Additional information is available in the medical literature (7).

50.2. Answer a.

For most patients with acute venous thromboembolism, thrombophilia testing is not recommended at the time of diagnosis, regardless of the presence of provoking factors, and has not been shown to affect outcomes. Acute thrombus and treatment with anticoagulation can confound results, lead to false-positive or false-negative results, and cause unnecessary harm and cost. If a patient has thrombosis in an atypical site, such as the portal venous system or arterial system, testing for antiphospholipid antibodies may be indicated with careful consideration as to whether testing will affect short- or long-term management. Testing is warranted for young patients, particularly those with a personal or family history that suggests inherited thrombophilia. In those rare instances when thrombophilia testing is warranted, testing should be delayed until after at least 3 months of anticoagulation and should be performed during a period when anticoagulation has been held. Additional information is available in the medical literature (14,15).

50.3. Answer a.

Placement of an IVC filter should be considered for patients who are deemed to have an ongoing risk for venous thromboembolism and a contraindication to anticoagulation or who require a prolonged interruption in anticoagulation. Data do not support the routine placement of IVC filters in patients who have PE and concomitant DVT or other clinical features that are concerning for decompensation. Patients with malignancy, depending on the site of the malignancy, may have an increased risk for bleeding, but routine placement of an IVC filter should be avoided. Regardless of a patient's risk category, IVC filters should not be routinely placed in patients who present with venous thromboembolism. Structured follow-up and frequent reevaluation of the need for an IVC filter are recommended because of the risk of complication and retrievable nature of modern IVC filters. Additional information is available in the medical literature (16).

50.4. Answer b.

Guidelines recommend dosing intravenous tPA according to the clinical scenario. With consideration of the risks and benefits, the ideal dose of alteplase is likely 25 to 100 mg (depending on the duration of the infusion). Current guidelines recommend dosing alteplase at either 100 mg over 2 hours or 0.6 mg/kg over 15 minutes. Higher doses and simultaneous heparin infusion are associated with an increased risk of major bleeding, including intracranial hemorrhage. Ultimately, tPA dosing should be decided on a case-by-case basis. Additional information is available in the medical literature (6,17,18).

50.5. Answer c.

Many patients with acute PE have shortness of breath and exercise limitation that persist beyond 3 months after initial presentation. On follow-up, CTEPH and CTED should be ruled out in symptomatic patients because either disease could affect management, so evaluation should include 1 or more of the following: transthoracic echocardiography, lung ventilation-perfusion scan, or pulmonary catheterization. Additional testing for other causes contributing to dyspnea may be warranted, and some patients may require cardiopulmonary exercise testing. Further study is needed to better understand what appears to be a spectrum of disease that contributes to symptoms in many patients after acute PE despite adequate treatment. Additional information is available in the medical literature (19,20).

References

1. Goldhaber SZ, Visani L, De Rosa M. Acute pulmonary embolism: clinical outcomes in the International Cooperative Pulmonary Embolism Registry (ICOPER). Lancet. 1999;353(9162):1386–9.
2. Kucher N, Rossi E, De Rosa M, Goldhaber SZ. Massive pulmonary embolism. Circulation. 2006; 113(4):577–82.
3. Laporte S, Mismetti P, Decousus H, Uresandi F, Otero R, Lobo JL, et al. Clinical predictors for fatal pulmonary embolism in 15,520 patients with venous thromboembolism: findings from the Registro Informatizado de la Enfermedad TromboEmbolica venosa (RIETE) Registry. Circulation. 2008;117(13):1711–6.
4. Rali PM, Criner GJ. Submassive pulmonary embolism. Am J Respir Crit Care Med. 2018;198(5):588–98.
5. Kearon C, Akl EA, Ornelas J, Blaivas A, Jimenez D, Bounameaux H, et al. Antithrombotic therapy for VTE disease: CHEST Guideline and Expert Panel Report. Chest. 2016;149(2):315–52.
6. Konstantinides SV, Meyer G, Becattini C, Bueno H, Geersing GJ, Harjola VP, et al. 2019 ESC Guidelines for the diagnosis and management of acute pulmonary embolism developed in collaboration with the European Respiratory Society (ERS). Eur Heart J. 2020;41(4):543–603.
7. Jaff MR, McMurtry MS, Archer SL, Cushman M, Goldenberg N, Goldhaber SZ, et al. Management of massive and submassive pulmonary embolism, iliofemoral deep vein thrombosis, and chronic thromboembolic pulmonary hypertension: a scientific statement from the American Heart Association. Circulation. 2011;123(16):1788–830.
8. Meyer G, Vicaut E, Danays T, Agnelli G, Becattini C, Beyer-Westendorf J, et al. Fibrinolysis for patients with intermediate-risk pulmonary embolism. N Engl J Med. 2014;370(15):1402–11.
9. Konstantinides SV, Vicaut E, Danays T, Becattini C, Bertoletti L, Beyer-Westendorf J, et al. Impact of thrombolytic therapy on the long-term outcome of intermediate-risk pulmonary embolism. J Am Coll Cardiol. 2017;69(12):1536–44.
10. Vanni S, Viviani G, Baioni M, Pepe G, Nazerian P, Socci F, et al. Prognostic value of plasma lactate levels among patients with acute pulmonary embolism: the thrombo-embolism lactate outcome study. Ann Emerg Med. 2013;61(3):330–8.
11. Reardon PM, Yadav K, Hendin A, Karovitch A, Hickey M. Contemporary management of the high-risk pulmonary embolism: the clot thickens. J Intensive Care Med. 2019;34(8):603–8.
12. Chaudhury P, Gadre SK, Schneider E, Renapurkar RD, Gomes M, Haddadin I, et al. Impact of multidisciplinary pulmonary embolism response team availability on management and outcomes. Am J Cardiol. 2019;124(9):1465–9.
13. Rosovsky R, Chang Y, Rosenfield K, Channick R, Jaff MR, Weinberg I, et al. Changes in treatment and outcomes after creation of a pulmonary embolism response team (PERT), a 10-year analysis. J Thromb Thrombolysis. 2019;47(1):31–40.
14. Christiansen SC, Cannegieter SC, Koster T, Vandenbroucke JP, Rosendaal FR. Thrombophilia, clinical factors, and recurrent venous thrombotic events. JAMA. 2005;293(19):2352–61.
15. Stevens SM, Woller SC, Bauer KA, Kasthuri R, Cushman M, Streiff M, et al. Guidance for the evaluation and treatment of hereditary and acquired thrombophilia. J Thromb Thrombolysis. 2016;41(1): 154–64.
16. Kaufman JA, Barnes GD, Chaer RA, Cuschieri J, Eberhardt RT, Johnson MS, et al. Society of Interventional Radiology Clinical Practice Guideline for Inferior Vena Cava Filters in the Treatment of Patients with Venous Thromboembolic Disease: Developed in collaboration with the American College of Cardiology, American College of Chest Physicians, American College of Surgeons Committee on Trauma, American Heart Association, Society for Vascular Surgery, and Society for Vascular Medicine. J Vasc Interv Radiol. 2020;31(10):1529–44.
17. Wang C, Zhai Z, Yang Y, Wu Q, Cheng Z, Liang L, et al. Efficacy and safety of low dose recombinant tissue-type plasminogen activator for the treatment of acute pulmonary thromboembolism: a randomized, multicenter, controlled trial. Chest. 2010;137(2):254–62.
18. Sharifi M, Bay C, Skrocki L, Rahimi F, Mehdipour M, Investigators M. Moderate pulmonary embolism treated with thrombolysis (from the "MOPETT" Trial). Am J Cardiol. 2013;111(2):273–7.
19. Pugliese SC, Kawut SM. The post-pulmonary embolism syndrome: real or ruse? Ann Am Thorac Soc. 2019;16(7):811–4.
20. Klok FA, van der Hulle T, den Exter PL, Lankeit M, Huisman MV, Konstantinides S. The post-PE syndrome: a new concept for chronic complications of pulmonary embolism. Blood Rev. 2014;28(6):221–6.

A 71-Year-Old Man With Dyspnea and Hypoxemia

51

Gregory R. Stroh, MD, and Hilary M. DuBrock, MD

Case Presentation

A 71-year-old man was referred for evaluation of a 10-year history of dyspnea and chronic hypoxic respiratory failure without cough, wheezing, sputum production, orthopnea, or lower extremity edema. He described having platypnea and did not use recommended supplemental oxygen. At a prior evaluation he had normal results on spirometry and a patent foramen ovale (PFO) with a right-to-left shunt. The PFO was closed 6 months before the current presentation; afterward he had partial symptomatic improvement and less need for supplemental oxygen.

His medical history included obstructive sleep apnea (treated with continuous positive airway pressure), monoclonal gammopathy of undetermined significance, erythrocytosis (treated with phlebotomy), stroke, multiple skin cancers, and PFO (now closed). He was a retired farmer with a remote smoking history of fewer than 10 pack-years. He rarely consumed alcohol and had no other occupational or environmental exposures. He had no family history of pulmonary parenchymal disease, vascular disease, venous thromboemboli, autoimmune disease, or hereditary hemorrhagic telangiectasia.

On physical examination he was thin and appeared chronically ill, but he was not in distress. His oxygen saturation was 76% while breathing room air. On auscultation his lungs were clear bilaterally. The jugular venous pressure was normal,

and he had no lower extremity edema. On cardiac auscultation he had a regular heart rate and rhythm without murmurs. His abdomen was soft without hepatosplenomegaly. He had telangiectases on his face, anterior chest, hands, and arms.

Chest radiography did not show any consolidation, pulmonary edema, cardiomegaly, or right atrial enlargement. Pulmonary function testing demonstrated borderline obstruction: Forced expiratory volume in the first second of expiration (FEV_1)/forced vital capacity was 60.9; FEV_1 was 3.55 L (115% of the predicted value); and the diffusing capacity of lung for carbon monoxide ($DLCO$) was 42% of the predicted value after correction for hemoglobin. Computed tomography (CT) of the chest did not show any evidence of pulmonary parenchymal disease, pulmonary emboli, pulmonary arteriovenous malformations (PAVMs), or adenopathy.

He had normal laboratory test results for a complete blood cell count, complete metabolic profile, and autoimmune serology cascade. The presence of a monoclonal immunoglobulin G-λ M-spike was similar to results 2 years earlier. The level of N-terminal pro–brain natriuretic peptide was mildly elevated (174 pg/mL; reference range ≤103 pg/mL). With the patient breathing room air, arterial blood gas results were pH 7.44, $PaCO_2$ 27.8 mm Hg, and PaO_2 49 mm Hg. With the patient breathing 100% oxygen, arterial blood gas results were pH 7.38, $PaCO_2$ 34 mm Hg, and PaO_2 193 mm Hg.

Questions

Multiple Choice (choose the best answer)

51.1. What is the most likely mechanism of the patient's hypoxia?
a. Right-to-left shunting
b. Chronic obstructive pulmonary disease (COPD)
c. Obesity-hypoventilation syndrome
d. Pulmonary embolism
e. Ventilation-perfusion ($\dot{V}$/Q) mismatch

51.2. Which test would be most appropriate to perform next?
a. Stress echocardiography
b. Coronary angiography
c. Measurement of exhaled nitric oxide
d. Peripheral smear
e. Echocardiography with a contrast agent (bubble study)

51.3. What study should be performed to differentiate intracardiac shunting from intrapulmonary shunting?
a. Transesophageal echocardiography (TEE)
b. Arterial blood gas testing at rest and with exercise
c. Technetium-labeled macroaggregated albumin lung perfusion scan
d. Cardiac magnetic resonance imaging
e. Positron emission tomographic CT scan

51.4. Which of the following conditions is *not* associated with intrapulmonary shunting?
a. Hepatopulmonary syndrome
b. Hereditary hemorrhagic telangiectasia (HHT)
c. TEMPI syndrome (telangiectasias, erythrocytosis with elevated erythropoietin, monoclonal gammopathy, perinephric fluid collections, and intrapulmonary shunting)
d. Eisenmenger syndrome
e. Schistosomiasis

51.5. Why did this patient's symptoms improve partially after PFO closure?
a. Reduced right ventricular preload
b. Increased left ventricular preload
c. Reduction in total shunt fraction
d. Reduced left ventricular afterload
e. Improved alveolar gas exchange

Case Follow-up and Outcome

A transthoracic echocardiogram showed normal left and right ventricular size and function, an estimated right ventricular systolic pressure of 37 mm Hg, a small left-to-right shunt across the atria, and a small intrapulmonary shunt. On TEE, saline contrast medium entered the left side of the heart from all 4 pulmonary veins without intracardiac shunting at rest or with the Valsalva maneuver. The patient underwent abdominal ultrasonography, which was negative for signs of cirrhosis or portal hypertension. Erythropoietin levels were elevated (262 mIU/mL; reference range, 2.6-18.5 mIU/mL). Pulmonary angiography showed dilated pulmonary vasculature, but no PAVMs were identified.

The constellation of telangiectases, erythrocytosis, monoclonal gammopathy, and intrapulmonary shunting prompted consideration of TEMPI syndrome as an underlying cause of the patient's presentation. This syndrome is a rare plasma cell dyscrasia that causes a multisystem paraneoplastic syndrome with the manifestations listed above.

The patient was referred to a hematologist who confirmed the diagnosis, and therapy was initiated with daratumumab (an anti-CD38 monoclonal antibody typically used to treat multiple myeloma). At follow-up he had symptomatic improvement, decreased oxygen needs, and smaller and fewer telangiectases.

Discussion

This patient presented with hypoxia from an unclear cause that was ultimately determined to be a rare disease. The case demonstrates the need for a systematic approach in the evaluation of patients with hypoxia in order to classify the predominant cause and then make a final diagnosis. This process requires a thorough understanding of the different categories of hypoxia. These categories (excluding low barometric pressure and low inspired oxygen) include shunt, $\dot{V}/\dot{Q}$ mismatch, diffusion impairment, and hypoventilation.

A shunt occurs when deoxygenated blood moves from the systemic venous or pulmonary arterial circulation to the systemic arterial circulation without being oxygenated in the lungs. If the shunt is sufficiently large, the mixing of oxygenated and deoxygenated blood results in a lower total arterial oxygen content and hypoxemia. Intrapulmonary shunts are classically related to anatomical vascular abnormalities; however, some conditions with extreme $\dot{V}/\dot{Q}$ mismatch, such as acute respiratory distress syndrome, alveolar hemorrhage, airway obstruction, and pneumonia, may have the same physiologic effect as a shunt.

Anatomical right-to-left shunting can occur by numerous pathways, such as when blood travels across a cardiac septum (intracardiac shunts) or through PAVMs without capillary beds at the alveolar level (intrapulmonary shunts). Intracardiac shunts require, at least transiently, elevated pressures in the pulmonary arteries or in the right-sided cardiac chambers (or in both) to overcome the higher pressures of the left atrium or left ventricle.

The most common cause of an anatomical intrapulmonary shunt secondary to PAVMs is HHT, although PAVMs are often idiopathic (1). Hepatopulmonary syndrome (HPS) is another important cause of intrapulmonary shunting. HPS is characterized by the clinical triad of hypoxemia, intrapulmonary vasodilatation, and advanced liver disease. This condition results in pulmonary capillary and precapillary dilatation that impairs oxygen diffusion across the alveolus to the red blood cells. Although true PAVMs develop in some patients with HPS, those PAVMs are less common and are not a major contributor to hypoxemia in most patients (2,3).

Several findings suggested that a shunt was the primary cause of this patient's hypoxia. These included the unremarkable results on pulmonary imaging and pulmonary function testing, the normal cardiopulmonary examination findings, the presence of platypnea, and an inappropriate increase in the Pao_2 while the patient was breathing 100% oxygen.

An inappropriate response to supplemental oxygen is an important clue that suggests shunting is the mechanism for hypoxemia because the shunted blood is not exposed to the increased oxygen levels in the alveoli. This is because under normal conditions the transfer of oxygen from the alveoli to the blood is limited by perfusion (not diffusion), so the hemoglobin molecules within the red blood cells are fully bound with oxygen and the Pao_2 in the arterial blood is at equilibrium with the alveoli early in the passage across the capillary-alveolus interface (4). With high levels of supplemental oxygen, the alveolar partial pressure of oxygen (Pao_2) will be high and result in a higher Pao_2; however, this cannot overcome a shunt because Pao_2 is only a small component of the oxygen carrying capacity of the blood (Box 51.1), and the delivery of oxygen is primarily dependent on the oxygen bound to hemoglobin. The appropriateness of a patient's response to supplemental oxygen can be calculated with the alveolar gas equation and the alveolar-arterial gradient (Box 51.1) (5-7). Although an abnormal alveolar-arterial gradient in isolation can be present in other forms of hypoxemia, it should respond appropriately to supplemental oxygen.

Platypnea (shortness of breath that is worsened by sitting upright) is another important clue that a shunt may be present. Platypnea is often accompanied by *orthodeoxia* (worsening oxygenation in the upright position) (8) and is classically associated with hepatopulmonary syndrome (a complication of advanced liver disease), although it has also been reported to occur in patients with basally predominant interstitial lung disease (9,10). This phenomenon results from gravity-dependent increases in blood flow to the lower lobes of the lungs (where most intrapulmonary vasodilatation [in hepatopulmonary syndrome] or parenchymal abnormalities [in interstitial lung disease] are present) and is compounded by decreased ventilation in the lower lobes in the upright position, which results in worsening $\dot{V}/Q$ mismatch (8).

When a shunt is suspected, an important first test is transthoracic echocardiography performed with a bubble study (ie, with an injection of agitated saline). In addition to providing valuable information on the structure and function of the heart, visualization of bubbles appearing in the left atrium indicates the presence of a shunt because the lung capillaries normally filter out the microbubbles. In general, bubbles seen in the

---

Box 51.1

Oxygen Carrying Capacity of Blood and Response to Supplemental Oxygen

The *oxygen carrying capacity of blood* is calculated as follows:

Oxygen Carrying Capacity = $(1.39 \times$ [Hemoglobin] $\times Spo_2) + (Pao_2 \times 0.003)$,

where Spo_2 is the oxygen saturation as measured by pulse oximetry.

A patient's response to supplemental oxygen is measured with the following *alveolar gas equation*:

$Pao_2 = [Fio_2 \times (Patm - PH_2O)] - Paco_2/RQ$,

where Fio_2 is the fraction of inspired oxygen; Patm, atmospheric pressure; PH_2O, partial pressure of water; and RQ, respiratory quotient.

For example, consider a patient with the following results: Patm, 747 mm Hg; Fio_2, 1.0; $Paco_2$, 40 mm Hg; PH_2O, 47 mm Hg; and RQ, 0.8. The Pao_2 should normally be about 650 mm Hg, and the Pao_2 should be near 620 mm Hg. This patient's Pao_2 was 129 mm Hg, which represents an alveolar-arterial gradient of 534 (expected gradient, 22).

left ventricle within 1 to 3 cardiac cycles (or seen crossing the cardiac septum) indicate the presence of an intracardiac shunt, whereas bubbles seen at least 3 beats after injection of agitated saline indicate an intrapulmonary shunt (11). The degree of shunting can be quantified from the volume of bubbles in the left ventricle.

The use of contrast-enhanced echocardiography to differentiate an intracardiac shunt from an intrapulmonary shunt, in addition to quantifying the degree of the shunt, provides advantages over other tests that identify only the presence of a shunt or the degree of shunting (eg, shunt fraction calculation and albumin-labeled technetium Tc 99m radionucleotide scan). In some patients, differentiation of intracardiac and intrapulmonary shunting with transthoracic echocardiography is challenging, and TEE can help in better visualizing the source of microbubbles appearing in the left atrium.

After an intrapulmonary shunt is identified, CT of the chest with contrast should be performed to evaluate for PAVMs that could be embolized. PAVM embolization should be performed if feasible, even in asymptomatic patients, to prevent devastating complications, such as brain abscesses and strokes. Also, patients should be evaluated for an underlying cause of a PAVM, such as HHT.

The differential diagnosis is limited when a patient has intrapulmonary shunting in the absence of a PAVM, HHT, or liver disease, as in this patient. If a patient with pulmonary shunts from an unclear cause has erythrocytosis and monoclonal gammopathy, a diagnosis of TEMPI syndrome should be considered. TEMPI syndrome is a rare, newly recognized syndrome with specific clinical manifestations, including intrapulmonary shunting (12,13). Although this disorder is poorly understood, it can be treated with agents that are also used to treat multiple myeloma, such as daratumumab and bortezomib; autologous stem cell transplant has also been performed (14-18).

Summary

Hypoxemia is a common clinical issue that occasionally presents a diagnostic challenge to clinicians. An understanding of the underlying mechanisms of hypoxemia is essential to appropriately and effectively evaluate patients. When a patient has a rare underlying disease, an understanding of the mechanism of hypoxemia can assist with the diagnostic approach.

Answers

51.1. Answer a.

The presence of a right-to-left shunt is suggested by the patient's resting hypoxia in the absence of pulmonary parenchymal disease and the inappropriate increase in Pao_2 in response to 100% oxygen. Although the patient had mild obstruction on pulmonary function testing and a reduced DLCO, the lack of radiographic evidence of emphysema with a disproportionately low DLCO makes COPD an unlikely cause of the hypoxemia. He was not obese or hypercapnic, so obesity-hypoventilation syndrome is unlikely. Pulmonary embolism and other forms of $\dot{V}/Q$ mismatch could be considered, but they would not be expected to cause an inappropriate response to 100% oxygen. Additional information is available in the medical literature (19).

51.2. Answer e.

The most appropriate study to perform next would be echocardiography with a bubble study. Stress echocardiography and coronary angiography are more appropriate for investigating dyspnea related to cardiac ischemia and would not provide information on shunting. Exhaled nitric oxide levels are helpful when a patient has asthma or an asthmalike pulmonary condition, but neither condition was suggested by this patient's presentation. A peripheral smear would not be helpful on the basis of the patient's clinical presentation.

Additional information is available in the medical literature (4).

51.3. Answer a.

TEE is the most appropriate study to differentiate intrapulmonary shunting from intracardiac shunting. A lung perfusion scan can be used to quantify the severity of shunting but not to differentiate intracardiac from intrapulmonary shunting. The other studies do not assist in determining the relative contributions of an intracardiac shunt or an intrapulmonary shunt. Additional information is available in the medical literature (20).

51.4. Answer d.

Eisenmenger syndrome is a form of intracardiac shunting that results from severe pulmonary hypertension related to a congenital cardiac anomaly. All the other conditions cause intrapulmonary shunts. Additional information is available in the medical literature (21).

51.5. Answer c.

Before the PFO was closed, both intrapulmonary and intracardiac shunting were present. When the intracardiac shunt was closed, the total shunt fraction decreased. The impact on the afterload and preload of the ventricles would not greatly affect his symptoms, and increased preload is not necessarily beneficial. PFO closure would not affect alveolar gas exchange. Additional information is available in the medical literature (22).

References

1. Shovlin CL. Pulmonary arteriovenous malformations. Am J Respir Crit Care Med. 2014 Dec 1;190(11):1217–28.
2. Rodríguez-Roisin R, Krowka MJ. Hepatopulmonary syndrome: a liver-induced lung vascular disorder. N Engl J Med. 2008 May 29;358(22):2378–87.
3. Berthelot P, Walker JG, Sherlock S, Reid L. Arterial changes in the lungs in cirrhosis of the liver: lung spider nevi. N Engl J Med. 1966 Feb 10;274(6):291–8.
4. Wagner PD, West JB. Effects of diffusion impairment on O_2 and CO_2 time courses in pulmonary capillaries. J Appl Physiol. 1972 Jul;33(1):62–71.
5. Fenn WO, Rahn H, Otis AB. A theoretical study of the composition of the alveolar air at altitude. Am J Physiol. 1946 Aug;146:637–53.
6. Curran-Everett D. A classic learning opportunity from Fenn, Rahn, and Otis (1946): the alveolar gas equation. Adv Physiol Educ. 2006 Jun;30(2):58–62.
7. Mellemgaard K. The alveolar-arterial oxygen difference: its size and components in normal man. Acta Physiol Scand. 1966 May;67(1):10–20.
8. De Vecchis R, Baldi C, Ariano C. Platypnea-orthodeoxia syndrome: multiple pathophysiological interpretations of a clinical picture primarily consisting of orthostatic dyspnea. J Clin Med. 2016 Sep 23;5(10):85.
9. Takhar R, Biswas R, Arora A, Jain V. Platypnoea-orthodeoxia syndrome: novel cause for a known condition. BMJ Case Rep. 2014 Mar 7;2014:bcr2013201284.
10. Tenholder MF, Russell MD, Knight E, Rajagopal KR. Orthodeoxia: a new finding in interstitial fibrosis. Am Rev Respir Dis. 1987 Jul;136(1):170–3.
11. Velthuis S, Buscarini E, Gossage JR, Snijder RJ, Mager JJ, Post MC. Clinical implications of pulmonary shunting on saline contrast echocardiography. J Am Soc Echocardiogr. 2015 Mar;28(3):255–63.
12. Sykes DB, Schroyens W, O'Connell C. The TEMPI syndrome: a novel multisystem disease. N Engl J Med. 2011 Aug 4;365(5):475–7.
13. Mohammadi F, Wolverson MK, Bastani B. A new case of TEMPI syndrome. Clin Kidney J. 2012 Dec; 5(6):556–8.
14. Sykes DB, Schroyens W. Complete responses in the TEMPI syndrome after treatment with daratumumab. N Engl J Med. 2018 Jun 7;378(23):2240–2.
15. Jasim S, Mahmud G, Bastani B, Fesler M. Subcutaneous bortezomib for treatment of TEMPI syndrome. Clin Lymphoma Myeloma Leuk. 2014 Dec;14(6):e221–3.
16. Schroyens W, O'Connell C, Sykes DB. Complete and partial responses of the TEMPI syndrome to bortezomib. N Engl J Med. 2012 Aug 23;367(8):778–80.
17. Kwok M, Korde N, Landgren O. Bortezomib to treat the TEMPI syndrome. N Engl J Med. 2012 May 10;366(19):1843–5.
18. Kenderian SS, Rosado FG, Sykes DB, Hoyer JD, Lacy MQ. Long-term complete clinical and hematological responses of the TEMPI syndrome after autologous stem cell transplantation. Leukemia. 2015 Dec;29(12):2414–6.
19. Sarkar M, Niranjan N, Banyal PK. Mechanisms of hypoxemia. Lung India. 2017 Jan-Feb;34(1):47–60. Erratum in: Lung India. 2017 Mar-Apr;34(2):220.
20. Attaran RR, Ata I, Kudithipudi V, Foster L, Sorrell VL. Protocol for optimal detection and exclusion of a patent foramen ovale using transthoracic echocardiography with agitated saline microbubbles. Echocardiography. 2006 Aug;23(7):616–22.
21. Arvanitaki A, Giannakoulas G, Baumgartner H, Lammers AE. Eisenmenger syndrome: diagnosis, prognosis and clinical management. Heart. 2020 Nov;106(21):1638–45. Epub 2020 Jul 20: 1638–45.
22. De Cuyper C, Pauwels T, Derom E, De Pauw M, De Wolf D, et al. Percutaneous closure of PFO in patients with reduced oxygen saturation at rest and during exercise: short- and long-term results. J Interv Cardiol. 2020 Mar 20;2020:9813038.

Occupational and Environmental Diseases

A 91-Year-Old Man With a Pulmonary Nodule, Abdominal Pain, and Anorexia

Luiza Azevedo Gross, MD, and Alice Gallo de Moraes, MD

Case Presentation

A 91-year-old man presented to the pulmonary clinic with an incidental pulmonary nodule. He had initially presented to the gastroenterology clinic with abdominal pain, anorexia, and weight loss of 18 kg (40 lb) in the previous 6 months. His history included asbestosis, peptic ulcer disease (a Billroth II operation was performed when he

was in his 30s), cholecystectomy (performed when he was in his 70s), recurrent de novo choledocholithiasis, and cholangitis complicated by duodenal perforation related to endoscopic retrograde cholangiopancreatography performed elsewhere (2 years before).

Evaluation included computed tomography (CT) of the abdomen (Figure 52.1), which did not show any recent pathologic changes, and

Figure 52.1   CT of the Abdomen

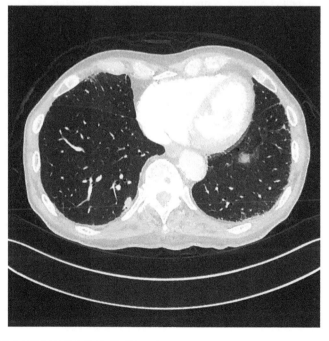

Axial view does not show any recent pathologic changes.

Figure 52.2   CT of the Chest

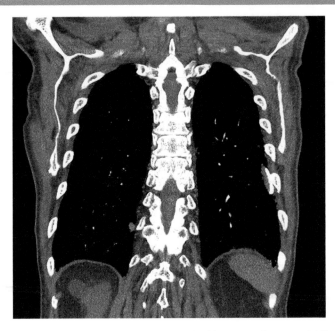

Coronal view shows a 15-mm nodule in the right lower lobe and mild, nonspecific interstitial fibrotic changes.

CT of the chest (Figure 52.2), which showed a 15-mm nodule in the right lower lobe and mild, nonspecific interstitial fibrotic changes. These findings were not present when CT was performed 3 years earlier. The presence of the nodule in the right lower lobe prompted referral to the pulmonary clinic. Ultrasonography of the mesenteric artery did not show a stenosis.

In the pulmonary clinic, the patient reported that he did not have dyspnea, chest pain, or hemoptysis. He did have throat discomfort and cough. Flexible laryngoscopy performed the previous day showed evidence of candidiasis.

Nystatin was prescribed, and a 2-week follow-up was scheduled; at that time, if his symptoms persisted, the plan was to consider use of fluconazole.

Otherwise, the patient reported having progressive fatigue, but he was relatively active and independent in his daily activities. A former smoker, he had a history of 35 pack-years but had not smoked for more than 40 years. He had a history of asbestos exposure, and pleural plaques on CT of the chest were consistent with asbestosis. He was not aware of any family history of malignancy.

Questions

Multiple Choice (choose the best answer)

52.1. What is required for the diagnosis of asbestosis in a patient who has a history of asbestos exposure and no other causes of parenchymal lung disease?
   a. Imaging or histologic evidence of structural change
   b. Lung tissue biopsy that shows interstitial fibrosis
   c. High-resolution CT (HRCT) showing pleural plaques
   d. Bronchioalveolar lavage that shows inflammation
   e. Abnormal results from pulmonary function testing (PFT) and decreased diffusing capacity

52.2. What is the best therapy for asbestosis?
   a. Corticosteroids
   b. Immunotherapy
   c. Preventive and supportive measures
   d. Nonsteroidal anti-inflammatory drugs
   e. Antifibrotic medications

52.3. What is the best way to monitor a patient after a diagnosis of asbestosis?
   a. Lung cancer and mesothelioma screening with annual low-dose CT, periodic colon cancer screening, and annual radiography of the chest and PFT
   b. Periodic screening for colon cancer and, every 3 to 5 years, radiography of the chest and PFT
   c. Lung cancer screening with annual low-dose CT, radiography of the chest, and PFT
   d. Mesothelioma screening with annual low-dose CT and periodic colon cancer screening
   e. Lung cancer and mesothelioma screening with annual low-dose CT and radiography of the chest and PFT every 3 to 5 years

52.4. What is the best management for the 15-mm lung nodule in this patient?
   a. Resection
   b. No routine follow-up
   c. Tissue sampling at 6 months
   d. Positron emission tomography (PET)-CT at 6 months
   e. CT at 3 months

52.5. Which of the following CT features of a lung nodule would be most indicative of malignancy?
   a. Solid type
   b. Spiculation
   c. Calcification
   d. Location in the lower lung
   e. Perifissural

Case Follow-up and Outcome

The patient returned for annual follow-up evaluations, and his condition remained stable.

Discussion

The spectrum of pleuropulmonary disorders associated with asbestos exposure includes asbestosis, pleural disease, and malignancies. Asbestos exposure is classically associated with mining and milling of asbestos fibers; work with textiles, cement, and friction materials; shipbuilding; exposure to insulation material; and nonoccupational exposure to airborne asbestos. Patients rarely become symptomatic until at least 20 years after exposure, and the earliest symptom is shortness of breath on exertion (1).

Diagnosis is made from the exposure history, definite evidence of interstitial fibrosis, and the absence of other causes of parenchymal lung disease. Conclusive evidence of structural change may be found with imaging or histology. A patient with interstitial fibrosis would be expected to have end-expiratory crackles on pulmonary auscultation and clubbing. Functional impairment would be indicated by symptoms and signs, such as those described above, and decreased lung volumes or diffusing capacity of lung for carbon monoxide (2). Typical findings of asbestosis on HRCT are pleural plaques (in 85% of patients), interstitial lines (in 84%), parenchymal bands (in 76%), architectural distortion of secondary pulmonary lobules (in 56%), basilar and dorsal lung parenchymal fibrosis, honeycombing in advanced disease, and subpleural lines (ie, linear densities that are parallel to the pleura). Tissue sampling is rarely needed to establish a diagnosis (3,4).

Asbestosis has no specific treatment. Therefore, management should include preventive and supportive measures, such as smoking cessation, supplemental oxygen if the patient has hypoxemia, elimination of further exposure, pneumococcal and influenza virus vaccination, and management of concurrent respiratory disease and other diseases. After receiving a diagnosis of asbestosis related to work, the patient should be informed about options for compensation, and the occupational disease should be reported to the appropriate authority as required by law. The patient should also undergo functional impairment assessment with PFT. Asbestosis monitoring consists of radiography of the chest and PFT every 3 to 5 years, and colon cancer screening and observation. Vigilance should be maintained for lung cancer, but there is no indication for screening for lung cancer, mesothelioma, or other cancers besides colon cancer (2).

A serious complication of asbestosis is malignancy. Asbestos exposure increases the risk of lung cancer, malignant mesothelioma, cancer in the gastrointestinal tract, and laryngeal cancer. In a study of a Dutch cohort with more than 58,000 patients, asbestos exposure was associated with a relative risk of 3.5 for lung cancer (5). Asbestosis in combination with tobacco smoking markedly increases the risk of lung cancer. In comparisons with nonsmokers without asbestos exposure, the odds ratios for lung cancer developing in persons with asbestos exposure are 1.7 for nonsmokers and 8.7 for smokers (6). Also, among patients with asbestos exposure, the risk of dying of lung cancer increases 16-fold for smokers compared to nonsmokers (7).

In contrast, smoking does not increase the prevalence of malignant mesothelioma, which is classically associated with asbestos exposure. Most cases of diffuse malignant mesothelioma (80%) occur in men exposed to asbestos in the workplace (8) because the only risk factor associated with malignant mesothelioma is asbestos exposure. If a lung nodule is found in a patient who has asbestosis and a smoking history of more than 30 pack-years, the possibility of malignancy is greatly increased.

For patients with lung nodules found incidentally, the current guidelines recommend follow-up according to nodule type, size, and quantity and the patient's baseline risk factors. Nodule type is classified as nonsolid or ground-glass and as partially solid or solid. The risk of malignancy is increased for patients with partially solid nodules, decreased for patients with nonsolid or ground-glass nodules, and neutral for patients with solid nodules. Nodule size is categorized as less than 6 mm, 6 to 8 mm, and greater than 8 mm. Most lung nodules smaller than 6 mm do not require routine follow-up if patients have low risk, but nodules larger than 8 mm usually require follow-up imaging at 3 to 6 months. The risk of primary cancer increases as the total nodule count increases from 1 to 4 but decreases if more than 4 nodules are present because multiple small nodules tend to be associated with an infectious process. Specific features of nodules indicate higher risk (eg, spiculation), whereas other features indicate a benign cause (eg, popcorn calcifications, which are consistent with hamartomas) (9-11).

Patient characteristics are also useful in considering the probability that an incidental lung nodule may be malignant. For example, the risk of primary lung cancer is greater among patients who are older, who have a family history of lung cancer, a history of tobacco smoking, or a history of exposure to other inhaled carcinogens, such as asbestos, and sex has been debated as an isolated risk factor, although most authors believe that women have an increased risk for cancer (9-11).

Summary

Asbestosis is an interstitial lung disease that is associated with an increased risk of malignancy. That risk is even higher if patients smoke tobacco. There are no lung cancer screening recommendations for patients who have asbestosis. However, the suspicion for malignancy should be low. Patients with asbestosis and an incidental lung nodule are definitely at high risk, and a nodule larger than 8 mm warrants follow-up CT at 3 to 6 months.

Answers

52.1. Answer a.

The diagnostic criteria for nonmalignant lung disease related to asbestos, according to the 2004 guidelines from the American Thoracic Society, are shown in Table 52.A1.

Table 52.A1	Criteria for Diagnosis of Nonmalignant Lung Disease Related to Asbestos	
Criterion	**Source of evidence**
Evidence of structural change	Imaging[a] Histology
Evidence of plausible causation	Occupational and environmental history of exposure with plausible latency[b] Markers of exposure (eg, pleural plaques) Recovery of asbestos bodies in lung tissue
Exclusion of alternative diagnosis	Other causes of parenchymal lung disease
Evidence of functional impairment	Signs and symptoms (bibasilar, fine end-expiratory crackles and clubbing) Change in ventilatory function (restrictive, obstructive patterns in context or disease history) Impaired gas exchange (eg, reduced diffusing capacity) Inflammation (eg, by bronchoalveolar lavage) Exercise testing

[a] According to Banks et al (12), chest radiographs with small irregular opacities with a profusion level of at least 1/1 or HRCT in the prone position at the lung bases are useful for the diagnosis of asbestosis in patients who do not have lung disease. On chest radiography, small irregular opacities with a profusion level of 1/0 are useful for screening but lack specificity for an accurate diagnosis of asbestosis. The use of HRCT increases the specificity of the chest radiographic findings.

[b] According to Banks et al (12), this would be necessary in the absence of pathologic examination of lung tissue.

Data from American Thoracic Society (2).

According to the 2004 guidelines, although functional assessment is not required for diagnosis, it is recommended for a thorough evaluation. Usually the first step in the evaluation of asbestosis is PFT to assess the severity and pattern of lung impairment. This functional assessment is diagnostically useful in defining the disease activity and the resulting impairment. Additional information is available in the medical literature (2,12).

52.2. Answer c.

Management of asbestosis should focus on preventive and supportive measures, such as smoking cessation (which is primary prevention for smoking-related disorders), elimination of further excessive exposure, use of supplemental oxygen if the patient has hypoxemia at rest or exercise-induced oxygen desaturation, prompt treatment of respiratory infections, and pneumococcal and influenza virus vaccinations. The patient should also be informed about compensation options for work-related illness, and the occupational disease should be reported to the appropriate authority as required by law. Additional information is available in the medical literature (2).

52.3. Answer b.

After a patient receives a diagnosis of asbestosis, recommendations include monitoring with chest radiography and PFT every 3 to 5 years, active monitoring (with periodic screening) for colon cancer, and observation. Vigilance should be maintained for lung cancer, but there is no indication for screening for lung cancer, mesothelioma, or other cancers besides colon cancer. Additional information is available in the medical literature (2).

52.4. Answer e.

According to the Fleischner Society 2017 guidelines for the management of incidentally detected pulmonary nodules in adults, the 2 most important features of a nodule for predicting risk are nodule size and morphology. For solid nodules larger than 8 mm, the recommendations are CT at 3 months, PET-CT, or tissue sampling. For subsolid nodules that are 6 mm or larger, CT should be performed at 6 to 12 months to confirm persistence and then every 2 years for 5 years if the nodule is the ground-glass subtype. For partially solid nodules, CT should be performed at 3 to 6 months and then annually for 5 years.

For the patient described above, nodule morphology was indeterminate. However, given his age, smoking history, and larger nodule size, it would be reasonable to consider that he had a high risk for malignancy. The only feature that would decrease his risk is the location in an area other than the upper lobe. Given that risk assessment and the above recommendations, the most appropriate follow-up would be CT in 3 months. Additional information is available in the medical literature (9).

52.5. Answer b.

A model has been created for predicting the probability of malignancy of lung nodules. When present in the first screening low-dose CT, predictors of cancer are location of the nodule in the upper lobe, part-solid nodule type, lower nodule count, and spiculation. Additional information is available in the medical literature (11).

References

1. Wagner GR. Asbestosis and silicosis. Lancet. 1997 May 3;349(9061):1311–5.
2. American Thoracic Society. Diagnosis and initial management of nonmalignant diseases related to asbestos. Am J Respir Crit Care Med. 2004 Sep 15;170(6): 691–715.
3. Gamsu G, Salmon CJ, Warnock ML, Blanc PD. CT quantification of interstitial fibrosis in patients with asbestosis: a comparison of two methods. AJR Am J Roentgenol. 1995 Jan;164(1):63–8.
4. Muller NL, Miller RR. Computed tomography of chronic diffuse infiltrative lung disease. Part 1. Am Rev Respir Dis. 1990 Nov;142(5):1206–15.
5. van Loon AJ, Kant IJ, Swaen GM, Goldbohm RA, Kremer AM, van den Brandt PA. Occupational exposure to carcinogens and risk of lung cancer: results from The Netherlands cohort study. Occup Environ Med. 1997 Nov;54(11):817–24.
6. Ngamwong Y, Tangamornsuksan W, Lohitnavy O, Chaiyakunapruk N, Scholfield CN, Reisfeld B, et al. Additive synergism between asbestos and smoking in lung cancer risk: a systematic review and meta-analysis. PLoS One. 2015 Aug 14;10(8):e0135798.
7. Hammond EC, Selikoff IJ, Seidman H. Asbestos exposure, cigarette smoking and death rates. Ann N Y Acad Sci. 1979;330:473–90.
8. Mossman BT, Gee JB. Asbestos-related diseases. N Engl J Med. 1989 Jun 29;320(26):1721–30.
9. MacMahon H, Naidich DP, Goo JM, Lee KS, Leung ANC, Mayo JR, et al. Guidelines for Management of Incidental Pulmonary Nodules Detected on CT Images: from the Fleischner Society 2017. Radiology. 2017 Jul;284(1):228–43.
10. Midthun DE, Swensen SJ, Jett JR. Approach to the solitary pulmonary nodule. Mayo Clin Proc. 1993 Apr;68(4):378–85.
11. McWilliams A, Tammemagi MC, Mayo JR, Roberts H, Liu G, Soghrati K, et al. Probability of cancer in pulmonary nodules detected on first screening CT. N Engl J Med. 2013 Sep 5;369(10):910–9.
12. Banks DE, Shi R, McLarty J, Cowl CT, Smith D, Tarlo SM, et al. American College of Chest Physicians consensus statement on the respiratory health effects of asbestos: results of a Delphi study. Chest. 2009 Jun;135(6):1619–27.

A 23-Year-Old Man With Dyspnea and Pleural Effusions

Jamie R. Felzer, MD, MPH, and Ashley M. Egan, MD

Case Presentation

A 23-year-old male college student who had a history of asthma and a recent diagnosis of esophagitis presented to another hospital with fevers and abdominal pain. He had diffuse lymphadenopathy and underwent biopsy of mediastinal and inguinal lymph nodes and bone marrow. Biopsy results showed a reactive or inflammatory hyperproliferative process with nonclonal lymphocytes. A complete infectious and autoimmune evaluation yielded unremarkable results, including negative results for HIV and human herpesvirus 8 (HHV-8). At that time, pulmonary emboli and a portal vein thrombus were also diagnosed, and he began receiving therapeutic anticoagulation. Temporary chest tubes were placed bilaterally for pleural effusions. The diagnosis was presumed multicentric Castleman disease (MCD); therapy was begun with prednisone, which provided some symptomatic relief and allowed for the patient to be discharged to his home briefly after a prolonged hospitalization.

The patient's shortness of breath worsened, and lower extremity edema developed. Radiography of the chest showed moderate-sized pleural effusions, and he subsequently underwent thoracentesis. His triglyceride level exceeded 2,000 mg/dL, which was consistent with chylothoraces. Chest tubes were placed bilaterally for drainage. Cytology of the pleural fluid was unremarkable and did not show growth of any organisms. Transthoracic echocardiography showed a new, large anterior pericardial effusion with physiologic changes consistent with tamponade; the effusion was therefore drained. The appearance of the pericardial fluid resembled milk, which was consistent with a chylous pericardial effusion. Follow-up computed tomography showed that the patient still had bulky lymphadenopathy in addition to a pelvic mass. Subsequent biopsy results showed mesothelial proliferation with chronic inflammation and negative results on flow cytometry.

Questions

Multiple Choice (choose the best answer)

53.1. Which of the following is *false* about Castleman disease?
a. Castleman disease is a benign disease that is not associated with malignancy
b. The survival rate of patients with multicentric disease is 60%
c. Multicentric disease occurs most commonly in patients who have HIV and HHV-8 infection, and it carries a poor prognosis
d. The typical presentation includes lymphadenopathy, fevers, night sweats, weight loss, and fatigue
e. Treatment options include surgery or rituximab

53.2. What results would you expect with pleural fluid analysis of chylothorax?
a. pH, 7.0; lactate dehydrogenase (LDH), 431 U/L; protein, 5.2 g/dL; appearance, serous or milky; odor, putrid
b. pH, 7.4; LDH, 140 U/L; protein, 2.1 g/dL; appearance, serous
c. pH, 7.3; LDH, 431 U/L; protein, 5.2 g/dL; appearance, serous or milky
d. pH, 7.35; LDH, 350 U/L; protein, 3.7 g/dL; appearance, serosanguinous
e. pH, 7.25; LDH, 431 U/L; protein, 5.2 g/dL; appearance, sanguinous

53.3. What is the most common site of mesothelioma in the general population?
a. Peritoneum
b. Pericardium
c. Pleura
d. Tunica vaginalis
e. Synovium

53.4. Which of the following is *false* about chylothorax?
a. Chyle production can be decreased with dietary measures, including total parental nutrition or low-fat diet with medium-chain triglyceride supplementation
b. Some patients require thoracic duct ligation and pleurodesis
c. An increased level of triglycerides in the pleural fluid is diagnostic
d. Outcomes are better with surgical therapy than with conservative measures
e. Patients with nontraumatic causes of chylothorax have worse outcomes than those with traumatic causes

53.5. Which of the following is most closely associated with the development of mesothelioma?
a. Cigarette smoke
b. Ionizing radiation
c. No known exposure
d. Sequence variations in the *BRCA* gene
e. Lead exposure

Figure 53.1   PET Findings

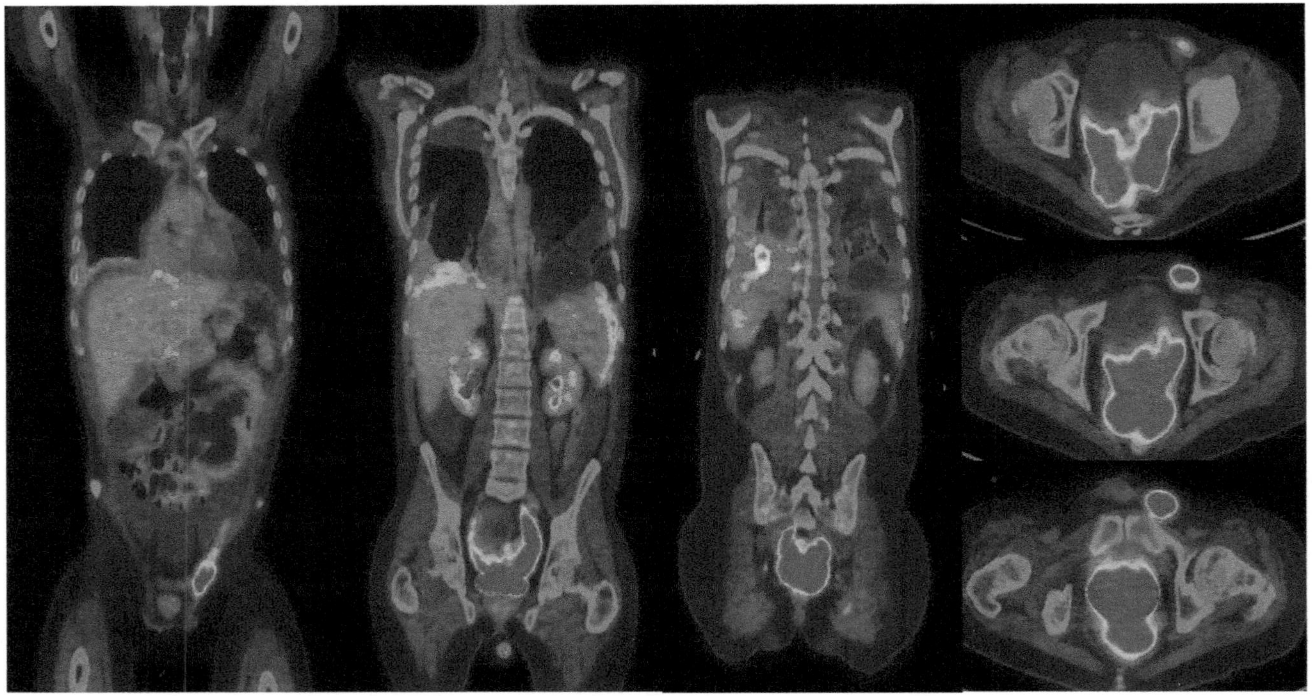

Extensive FDG-avid uptake occurred, especially in the iliac region.

Case Follow-Up and Outcome

The patient was transferred to a quaternary care center for further evaluation. Fluid characteristics from a follow-up thoracentesis were as follows: appearance, milky; pH, 7.44; glucose, 105 mg/dL; total nucleated cells, 215/μL; lymphocytes, 61%; and triglycerides, 1,714 mg/dL. Cytologic examination of the pleural fluid showed reactive mesothelial cells but no malignant cells. Positron emission tomography (PET) showed extensive uptake of fluorodeoxyglucose F 18 (FDG) throughout, most notably in the iliac region with involvement of the sigmoid colon and bladder, FDG-avid ascites with possible serosal and omental involvement, and widespread FDG-avid lymphadenopathy (Figure 53.1). Biopsy findings from the FDG-avid mass in the inguinal region were consistent with the epithelioid type of malignant mesothelioma. Staining showed reactivity for the OSCAR cytokeratin and calretinin but not for other markers (Figure 53.2). Results of the previous lymph node biopsy at the other hospital showed atypical mesothelial proliferation. In a follow-up evaluation for an infectious cause, results were again negative for HIV and HHV-8. Results were also negative for BRCA-associated protein 1 (BAP1).

Lymphangiography showed leakage of the contrast material with extrinsic compression of the thoracic duct, which prompted thoracic duct embolization with coils and glue. The patient was given total parental nutrition with nothing by mouth to decrease the accumulation rate of the chylothorax. However, drainage from the multiple chest tubes was difficult because of loculations even with intrapleural lytic therapy. He underwent bilateral video-assisted thoracic surgery decortication for better management of the loculated effusions and for mediastinal staging because of the extreme rarity of the presentation. Diffuse loculated effusions with adhesions were found intraoperatively.

Recurrent ascites developed that was initially serous but became chylous. The patient was treated appropriately for spontaneous bacterial peritonitis.

Chemotherapy was initiated with pemetrexed and carboplatin. Initially the patient's condition improved, but he required medication for pain control. When remission was not achieved, his therapy was transitioned to nivolumab, which did not provide therapeutic benefit. Approximately 1 year after his diagnosis, his condition continued to worsen, and he was eventually given hospice care. He died at age 24 years.

Discussion

Malignant mesothelioma is extremely rare. Approximately 3,000 cases occur annually, and 8% to 15% are peritoneal (1). The incidence is expected to increase because of previous exposures to asbestos and a latency of 13 to 70 years. Malignant pleural mesothelioma arises from mesothelial cells in the parietal pleura and spreads into the visceral pleura. Mesothelioma can also arise from mesothelial cells in the pericardium, peritoneum, or tunica vaginalis. Mesothelioma has been linked to multiple industrial pollutants and mineral exposures; the most well-known, asbestos, accounts for 80% of cases. Asbestos is a natural mineral that was used in many commercial applications for fireproofing, building materials, blackboards, pipes, and insulation. It was also previously used on submarines, but its use is now generally banned because of the associated health hazards (2). Asbestos can break into small fibers, which can be inhaled and cause pulmonary disease. These fibers can lead to the development of mesothelioma, but often the latency period is 20 to 40 years. Although development of mesothelioma may be related to cumulative exposure, there is not a clear dose-response relationship. Among men and women who have mesothelioma, men are twice as likely to have been exposed to asbestos. Additionally, although asbestos exposure can lead to pleural plaques and mesothelioma independently, plaques do not transform into malignant mesothelioma. Plaques often have a shorter

Figure 53.2   Left Inguinal Biopsy Findings in Malignant Mesothelioma

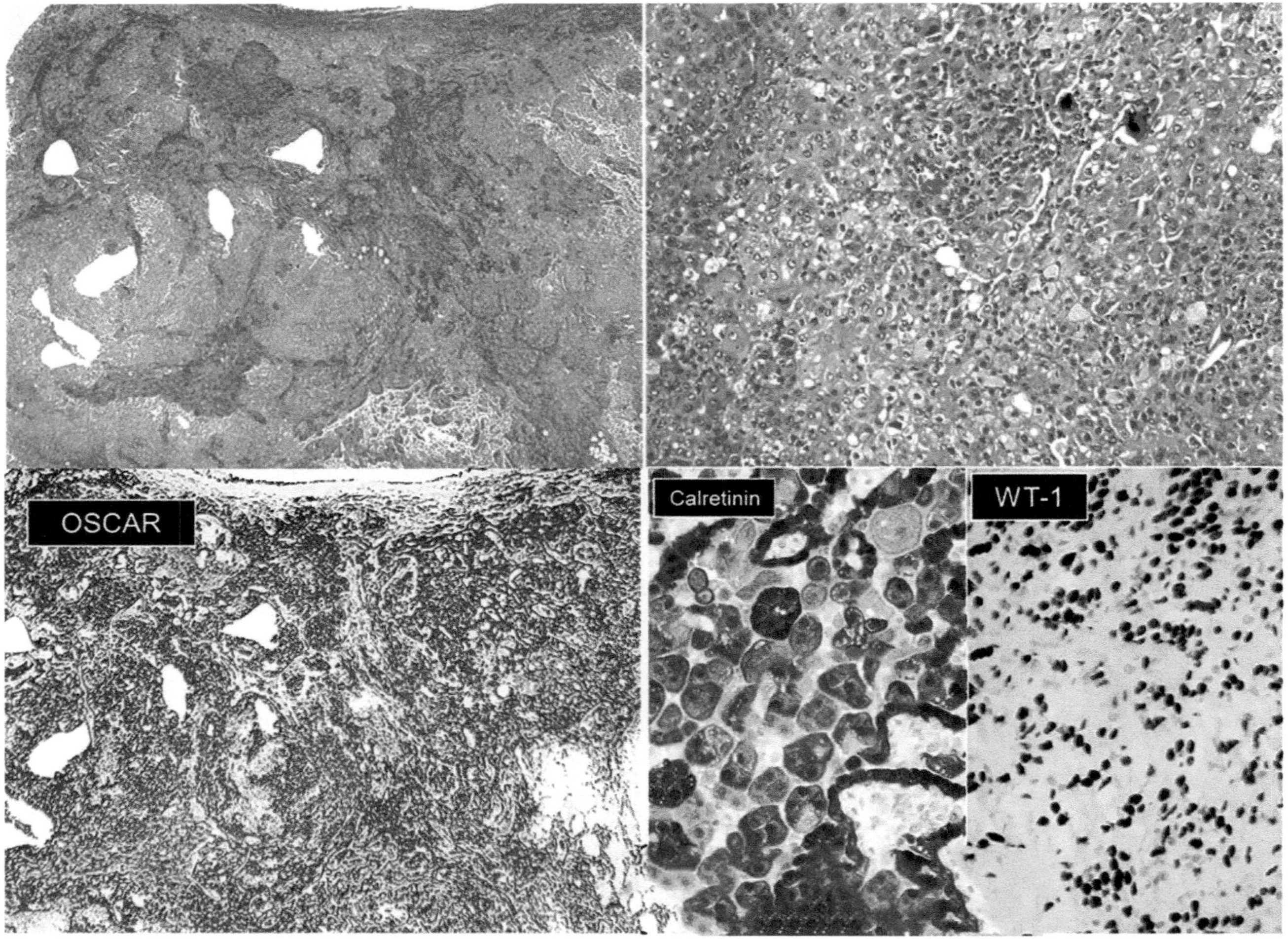

Staining for BAP (not shown) indicated that BAP1 was retained in the nucleus. Upper panels, Staining with hematoxylin–eosin showed atypical mesothelial proliferation. Lower panels, Staining showed reactivity for the OSCAR cytokeratin and calretinin but not for other markers, including WT-1, S100, SALL4, glypican 3, MOC31, and brachyury.

latency period and therefore may appear before mesothelioma.

Other minerals involved in the development of mesothelioma are erionite, thorium, and mica. Mesothelioma may also be associated with ionizing radiation, simian virus, and chronic pleural disease. Smoking itself does not contribute to the development of mesothelioma, but smoking in combination with asbestos increases the risk of lung cancer (1). Furthermore, some genetic associations occur with BAP1, which our patient did not have.

The median age at diagnosis is 74 years; only 2% to 15% of affected patients are younger than 40 years (3). Among younger patients, the distribution between sexes is equal, but in the general population mesothelioma is nearly 3 to 5 times more likely to develop in men than in women (4,5). Interestingly, in the current incident populations, the distribution between sexes is equal. In the general population, the most common site is the pleura (85%); the second most common site is the peritoneum (15%). However, in patients younger than 40 years, mesothelioma is equally common in the pleura and the peritoneum (4). In the US, the distribution of malignant peritoneal mesothelioma is equal between the sexes (4).

Presentation is often vague and varies according to the primary site of involvement, so diagnosis may be delayed up to an estimated 4 to 6 months after symptom onset (6). When the disease is in the pleural space, as is most common, patients often have dyspnea, cough, and pain in the chest wall. If the peritoneum is involved, the patient typically has abdominal distention or pain or, rarely, bowel obstruction. Other early symptoms include early satiety, fatigue, fever, weight loss, and nausea (4). Serum chemistry and markers have limited diagnostic utility. Typically, computed tomography shows a heterogenous soft tissue mass with irregular margins that enhances with a contrast agent. The mass is usually expansive and not infiltrative, and it does not involve lymph nodes, which helps in differentiating it from other malignancies (4). Malignant pleural mesothelioma can be distinguished from benign processes when the pleura is thicker than 1 cm and has nodularity with mediastinal pleural involvement (7). Magnetic resonance imaging can be helpful in distinguishing the soft tissue planes. On PET, more FDG uptake is associated with a worse prognosis. Cytology cannot be used for the diagnosis of mesothelioma.

The prognosis for patients with mesothelioma is poor; without treatment, the survival rate is less than 1 year. The 5-year survival rate is less than 5%. Patients with sarcomatoid or biphasic histologic subtypes have a worse prognosis, whereas those with the epithelioid subtype generally have a more favorable prognosis (4). Lymph node involvement is quite rare, and its presence is a poor prognostic factor. Average survival for patients with lymph node involvement is 6 months, whereas for patients without lymph node involvement it is 59 months. Older age and male sex are also poor prognostic factors (8). Mesothelioma in patients with BAP1, which this patient did not have, is often less aggressive clinically and carries a longer survival, but the person is more susceptible to other tumors such as uveal melanoma, cutaneous melanoma, and renal cell carcinoma. BAP1 sequence variants are frequently present in peritoneal disease.

Malignant mesothelioma is so rare that treatment is generally undertaken with a multidisciplinary team that includes an oncologist, pulmonologist, radiologist, pathologist, thoracic surgeon, and cancer nurse. Recurrent pleural effusions and ascites should be controlled because, when present, they greatly affect the patient's quality of life. Pleural effusions can be managed with mechanical decortication if the patient can undergo surgery. Otherwise, chemical pleurodesis is an option. If neither option is possible, a tunneled pleural catheter can be placed for daily drainage.

Chemotherapy should be used when patients have a good performance status. The standard for many years has been the use of pemetrexed and cisplatin with the possible addition of bevacizumab, which can be especially useful for patients with low levels of vascular endothelial growth factor (9). The use of nivolumab in combination with ipilimumab was recently shown to improve survival compared with the use of standard chemotherapy and is now recommended as a first-line therapy (1,10). However, these options are often palliative because of the poor prognosis despite chemotherapy. Bevacizumab was considered for the patient described above in the Case Presentation, but it was not used because of the patient's high risk for bleeding.

The benefit of surgery is unclear, but if undertaken the procedure would most likely include extrapleural pneumonectomy, pleurectomy with decortication, or debulking through cytoreductive surgery in conjunction with chemotherapy (4,5). Extrapleural pneumonectomy has not been performed except in clinical trials, however, so pleurectomy decortication is the procedure of choice. Generally, these procedures are undertaken for palliation because curative surgery is difficult to successfully perform (7). The current Mesothelioma and Radical Surgery 2 (MARS2) trial (NCT02040272) in the UK is expected to provide further guidance on whether extended pleurectomy decortication in addition to chemotherapy can increase survival and improve quality of life. Radiotherapy is sometimes performed as an adjunct to surgery or with chemotherapy, but it has limited efficacy and is usually used as a palliative option for symptom relief. It has not been shown to prolong survival (7). When the disease is unresectable, radiotherapy should not be administered to the entire hemithorax because it is difficult to avoid vital thoracic organs (1).

The findings for the patient described above are unusual for several reasons. Chylothorax has rarely been described as the initial presentation in mesothelioma, and the presence of bilateral chylothoraces is even rarer. For the patient described above, the previous comprehensive evaluation showed only reactive mesothelial cells, but the findings suggested the possibility of an underlying malignancy.

Chylothorax results from the accumulation of chyle in the pleural space when the thoracic duct or other tributaries have been blocked. The thoracic duct is the main lymphatic vessel that transports chyle from the abdomen to the venous system. It is a cause of a lymphocytic-predominant exudative effusion (11). The most common causes of chylothorax are lymph blockage from lymphoma or solid tumors, subclavian vein thrombosis, portal hypertension, radiotherapy, or surgery for pneumonectomy, lung or heart transplant, esophageal resection, and neck dissection (12,13). Presumedly mesothelioma spreads through lymphatic structures and causes lymph blockage, eventually leading to chylothorax as in the patient described above. Chylothorax is diagnosed with the finding of an exudative, lymphocyte-predominant effusion with high levels of triglycerides. Alternatively, chylomicrons can be found if the triglyceride level is low, as in a fasting patient. Lymphangiography may be performed to determine the location of the leak, but the use of such information does not seem to affect outcomes. Treatment includes conservative management with dietary measures, such as the use of a high-protein, low-fat diet supplemented with medium-chain triglycerides or total parenteral nutrition; repeated thoracenteses; or placement of a thoracostomy tube. More invasive surgical measures include talc pleurodesis, thoracic duct ligation, mechanical pleurodesis, and pleurectomy. Recurrence is higher for patients if the cause of the chylothorax was nontraumatic despite the use of various types of management (12).

Summary

Malignant mesothelioma is a rare disease that is more common in older male patients who have been exposed to asbestos, but it can occur in younger patients without asbestos exposure. Symptoms are nonspecific and may include fever, weight loss, pain, and lymphadenopathy. Diagnosis should be made from biopsy of the mass. The prognosis is poor overall, but surgery and chemotherapy are options.

53.1. Answer a.

Castleman disease is a nonmalignant lymphoproliferative disorder, but it can present with concomitant malignancies, including Kaposi sarcoma or primary effusion lymphoma. The 2 types of Castleman disease are unicentric and MCD. Unicentric disease usually occurs in younger patients and carries a better prognosis than MCD. MCD is associated with HIV and HHV-8 infection, which occurs in HIV-positive patients and in HIV-negative patients. Patients with MCD are older at presentation and have poorer outcomes. The presentation includes fever, an increased level of C-reactive protein, and at least 3 of the following: peripheral lymphadenopathy, splenomegaly, edema, pleural effusion, ascites, cough, nasal obstruction, xerostomia, rash, central neurologic symptoms, jaundice, and autoimmune hemolytic anemia. Patients also typically have systemic inflammatory symptoms of fevers, night sweats, weight loss, and fatigue. It can mimic many other diseases, commonly lymphoma or autoimmune disorders, so they should be excluded in the evaluation. Surgical resection in unicentric disease is often curative. In HIV-associated MCD, initiation of antiretrovirals is important with the eventual addition of rituximab, often as monotherapy but sometimes with additional chemotherapy agents such as etoposide, vinblastine, cyclophosphamide, cladribine, chlorambucil, or liposomal doxorubicin. In cases associated with HHV-8, therapy with antivirals such as valganciclovir or ganciclovir should be initiated as well. Glucocorticoids can be used as adjunctive therapy but are rarely curative. Additional information is available in the medical literature (14,15).

53.2. Answer c.

Chylothorax is a rare type of pleural effusion that is an exudative, lymphocytic effusion. The increased triglyceride levels in chylothoraces can be useful in differentiating them from pseudochylothoraces. To distinguish between an empyema and a lipid effusion, the sample can be centrifuged. If the supernatant is clear, the cloudy appearance was due to cellular debris, and the effusion is most likely an empyema. If the supernatant is still turbid, the effusion is a chylothorax. The pleural fluid with a putrid odor and low pH (answer choice *a*) is most likely from an empyema. Answer choice *b* describes a transudative effusion, with the most common cause being heart failure or cirrhosis. Answer choices *d* and *e* describe exudates; *e* most likely indicates a hemothorax, but the cause could be malignancy, a parapneumonic effusion, postsurgical inflammatory changes, or autoimmune pleuritis. Additional information is available in the medical literature (11).

53.3. Answer c.

The pleura is the site of mesothelioma in 80% of patients. Mesothelioma arises from mesothelial cells and therefore can arise from any surface that has a mesothelium, including the peritoneum (about 8% of patients), pericardium, and tunica vaginalis testis. Synovial membranes do not contain mesothelial cells. Additional information is available in the medical literature (1).

53.4. Answer d.

Chylothorax is a rare cause of pleural effusion, and the diagnosis is made with the results of pleural fluid studies that show an exudative, milky pleural effusion with an increased triglyceride level. Management can be conservative with a low-fat diet or total parenteral nutrition, typically with concurrent chest tube drainage. Management may need to be more invasive and include pleurodesis or thoracic duct ligation if the chylothorax does not resolve with conservative measures or if it is relatively severe with large-volume effusions. Invasive strategies do not necessarily have higher success rates, and it has been shown that regardless of the initial strategy used, it is successful only about half the time. Patients with a chylothorax from a non-traumatic cause have worse outcomes overall, and a nontraumatic chylothorax often recurs, whereas surgical or trauma-related chylothoraces can be treated. Additional information is available in the medical literature (12).

53.5. Answer b.

Chemical exposures, asbestos, and ionizing radiation are most commonly associated with mesothelioma development. The minerals erionite, thorium, and mica are also known to be involved in the development of mesothelioma. Mesothelioma can also be associated with simian monkey virus and chronic pleural disease. Cigarette smoke is not correlated with development of mesothelioma but can contribute to lung cancer. Although some patients have not had clear exposure to any of these factors, many cases can be traced back to a certain exposure with asbestos, which accounts for about 80% of cases. Less commonly, a genetic association to BAP1 may be involved. Additional information is available in the medical literature (1).

References

1. Network NCC. NCCN Clinical Practice Guidelines in Oncology: malignant pleural mesothelioma 2021 Available from: NCCN.org2021.

2. Zarogoulidis P, Orfanidis M, Constadinidis TC, Eleutheriadou E, Kontakiotis T, Kerenidi T, et al. A 26-year-old male with mesothelioma due to asbestos exposure. Case Rep Med. 2011;2011:951732.

3. Perez-Guzman C, Barrera-Rodriguez R, Portilla-Segura J. Malignant pleural mesothelioma in a 17-year old boy: a case report and literature review. Respir Med Case Rep. 2016;17:57–60.

4. Kim J, Bhagwandin S, Labow DM. Malignant peritoneal mesothelioma: a review. Ann Transl Med. 2017;5(11):236.

5. British Thoracic Society Standards of Care Committee. BTS statement on malignant mesothelioma in the UK, 2007. Thorax. 2007;62 Suppl 2:ii1–ii19.

6. Kaya H, Sezgi C, Tanrikulu AC, Taylan M, Abakay O, Sen HS, et al. Prognostic factors influencing survival in 35 patients with malignant peritoneal mesothelioma. Neoplasma. 2014;61(4):433–8.

7. Kondola S, Manners D, Nowak AK. Malignant pleural mesothelioma: an update on diagnosis and treatment options. Ther Adv Respir Dis. 2016;10(3):275–88.

8. Wolf AS, Richards WG, Tilleman TR, Chirieac L, Hurwitz S, Bueno R, et al. Characteristics of malignant pleural mesothelioma in women. Ann Thorac Surg. 2010;90(3):949–56; discussion 56.

9. Kindler HL, Karrison TG, Gandara DR, Lu C, Krug LM, Stevenson JP, et al. Multicenter, double-blind, placebo-controlled, randomized phase II trial of gemcitabine/cisplatin plus bevacizumab or placebo in patients with malignant mesothelioma. J Clin Oncol. 2012;30(20):2509–15.

10. Baas P, Scherpereel A, Nowak AK, Fujimoto N, Peters S, Tsao AS, et al. First-line nivolumab plus ipilimumab in unresectable malignant pleural mesothelioma (CheckMate 743): a multicentre, randomised, open-label, phase 3 trial. Lancet. 2021; 397(10272):375–86.

11. Hooper C, Lee YC, Maskell N; Group BTSPG. Investigation of a unilateral pleural effusion in adults: British Thoracic Society Pleural Disease Guideline 2010. Thorax. 2010;65 Suppl 2:ii4–17.

12. Maldonado F, Cartin-Ceba R, Hawkins FJ, Ryu JH. Medical and surgical management of chylothorax and associated outcomes. Am J Med Sci. 2010;339(4): 314–8.

13. Darley DR, Granger E, Glanville AR. Chest pain and recurrent chylothorax: an unusual presentation of malignant pleural mesothelioma. Respirol Case Rep. 2017;5(5):e00250.

14. Abramson JS. Diagnosis and Management of Castleman Disease. J Natl Compr Canc Netw. 2019; 17(11.5):1417–9.

15. Soumerai JD, Sohani AR, Abramson JS. Diagnosis and management of Castleman disease. Cancer Control. 2014;21(4):266–78.

A 68-Year-Old Man With Chronic Cough[a]

Jennifer D. Duke, MD, and Cameron M. Long, MD, MS

Case Presentation

A 68-year-old man was referred to our clinic for evaluation of chronic cough and pulmonary nodules. The patient described a daily cough that began 2 years earlier and produced yellow sputum without hemoptysis. He had no wheeze or history of asthma, and he had never smoked. He maintained his activity level while working on his ranch, and he reported that his exercise capacity was stable; that he did not have joint pain, swelling, or redness; and that he did not have night sweats, fevers, or chills. He had no personal or family history of autoimmune disease, and he did not have muscle weakness or skin changes on his hands or fingernails.

He had worked as a sandblaster and painter for 30 years with inconsistent use of personal protective equipment, and he had raised livestock for 15 years. He was exposed to hay and grass on the ranch, to mold in his house, and, for the past 8 years, to a pet dog. He did not have exposure to asbestos or to anyone with tuberculosis.

On presentation, his vital signs were within normal limits, and oxygen saturation as measured by pulse oximetry was 91%. He appeared well and comfortable while breathing room air. Crackles were heard bilaterally without wheezing or rhonchi. Findings on cardiac and neurologic examinations were normal. He did not have evidence of joint disease, skin thickening or tightening, or rashes. Serologic testing showed the following: rheumatoid factor, 1,054 IU/mL; antinuclear antibody titer 1:1280; positive histone antibody, 7.9 U/mL; and human leukocyte antigen–B27 greater than 805 molecules of equivalent soluble fluorochrome (MESF). Results were negative for the remainder of the autoimmune evaluation, including double-stranded DNA, antineutrophil cytoplasmic autoantibody, ribonucleoprotein antibodies, anti–cyclic citrullinated peptide antibodies, and anti-Scl-70. Results were also negative for hepatitis B core antibody and hepatitis C antibody.

Computed tomography (CT) of the chest showed diffuse pulmonary nodules, which were most prominent in the upper lung lobes, and pleural thickening bilaterally (Figures 54.1–54.6). Peripheral and lower lobe reticular opacities were also seen with scattered ground-glass opacities throughout and partially calcified mediastinal and hilar lymphadenopathy (Figures 54.6 and 54.7). Honeycombing was absent.

Results of pulmonary function tests showed total lung capacity, 63% predicted; ratio of forced expiratory volume in the first second of expiration (FEV_1) to forced vital capacity (FVC), 68.9; FEV_1, 67% predicted; FVC, 73% predicted; and diffusion capacity, 53% predicted.

---

[a] Portions of this case were published in Krefft S et al (22); used with permission.

Figure 54.1   Calcified Pulmonary Nodules

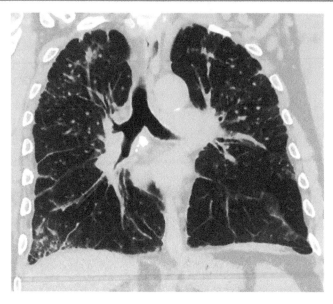

CT of the chest, coronal view, shows innumerable and variable calcified pulmonary nodules with no clear craniocaudal gradient.

Figure 54.2   Coalescent Pulmonary Nodules

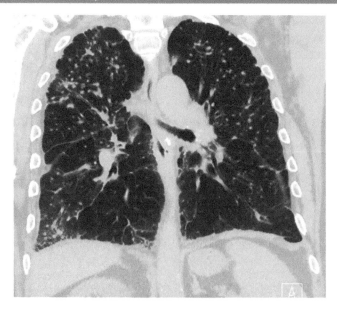

CT of the chest, coronal view, shows somewhat coalescent nodules in the apical and basal lung zones with architectural distortion.

Figure 54.3   Pneumoconiosis

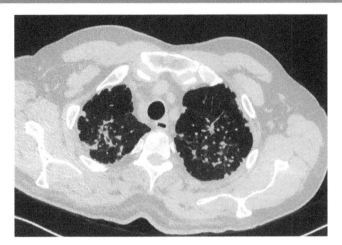

CT of the chest, axial view, shows diffuse lung disease consistent with pneumoconiosis.

Figure 54.4   Silicosis

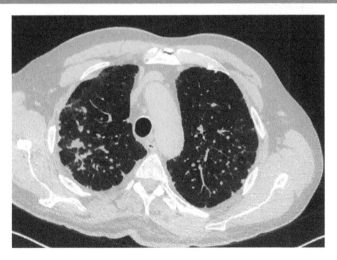

CT of the chest, axial view, is consistent with silicosis.

Figure 54.5   Silicosis

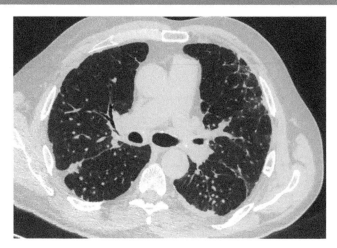

CT of the chest, axial view, is consistent with silicosis.

Figure 54.6   Silicosis

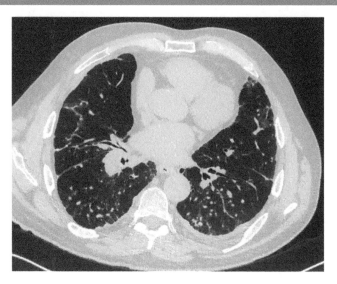

CT of the chest, axial view, shows calcified pulmonary nodules with a slight posterior predominance, which is consistent with silicosis.

Figure 54.7   Pneumoconiosis

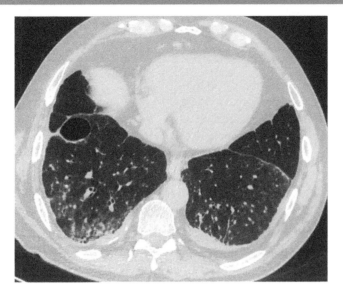

CT of the chest, axial view, shows cystic and varicoid bronchiolectasis in the context of diffuse lung disease, which is most compatible with pneumoconiosis.

Questions

Multiple Choice (choose the best answer)

54.1. Which of the following diagnoses is most consistent with the CT findings from the patient described in the Case Presentation above?
   a. Fibrotic hypersensitivity pneumonitis
   b. Idiopathic pulmonary fibrosis
   c. Nontuberculous mycobacteria
   d. Silicosis
   e. Asbestosis

54.2. Which specific classification best fits the disease of the patient described in the Case Presentation above?
   a. Acute silicosis
   b. Progressive massive fibrosis (PMF)
   c. Accelerated silicosis
   d. Chronic silicosis
   e. Acute-on-chronic silicosis

54.3. Which of the following procedures is needed to establish the most likely diagnosis?
   a. Bronchoalveolar lavage
   b. Transbronchial lung biopsy
   c. Surgical lung biopsy
   d. Positron emission tomography (PET)
   e. No additional testing

54.4. Which of the following is a complication associated with silicosis?
   a. Mycobacterial disease
   b. Mesothelioma
   c. Amyloidosis
   d. Lymphoma
   e. Colon cancer

54.5. Which of the following is the best method to prevent the development of silicosis?
   a. Prophylactic antibiotics before exposure
   b. Wearing of personal protective equipment
   c. Bronchodilators before exposure
   d. Chest physiotherapy
   e. Oxygen administration

Case Follow-up and Outcome

The patient underwent a video-assisted thoracoscopic lung biopsy, which showed severe lung adhesions to the chest wall. Pathologic evaluation of the wedge resection from the right lower lung lobe showed chronic, fibrosing, interstitial lung disease with moderate lymphoplasmacytic infiltrates, chronic bronchiolitis with prominent bronchiolization, marked pleural thickening, and a single dust-laden hyalinized nodule suggestive of a silicotic nodule. The diagnosis was chronic silicosis according to the characteristic CT findings and history. Results were negative for tuberculosis blood testing and for sputum cultures for bacteria, acid-fast bacilli, and fungi. A rheumatology consultation suggested that the patient had a low likelihood of underlying connective tissue disease because he did not have clinical manifestations of rheumatologic disease that corresponded with the nonspecific positive serologic test results.

Discussion

Occupational lung diseases arise from work-related pulmonary irritants such as smoke, dust, fumes, and biologic agents (1). The most common of these diseases are asthma, bronchitis, bronchiolitis, hypersensitivity pneumonitis, acute toxic inhalant syndromes, pneumoconiosis, and tumors. The patient described above had pneumoconiosis, a reaction of the lung to inhalation and subsequent deposition of inorganic particles and dust (2).

Silicosis, a type of pneumoconiosis, often results from occupational inhalation of free crystalline silica in the form of silicon dioxide. While the mechanism of injury is not fully understood, the injury is thought to be due to generation of free radicals as the particles interact with pulmonary cells such as macrophages. This injury potentiates a cytokine-mediated reaction

that can lead to inflammation and fibrosis in the lungs (3).

Industrial workers in mining, stone cutting or quarrying, sandblasting, glass manufacturing, and other fields may be at risk for the disease. In the US, an estimated 2 million workers are exposed to silicon dioxide (4,5). The disease severity generally correlates with the degree of exposure and with additional factors such as race (6). Although the number of cases of silicosis has decreased over time with new workplace protection regulations, the Centers for Disease Control and Prevention (CDC) reported 84 deaths from silicosis in 2014 and a total of 1,167 deaths in 2005 through 2014 (5).

The spectrum of silicosis can be subdivided into *acute, accelerated,* and *chronic. Acute silicosis,* or *acute silicoproteinosis,* is a rare presentation but typically presents as a constellation of symptoms that include cough, dyspnea, weight loss, and fatigue that occur within weeks to a few years after exposure (7). Although acute silicosis is a clinical diagnosis of exclusion, the hallmarks of the disease include a history of exposure to a high dose of silica, imaging findings that show diffuse nodular and patchy consolidative opacities, and a milky, lipoproteinaceous bronchoalveolar lavage effluent. The treatment is supportive care, and patients with this presentation tend to have a poor prognosis (8).

Accelerated silicosis is characterized by symptom onset within 5 to 10 years after exposure (9). The clinical presentation is variable, but imaging findings are consistent with those in chronic silicosis. Treatment involves supportive measures, including avoidance of additional exposure, smoking cessation, vaccinations for pulmonary diseases, supplemental oxygen, and bronchodilators if needed.

Chronic silicosis typically appears within 10 to 30 years after initial exposure, and the clinical presentation varies. Patients may be asymptomatic but have abnormal findings on imaging, or they may have chronic cough and dyspnea on exertion (9). Like the other forms of silicosis, chronic silicosis is suspected if the patient has a history of occupational exposure, and the disease is confirmed with typical findings on imaging of the chest.

Laboratory testing is not needed to make the diagnosis of chronic silicosis, although flexible bronchoscopy with lavage may be used to exclude infection and malignancy. Abnormal findings on pulmonary function testing tend to mirror worsening radiographic abnormalities and can show mixed obstructive and restrictive ventilatory impairment. In a study of 1,028 foundry workers who did not have abnormal findings on imaging, the workers had an annual 1.1-mL decrease in FEV_1 for each milligram per cubic meter of mean silica exposure (10).

Chronic silicosis can be classified as simple silicosis or PMF according to the radiographic features and the severity of clinical symptoms. In simple silicosis, innumerable, small, rounded opacities are present predominantly in the upper lung zones (11). In PMF, the smaller, rounded opacities coalesce into areas larger than 10 mm in diameter. These areas can result in asymmetric fibrosis in the upper lobes and hyperinflation in the lower lobes. A small portion of patients have hilar lymphadenopathy. High-resolution CT (HRCT) is not necessary but may improve diagnostic sensitivity (12).

Although a lung biopsy is often not needed for diagnosis, surgical lung biopsy may be needed rarely (13). Transbronchial lung biopsy is not recommended because of the increased risk of pneumothorax (14). Histopathology shows dust-laden macrophages and loose reticulin fibers in the peribronchial, perivascular, and paraseptal or subpleural areas (15). Over time, nodules that appear to spiral with hyalinized concentrically arranged collagen fibers at the core (ie, *silicotic nodules*) are seen as the pathologic hallmark of the disease (3).

No proven treatment exists for chronic silicosis. Management focuses on removing the exposing agent and supportive respiratory care, including smoking cessation and preventive care with vaccinations for influenza and pneumococcal pneumonia. Lung transplant may be a curative option for some patients (16-18).

Summary

Occupational pneumoconiosis is a reaction of the lung to inhalation and subsequent deposition of inorganic particles and dust. Silicosis is caused by the inhalation of silicon dioxide, which can lead to lung inflammation and fibrosis across a spectrum of severity. No proven treatment exists for silicosis, and lung transplant may be required.

Answers

54.1. Answer d.

Patients with silicosis have variable findings on HRCT. The chest imaging findings in simple silicosis include bilateral reticulonodular opacities that are typically predominant in the upper lobes, although linear interstitial opacities may occur in the lower lobes. Multiple small pulmonary nodules with perilymphatic distribution are commonly seen, as in the imaging for the patient described above in the Case Presentation. Pleural thickening or, less commonly, pleural effusion may be present. PMF is diagnosed by the presence of large opacities on chest radiography or with the finding of conglomerate opacities, typically with calcifications and fibrosis, on HRCT of the chest. Fibrotic hypersensitivity pneumonitis is characterized by coarse reticulations with lung distortion and often nonpredominant traction bronchiectasis and honeycombing. Idiopathic pulmonary fibrosis is characterized by honeycombing cysts and reticular septal thickening with subpleural and posterior basal predominance. The most common CT finding for nontuberculous mycobacteria is the presence of bronchiectasis and ill-defined nodules without cavities. Asbestosis can present with centrilobular dot-like opacities, intralobular linear opacities, and subpleural lines, which are often curvilinear. Additional information is available in the medical literature (19-21).

54.2. Answer d.

Acute, chronic, and accelerated silicosis phenotypes may share overlapping pulmonary histopathologic features of silicoproteinosis and interstitial fibrosis. Classification focuses on symptom onset. Symptoms of chronic silicosis include cough and dyspnea, which begin within 10 to 30 years after initial exposure. Symptom onset in acute silicosis occurs within weeks to a few years after exposure to high concentrations of the substance. The major distinction between accelerated silicosis and acute or chronic silicosis is disease latency. The onset of accelerated disease is within 5 to 10 years after exposure, and disease progression is more rapid than in chronic silicosis. Acute-on-chronic silicosis is not a classification commonly used. Additional information is available in the medical literature (22).

54.3. Answer e.

The diagnosis of silicosis is based on history and imaging findings that are consistent with the diagnosis. Additional testing may be helpful when the diagnosis is questionable. The use of bronchoalveolar lavage can exclude an additional explanation for abnormal CT findings (eg, infection). Transbronchial lung biopsy is not recommended for diffuse parenchymal lung disease because of an increased risk of pneumothorax associated with the procedure. Surgical lung biopsy is not required but may be helpful if the diagnosis is uncertain. PET would not help to distinguish silicosis from other diseases in the differential diagnosis, such as malignancy and infection. Additional information is available in the medical literature (23).

54.4. Answer a.

Mycobacterial infection, both tuberculous and nontuberculous, has long been recognized as a complication of silicosis and poses important challenges to global lung health. Specific mechanisms and risk factors for mycobacterial lung infection in workers exposed to silica are not well understood, although the risk is increased among persons with underlying HIV infection, previous tuberculosis, or more years with more intense exposure to respirable crystalline silica. A diagnosis of silicosis lowers the threshold for a positive qualitative result on a tuberculin skin test to 10 mm, and the CDC recommends treatment of latent tuberculosis in most workers with silica exposure. Treatment of mycobacterial lung infection in patients with silicosis is challenging; in 1 randomized clinical trial, sputum culture results were negative after 2 months in only 80% of patients. Mesothelioma, amyloidosis, lymphoma, and colon cancer are not associated with silicosis. Additional information is available in the medical literature (22,24).

54.5. Answer b.

Primary prevention with avoidance of exposure to silica is the best strategy to prevent silicosis, an untreatable and often devastating fibrotic lung disease. Although primary prevention is key, recent epidemics of acute and accelerated silicosis highlight the importance of the clinician's role in secondary and tertiary prevention strategies. The use of prophylactic antibiotics before known exposures is not recommended because it would be ineffective in preventing the disease or complications associated with exposure. Bronchodilators, chest physiotherapy, and oxygen administration may be used as supportive therapy after silicosis develops, but they would not prevent its development. Additional information is available in the medical literature (22).

References

1. Tarlo SM CP, Nemery B. Occupational and environmental lung diseases. Chichester; Hoboken (NJ): Wiley; 2010. 468 p.
2. Akira M, Kozuka T, Yamamoto S, Sakatani M, Morinaga K. Inhalational talc pneumoconiosis: radiographic and CT findings in 14 patients. AJR Am J Roentgenol. 2007;188(2):326–33.
3. Rimal B, Greenberg AK, Rom WN. Basic pathogenetic mechanisms in silicosis: current understanding. Curr Opin Pulm Med. 2005;11(2):169–73.
4. Rosenman KD, Reilly MJ, Kalinowski DJ, Watt FC. Silicosis in the 1990s. Chest. 1997;111(3):779–86.
5. Bang KM, Mazurek JM, Wood JM, White GE, Hendricks SA, Weston A, et al. Silicosis mortality trends and new exposures to respirable crystalline silica: United States, 2001-2010. MMWR Morb Mortal Wkly Rep. 2015;64(5):117–20.
6. Cohen RA, Go LHT. Artificial stone silicosis: removal from exposure is not enough. Chest. 2020;158(3):862–3.
7. Goodman GB, Kaplan PD, Stachura I, Castranova V, Pailes WH, Lapp NL. Acute silicosis responding to corticosteroid therapy. Chest. 1992;101(2):366–70.
8. Marchiori E, Ferreira A, Saez F, Gabetto JM, Souza AS Jr, Escuissato DL, et al. Conglomerated masses of silicosis in sandblasters: high-resolution CT findings. Eur J Radiol. 2006;59(1):56–9.
9. Wang XR, Christiani DC. Respiratory symptoms and functional status in workers exposed to silica, asbestos, and coal mine dusts. J Occup Environ Med. 2000;42(11):1076–84.
10. Hertzberg VS, Rosenman KD, Reilly MJ, Rice CH. Effect of occupational silica exposure on pulmonary function. Chest. 2002;122(2):721–8.
11. Talini D, Paggiaro PL, Falaschi F, Battolla L, Carrara M, Petrozzino M, et al. Chest radiography and high resolution computed tomography in the evaluation of workers exposed to silica dust: relation with functional findings. Occup Environ Med. 1995;52(4):262–7.
12. Meijer E, Tjoe Nij E, Kraus T, van der Zee JS, van Delden O, van Leeuwen M, et al. Pneumoconiosis and emphysema in construction workers: results of HRCT and lung function findings. Occup Environ Med. 2011;68(7):542–6.
13. Poletti V, Ravaglia C, Gurioli C, Piciucchi S, Dubini A, Cavazza A, et al. Invasive diagnostic techniques in idiopathic interstitial pneumonias. Respirology. 2016;21(1):44–50.
14. Sindhwani G, Shirazi N, Sodhi R, Raghuvanshi S, Rawat J. Transbronchial lung biopsy in patients with diffuse parenchymal lung disease without 'idiopathic pulmonary fibrosis pattern' on HRCT scan: experience from a tertiary care center of North India. Lung India. 2015;32(5):453–6.
15. Hoffmann EO, Lamberty J, Pizzolato P, Coover J. The ultrastructure of acute silicosis. Arch Pathol. 1973;96(2):104–7.
16. Hayes D, Jr., Hayes KT, Hayes HC, Tobias JD. Long-term survival after lung transplantation in patients with silicosis and other occupational lung disease. Lung. 2015;193(6):927–31.
17. Rosengarten D, Fox BD, Fireman E, Blanc PD, Rusanov V, Fruchter O, et al. Survival following lung transplantation for artificial stone silicosis relative to idiopathic pulmonary fibrosis. Am J Ind Med. 2017;60(3):248–54.
18. Singer JP, Chen H, Phelan T, Kukreja J, Golden JA, Blanc PD. Survival following lung transplantation for silicosis and other occupational lung diseases. Occup Med (Lond). 2012;62(2):134–7.
19. Bergin CJ, Muller NL, Vedal S, Chan-Yeung M. CT in silicosis: correlation with plain films and pulmonary function tests. AJR Am J Roentgenol. 1986;146(3):477–83.
20. Arakawa H, Honma K, Saito Y, Shida H, Morikubo H, Suganuma N, et al. Pleural disease in silicosis: pleural thickening, effusion, and invagination. Radiology. 2005;236(2):685–93.
21. Kim KI, Kim CW, Lee MK, Lee KS, Park CK, Choi SJ, et al. Imaging of occupational lung disease. Radiographics. 2001;21(6):1371–91.
22. Krefft S, Wolff J, Rose C. Silicosis: an update and guide for clinicians. Clin Chest Med. 2020;41(4):709–22.
23. Duchange L, Brichet A, Lamblin C, Tillie I, Tonnel AB, Wallaert B. [Acute silicosis. Clinical, radiologic, functional, and cytologic characteristics of the broncho-alveolar fluids. Observations of 6 cases]. Rev Mal Respir. 1998;15(4):527–34.
24. Yew WW, Leung CC, Chang KC, Zhang Y, Chan DP. Can treatment outcomes of latent TB infection and TB in silicosis be improved? J Thorac Dis. 2019;11(1):E8–E10.

Index

For the benefit of digital users, indexed terms that span two pages (e.g., 52–53) may, on occasion, appear on only one of those pages.

Tables, figures, and boxes are indicated by *t*, *f*, and *b* following the page number